AF711132

Risk Factors for Senility

Risk Factors for Senility

Edited by
Henry Rothschild, M.D., Ph.D.
Professor of Medicine and Anatomy
Louisiana State University School of Medicine

Coordinating Editor
Charles F. Chapman

New York Oxford
OXFORD UNIVERSITY PRESS
1984

Copyright © 1984 by Oxford University Press, Inc.

Library of Congress Cataloging in Publication Data
Main entry under title:

Risk factors for senility.

Bibliography: p.
Includes index.
1. Age factors in disease. 2. Senile dementia—Etiology. 3. Aging. I. Rothschild, Henry, 1932– II. Chapman, Charles Frederick, 1929– [DNLM: 1. Dementia, Senile. 2. Aging. 3. Nervous system diseases—In old age. WT 150 R595]
RB210.R57 1984 616.89′83071 83-22058
ISBN 0-19-503371-X

Printing (last digit): 9 8 7 6 5 4 3 2 1

Printed in the United States of America

To Fanny, who retains her youthful vigor with age

Preface

If control over the mental and physical deterioration that occurs with age is a worthy goal, then knowledge of the physiological basis of aging is appropriate as a step toward that goal.

Today the study of aging is approaching the stage that molecular biology achieved in the 1950s—at the fast-cutting edge of scientific investigation. Information is accumulating at a rapid rate concerning the specific factors implicated in the aging process: nutrition, physical activity, metabolic and endocrine functions, mental stimulation vs. stimulus deprivation, drug use, and life-style. Insights foreshadowing this information explosion have sometimes occurred despite the want of valid scientific data. For example, anticipating the experiments of Masoro (Chapter 14), Sir Thomas Elyot gave this advice in his book *Castel of Helthe* in 1524: "Always remember that aged men should eat often, and but little at every time, for it fareth by them as it doth by a lamp, the light whereof is almost extinct, which by pouring oil and little is kept long burning, but with much oil poured in it at once, it is put out." And Benjamin Rush, a physician and a signer of the Declaration of Independence, anticipated the data of King and Locke (Chapter 9) in his *Medical Inquiries and Observations* when he stressed "heredity, temperance, mental vigor, equanimity, and marriage" as factors in longevity.

Presented here are data not previously brought together in a compendium. This book attempts to give the latest scientific information available on the many aspects of aging, from the neurobehavioral to the physical. Where data are available, the authors have focused on practical strategies for risk assessment, risk-factor reduction, and disease prevention as related to aging. Delineating associations may give some insight into risk factors, even though such factors may not now be specific. New knowledge relating to aging—from molecular biology through epidemiology—should help illuminate important findings, changes, and trends in gerontology. Through this compendium, we look to stimulate interest in, and highlight the need for, collecting additional appropriate data to analyze the manifold factors specific to the risk factors for senility.

Because this subject is important in a wide range of disciplines related to human biology and health, this book is interdisciplinary, with contributors representing a diversity of approaches and areas of expertise. We have tried wherever possible to retain each contributor's style and individuality while shaping the whole into a timely, readable, and cohesive text.

New Orleans H. R.
October 1983 C. C.

Contents

BACKGROUND

NEUROBIOLOGICAL AGING

GENERAL SENESCENCE

Contributors

Fred Allison Jr., M.D., Edgar Hull Professor and Head, Department of Medicine, Louisiana State University Medical Center, New Orleans

F. William Black, Ph.D., Associate Professor of Neurology, Director of Neuropsychology Laboratory, Louisiana State University Medical Center, New Orleans

Kenneth R. Brizzee, M.D., Ph.D., Professor and Head, Division of Biomedical Science, Tulane University, New Orleans

Jacob A. Brody, M.D., Associate Director for Epidemiology, Demography, and Biometry Program, National Institute on Aging, Bethesda, Md.

Charles F. Chapman, Ph.B., Coordinator, Editorial Office, Louisiana State University, New Orleans

Fred B. Charatan, M.D., Chief of Psychiatry, Jewish Institute for Geriatric Care, New Hyde Park, N.Y.

Herbert A. deVries, Ph.D., Director, Physiology of Exercise Laboratory, Ethel Andrus Gerontology Center, University of Southern California, Los Angeles

Seymour Eisenberg, M.D., Professor of Medicine and Chief, Geriatric Medicine Division, Department of Internal Medicine, The University of Texas Health Science Center and Southwestern Medical School at Dallas; Chief, Geriatric Medicine, Office of VA, Dallas VA Medical Center, Dallas

D. Carleton Gajdusek, M.D., Chief, Nervous System Studies Laboratory, National Institute of Neurological Diseases and Stroke, National Institutes of Health, Bethesda, Md.

Ralph M. Garruto, Ph.D., Senior Research Biologist, National Institute of Neurological and Communicative Disorders and Stroke, National Institutes of Health, Bethesda, Md.

Leonard Hayflick, M.D., Director, Center for Gerontological Studies, University of Florida, Gainesville

Haitung King, Ph.D., Senior Research Scientist, Biometry Branch, National Cancer Institute, Bethesda, MD; Clinical Professor of Community Medicine and Family Health, Georgetown University Medical School, Washington, D.C.

Frances B. Locke, M.S., Statistician (Health), National Cancer Institute, National Institutes of Health, Bethesda, Md.

Alfredo Lopez-S, M.D., Ph.D., Professor of Medicine, Louisiana State University Medical Center, New Orleans

Edward J. Masoro, Ph.D., Professor and Chairman, Department of Physiology, University of Texas Health Science Center, San Antonio

Richard M. Paddison, M.D., Professor of Neurology, Louisiana State University Medical Center, New Orleans

Erdman B. Palmore, Ph.D., Professor of Medical Sociology, Duke University, Durham, N.C.

Norman W. Pedigo Jr., Ph.D., Assistant Professor of Pharmacology, Louisiana State University Medical Center, New Orleans

Henry Rothschild, M.D., Ph.D., Professor of Medicine and Anatomy, Louisiana State University Medical Center, New Orleans

David M. Schnarch, Ph.D., Director, Sexual and Marital Health Clinic; Associate Professor of Urology, Louisiana State University Medical Center, New Orleans

Lon R. White, M.D., Acting Chief, Epidemiology Section, Epidemiology, Biometry and Demography Program, National Institute on Aging, National Institutes of Health, Bethesda, Md.

Risk Factors for Senility

1 The Biology of Aging

Henry Rothschild

PRESENT CONCEPTS

Gerontologists generally regard aging as a progressive decline in an adult's body function which reduces the capacity to adjust to a dynamic environment and ends ultimately at death. Individuals within a species vary considerably in both the rate and the magnitude of age-related adaptive changes in cells, tissues, and organs. A common observation is that some people "burn themselves out" rapidly whereas others remain "well preserved." This observation and individual differences in longevity, and the wide variations in performance by persons of the same chronological age have led to the concept of biological functional aging as distinguished from chronological aging. At any given time, those who age rapidly are closer to death and, on the average, perform less well on age-related measures of functioning than do those who age slowly. These rapidly aging persons will be functionally older than their chronological-age peers.

Various tests have been used to assess age-associated physiological decrements. All are based on the biological, anthropomorphic, and psychological functions found to be decreased or increased in most older persons (Table 1-1). The commonly used tests for aging either measure baseline performances of a given function at rest or estimate the progressive reduction of the reserve capacity of a given organ or system, e.g., loading tests. The latter are often more sensitive to age change, and their results can be considered indices of adaptability of the function in question. Heron and Chown (*1*) identified eight variables that showed a linear relation with chronological age and created a functional-age profile on eight separate measures: forced expiratory volume, grip strength, sitting height, nonverbal intelligence, perceptual maze performance, digit coding, systolic blood pressure, and hearing loss. The

Table 1-1. Some Commonly Used Anthropometric, Physiological, and Psychometric Tests of Human Senescence

Anthropometric measures	Physiological tests
Standing height	Vital capacity
Sitting height	Tidal volume
Trunk height	Maximum breathing capacity
Biacromial diameter	Forced expiratory volume
Anteroposterior diameter of the thorax	Basal oxygen consumption
Weight	Systolic blood pressure
Fat-free weight	Hand-grip strength
Humeral (triceps) skinfold	Skin elasticity
Subscapular skinfold	Visual acuity
Paraumbilical skinfold	Critical flicker frequency
Dorsal skinfold of the hand	Dark adaptation
Hair graying score	Vibrometer
	Auditory threshold
Psychometric tests	Serum cholesterol
Wechsler's intelligence scale	Serum albumin and globulin
Raven's progressive matrices	Two-hour post-prandial blood glucose
Reaction time	Creatinine excretion
	Maximum rate of tapping

Source: Modified from Bourliere (*28*) and Shock (*29*).

authors did not combine these measures to form a functional-age score in years because they thought the diversity too great and the statistical correlation insufficient.

To be useful, however, a functional-age measure must predict performance that is influenced by aging with greater reliability and validity than chronological age itself. For example, if glomerular filtration rate (GFR) or vital capacity is the dependent measure, then one functional-age measure, whether it be a single test (such as the ability to accommodate to far or near vision) or a complex combination of several measures, must predict the GFR or vital capacity more accurately than age itself does.

The time of onset of age-dependent variables varies, as do the curves of change. The variables show three predominant patterns of change. Although most measures increase until adulthood, in several the decline is greatest between infancy and adulthood and negligible thereafter. Others decline more or less linearly with age throughout the entire life-span, and some others peak at adulthood and decline thereafter.

Deteriorative changes in one structure do not always signal the aging of the whole organism. Some functions show predictable decline with age: vital capacity, cardiac output, renal plasma flow, GFR, grip strength, and reaction time. In humans, most physiological functions, although subject to some individual variation, show a slow, nearly linear decline after about age 30. The rate constants for this linear loss seem to occur each year at about 0.8 to 0.9 per cent of the functional capacity present at age

30 (*2*). Other parameters, such as blood volume, osmotic pressure, pH, electrolyte content, and verbal intelligence, show no age-related changes.

With such time-related variables considered, aging may thus be defined to include the sum of all morphological and functional changes that occur in an organism and lead to function impairment, decreasing ability to survive stress, and, ultimately, death.

Pathological Processes

Superimposed on the basic biological changes that result from physiological decrements is an increasing vulnerability to disease. Disease-related causes of death should therefore be separated from the "normal" physiological decrements that give rise to the manifestations of old age. Such degenerative diseases as atherosclerosis, osteoporosis, and dementia may thus be considered separate from the aging process and their causes studied independently.

In most cases it is difficult to delineate where the normal aging processes terminate and pathology begins. However, aging can usually be distinguished from age-associated pathological changes by three criteria: progressiveness, intrinsicality, and universality. Although some authors also add decrementality, some functions, e.g., central nervous system activity and antidiuretic hormone release, may actually increase with age. Also, all-or-none phenomena, such as menopause, are difficult to explain by this criterion.

Furthermore, the pathological processes have, to a certain degree, been amenable to treatment. This is reflected in the *average* human life expectancy, which has increased greatly during the past century. The increase in life expectancy has been correlated with the control, elimination, and/or amelioration of these pathological processes by improved sanitation, nutrition, and drugs. In contrast, the *maximum* life-span (which may be considered a measure of the physiological variables and independent of disease) has not changed.

Mortality

The endpoint of the physiological decrements that encompass aging is death. The ultimate cause of most deaths in the elderly is not disease but the physiological decrements that make disease occurrence more probable. Except for that caused by accidents, death generally occurs when the capacity of the body to withstand a specific challenge has been surpassed. Furthermore, even though a given stress may not be sufficient to tax the body's tolerance, the functional impairments of old age may increase the frequency with which that stress is experienced. The loss of visual acuity, auditory perception, and muscle strength, for example, may predispose the elderly to accident or disease, which, in association with other physiological decrements, overtaxes their endurance. This predisposition is even more evident in animals. As soon as feral animals reach an age beyond sexual maturity, their declining capacities make them easier prey for predators and disease.

For example, pneumonia is not an uncommon cause of death in the elderly, whereas the same severity of lung infection caused by the same organism will be effectively resisted and overcome in a young person. The physiological decrements that may lead to death in this situation are the decrease in pulmonary function and reserve, and reduced immune function. Thus, pneumonia, a disease, is the proximate cause of death, but the physiological losses associated with aging are major determinants of the risk of dying.

Although aging may proceed linearly, the risk of mortality undergoes a sharp exponential increase with advancing years. For humans, the actuarial data, first analyzed by the English actuary Gompertz in the first quarter of the nineteenth century, show that mortality doubles every seven years beyond the age of 30—that is, after maturity, the rate and probability of dying are exponential with increasing age.

In summary, to understand the aging process, one must strive to distinguish between physiological decrements and superimposed pathological processes.

MODELS FOR STUDYING SENESCENCE

Many systems, from the cellular to the whole organism, each with its own inherent advantages and disadvantages, have been proposed as models for studying the human aging process.

Cultural Models

Among humans, the overall basic aging pattern is the same everywhere and the maximum life-span has not changed since the beginnings of recorded history. Nonetheless, significant differences in life expectancy do exist and differences in life-span have been reported. Claims of extreme longevity abound for particular ethnic groups (*3*). For example, investigators have frequently reported the claims of longevity with few debilitating diseases in three groups: one in the Andean village of Vilcabamba, in Ecuador; the second in the Hunza state in the Karakoram Mountains of the Pakistani region of Kashmir; and the third preponderantly in the Abkazia and Oestis regions in the Caucasus of the Georgian Republic of the Soviet Union.

Records supported by proper documentary evidence fix the highest age attained at about 120 years. To appreciate the magnitude of the claims made by these groups, one must realize that in other parts of the world the number of centenarians in the population is normally about two or three per 100 000. Yet in the three regions mentioned, not only are higher proportions of centenarians claimed, but many persons claim ages of 130 and even up to 160 years.

Although there is no question that many of the subjects in these areas are old, even centenarians, their exact age and their proportion in the total population have been questioned. The claims of superlongevity cannot be substantiated in any of these regions. Most records inevitably involve recording errors and suffer from the tendency of very elderly persons to exaggerate their age. The best-studied situation is that in the Soviet Union, where the spurious evidence was due to a combination of social mores, politics, and fraud. Nevertheless, many of the older persons in these ethnic groups were more vigorous than similarly aged persons in other areas. Various conclusions about genetic and environmental factors have been drawn from these unsubstantiated observations. Geographic, climatologic, dietary, genetic, and life-style situations were initially claimed as accounting for the increased life-span and vigor (*3*).

Human Diseases Associated with Premature Aging

Human diseases with accelerated aging phenotypes have been used to study aging. The major limitation of this approach is the rarity of patients with these syndromes.

1. Persons with *progeria* (Hutchinson-Gilford syndrome) show premature aging and bear an uncanny resemblance to one another. Characteristics of old age invariably present in childhood are short stature (comparable to loss of height in the aged), decreased weight for height, absence of sexual maturation, diminished subcutaneous fat, craniofacial disproportion, micrognathia, prominent scalp veins, alopecia, prominent eyes, delayed dentition, pyriform thorax, a wide-based and shuffling gait, and stiff joints. Persons with this syndrome have normal intelligence. The median age at death is 12 years, with more than 80 per cent of deaths attributed to cardiovascular disease. Widespread atherosclerosis and interstitial fibrosis of the heart are apparent at autopsy. Some features associated with aging, such as diabetes, increased frequency of tumors, cataracts, or osteoporosis, are not found.

   The incidence is about one in 8 million live births. Several families have had more than one child affected, and, in several, consanguinity has been documented (*4*). Both features are consistent with autosomal recessive transmission, but because of its rarity, its inheritance is still uncertain.

   A reduced in vitro cumulative cell population doubling has been reported for cultured fibroblasts derived from patients with progeria. Also, diminished DNA repair capacity after x-ray and ultraviolet radiation has been reported in cells from these patients.

2. *Cockayne's syndrome* is a rare autosomal recessive disease with some features of premature aging and some features that are not necessarily associated with senescence (*5*). After apparently normal early development, there is onset in late infancy of failure to grow, microcephaly, mental retardation, a peculiar facies and sunken eyes, prominent nose, prognathism, photosensitive dermatitis, pigmentary retinal degeneration, partial deafness, and a progressive neurological disorder characterized mainly by gait disturbance. Additional features include disproportionately long extremities with large hands and feet, limited joint movements, optic atrophy, cataracts, carious teeth, and thickened skull bones. Death usually occurs in late childhood or early adolescence (*6*).

   Fibroblasts taken from patients with this syndrome and grown in culture show increased sensitivity to ultraviolet irradiation but normal dimer excision, an important mechanism for repair of damaged DNA.

3. *Werner's syndrome,* a rare autosomal recessive disease, is characterized by growth retardation, short stature, premature graying and hair loss, juvenile cataracts, thin skin, thick subcutaneous tissue, leg ulcers, loss of teeth, osteoporosis, insulin-independent diabetes mellitus, and generalized atherosclerosis (*7*). The mean age of survival is 47 years, and the incidence of carcinomas and sarcomas is high.

   Cultured fibroblasts from these patients have reduced life-span but have normal levels of ultraviolet and x-irradiation damage repair capacity.

Animal Models

Much information on physiological aging derives from data obtained from feral, laboratory, and inbred vertebrates. The usefulness of mammalian model systems, from the molecular level to the whole organism, is proportional to their similarity to the human aging process. The advantage of some of these models is that the life-spans of those animals are shorter than our own (Table 1-2); the disadvantage lies in the complexities of extrapolating from one species to another. It is usually accepted that genetically controlled animals should be used, but no evidence has been presented that this need be so.

The appropriateness of the model system depends on the question to be studied. Primates have been useful in studying the neuropathological changes of aging (Chapter 3), and laboratory rodents, particularly rats and mice, have been used extensively to study the effects of nutrition on longevity (*8*) but are a poor model for studying the interaction between the physiological decline of aging and atherosclerosis. Other animal models may offer specific advantages. Specific genes, their products, and functions as related to aging can be isolated for study. The advantage of *Drosophila* as a model for aging is that it probably is the most widely

Table 1-2. Maximum Life-Span of Some Mammalian Species

Species	Maximum life-span (years)
Primates	
Human	115
Orangutan	50
Capuchin monkey	40
Brown lemur	31
Squirrel monkey	21
Rodents	
Norway rat	4
Pocket mouse	8
Gray squirrel	15
Carnivores	
Coyote	16
Brown bear	37
Bobcat	25
Ungulates	
Asiatic elephant	70
Syrian wild ass	36
Hippopotamus	51
Whales	
Finback	80
Pilot whale	50

Source: Modified from Rockstein et al. (*30*).

studied invertebrate, its genome being more thoroughly understood than that of any other animal. Also, its life-span is short, with one day in the life of a fly corresponding roughly to one year of human life. Its disadvantages are that it is not a mammal, its size is small, and it lacks somatic cell division after the pupa stage.

Relatively simple organisms with favorable genetic characteristics, such as the laboratory nematode *Caenorhabditis elegans,* are appealing to study because their ecology is well known and, unlike *Drosophila,* the sexes are readily differentiated. Furthermore, their life-span is short and their environment is readily manipulated.

Cells in Culture

Growing cells in culture has become a paradigm for the study of senescence. In his classic experiments, Hayflick (*9*) found, in contrast to the previously held theory, that cells grown in culture are mortal, that the ability of normal fibroblasts to replicate in cell culture is finite, and that the number of population doublings is universally related to donor age and longevity of the species. He advanced the hypothesis that the finite life-span of cells in vitro may be an expression of in vivo aging and, therefore, that such systems may be suitable models for the study of aging. He found that the life-span of a cell strain does not depend on chronological time but is a function of the number of potential population doublings that a particular cell strain may undergo. Human fibroblasts can proceed through an average of about 50 population doublings before a sharp decline in proliferation occurs.

Other evidence to support the validity of this system as a model for aging includes the following:

1. Cells from patients with progeria have curtailed life-spans in vitro relative to cells from age-matched controls;
2. Early-passage fibroblasts from old donors show the same characteristics of declining doublings as late-passage cells from embryos (*10*).

This model system lends itself to sophisticated manipulations. For instance, hybrids formed between either early- or late-passage anucleate cytoplasms (cytoplasts) and late-passage old cells with inactivated cytoplasm never progressed beyond a limited number of doublings, whereas hybrids involving early-passage cells with inactivated cytoplasms and cytoplasts of any passage survived doublings similar to those of early-passage controls. Furthermore, the study of cells as they age in culture has permitted investigation of cellular events independent of the complexity of the whole organism. However, the conditions of cells in culture are unphysiological and allow study only of a restricted class of cells. Other disadvantages of cells in culture are that the cells, once they double, are no longer the original cell but instead the progeny of the original cell and, most important, that cells in culture do not allow study of integrated functions that may be responsible for aging.

FACTORS INFLUENCING SENESCENCE

Two alternative views of the nature of senescence have arisen as a result of observations on these and other systems: first, that it is the result of random damage to cellular structures leading to tissue disorganization (this can be called the "wear-and-tear" theory) and, second, that it is a result of some programmed, hence controlled, time-dependent degeneration of the organism. However, though the evidence is scant at best, senescence probably reflects a complex interaction of hereditary and environmental influences.

Environmental Factors

To date, it has not been possible to document convincingly the action of any environmental factor on the rate of aging. Nevertheless, it has been suggested that three categories of environmental factors influence the rate of aging in humans:

1. Many investigators have implicated *physical and chemical components* of the environment as causing differential rates of aging. For instance, some experts have claimed that environmental pollutants, such as radiation, affect senescence. However, investigations in both laboratory animals and humans do not support this contention. For example, the life expectancy of radiologists, including the pioneer radiologists, many of whom suffered from such effects of overexposure as radiation dermatitis and skin cancer, is not reduced by their exposure to radiation. Comparisons of observed and expected numbers of deaths from all causes provide no evidence that occupational exposure to ionizing radiations leads to a detectable nonspecific shortening of the life expectation of radiologists. Nor do the Hiroshima survivors, who have an increased incidence of leukemia, show symptoms of premature aging. In this population Hollingsworth et al. (*11*) found no differences in age-related functions determined by periodic measurement of blood pressure, vital capacity, heart size, gastric achlorhydria, hearing acuity, skin elasticity, hair graying, and several immunological tests. Only hand grip strength as a measure of neuromuscular function varied significantly between exposure groups and control subjects. However, no significant association between grip strength and radiation dose was found in subjects within 2000 meters of the hypocenter.
2. Discussion of *biological factors* such as nutrition as probable causes of differential aging in humans is found in later chapters. *Pathogens and parasites* have been implicated in influencing the rate of human development and aging, more particularly in low-income groups and in tropical countries. Although they are important determinants of life expectancy (disease effect), there is no evidence that they influence senescence.
3. It is commonly thought that *socioeconomic factors,* such as any difficult life conditions of modern industrialized societies, be they bad housing, poor working conditions, or the stresses of life, accelerate the aging process. This acceleration may in fact occur, but it is difficult to confirm. Nonetheless, several studies have claimed to show that living under stress increases the rate of decline. For instance, Bourliere et al. (*12*), in their study of aging in subjects with long histories of peptic ulcer (which they assumed to be associated with stress), showed that performance of the ulcer group, in physical tests, was significantly lower than that of the controls, particularly with regard to muscle strength and maximum breathing capacity. In psychological tests, the ulcer group, showed (1) a more rapid decline in intellectual efficiency, (2) a greater frequency of disturbed personality, which was often associated with neurotic anxiety and depression, (3) a less satisfactory adaptation to the problems of aging, and (4) a greater susceptibility to occupational fatigue. They concluded that stressful living conditions—or a constitutional inability to cope with them—accelerates the aging process.

Many differences in the aging rates of our physical functions and mental abilities have been postulated to be a consequence of their disuse or misuse during childhood and adolescence. Also, regular physical activity by intellectuals and cultural activity by manual workers is generally considered to retard aging. Most studies, however, have produced no evidence in support of these statements. For instance, there is no clear-cut evidence to show either an advantage or a disadvantage resulting from the sustained practice of a sport. Clement (*13*) showed that cyclists 45 to 75 years of age had no greater maximum breathing capacity, greater resistance to fatigue, or better performance than did nonsporting subjects at all ages tested. Vital capacity, blood pressure, dark adaptation, performance at learning vocabulary, and digit symbol tests did not show significant differences between active and control subjects. The subjects' heart rates were slower and their reaction times a little shorter than those of controls. In the step test, the elderly persons who practiced some sport all their lives also tended to have a shorter recovery time after exercise than did less active controls.

Genetic Factors

Evidence that genetic factors play a role in aging is more substantial. No single mutation is known to increase life-span, but several mutations reduce it. It is unclear whether life-shortening mutations occur in specific longevity genes or whether the anomalies they produce only incidentally shorten life.

The principal evidence that aging, as expressed by life-span, is at least in part genetically determined derives from the following kinds of observations.

1. Species-specific life-spans Each species is characterized by its own pattern of aging and maximum (potential) life-span. The life-spans of multicellular organisms vary widely from a maximum of about 5000 years for the bristlecone pine in the White Mountains of California to a minimum of about one week for some species of rotifers.

Differences in life-spans of members of various animal groups argue strongly in favor of a species-specific genetic basis for longevity. Among mammals, the longevity ranges from that of humans, about 115 years, down to that of small rodents, about two years (*14*).

Selective factors do not seem to have played a role in species longevity. Few, if any, selective mechanisms favor long-lived members of a species. Beyond the age of sexual maturation longevous members have no selective advantage.

2. Hybrid vigor The effect of genetic constitution on longevity is perhaps best exemplified by those experiments in which hybrid vigor has been demonstrated. However, the increased longevity seen in hybrids does not exceed the maximum life-span characteristic of feral strains.

One of the earliest studies on longevity was by Hyde (*15*), who showed that when an inbred wild-type strain of *Drosophila* with a mean life-span of 37.4 days was crossed with a mutant strain truncate having a mean life-span of 21.4 days, the F_1 generation's life-span was 47.0 days, greater than that of either parent. In many similar studies using inbred, feral, and geographically isolated strains of *Drosophila,* the F_1 lived longer and had a less variable life-span when crossed than did its inbred parents. Most explanations of hybrid vigor suggest that recessive, harmful, but nonlethal mutations are produced by inbreeding; hence, hybrid vigor results from the reciprocal dominance between the wild-type alleles of one parental strain and the recessive, suboptimal genes of the other.

3. Sex In humans and most animals studied, the male is shorter-lived. For example, a white female born in the United States in 1974 can expect to outlive her male counterpart by 7.7 years (*16*). Hayflick (*17*) speculated that, if genes carried on the sex chromosomes indicate life-span, then genes on the X chromosome may decrease vulnerability to degenerative diseases. Contrariwise, genes on the Y chromosome may exert life-shortening effects that are incidental to their main function. Although the male is the shorter-lived in most species, the opposite is true in some mouse, rat, and *Drosophila* strains.

4. Parental age Persons with older parents have a greater life expectancy than persons whose parents died early. Pearl and Pearl (*18*) found that the summed ages at death of the six immediate ancestors of centenarians and nonagenarians were significantly greater than those of persons in a control series. Persons older than 70 had at least one long-lived parent. Of nonagenarians, 48.5 per cent had two such parents, and of centenarians, 53.4 per cent had two long-lived parents. All these figures are significantly higher than those found in control groups.

5. Twin studies The mean difference in life-span for monozygotic twins has been found to be consistently less than that for dizygotic twins (*19*). As twins age, however, the differences decrease, due perhaps to the approaching maximum life-span. Dizygotic twins show more variation in age at death than do monozygotic twins, but the difference was significant only in younger females. Thus, individual genetic factors may shorten life expectation rather than increase it.

THEORIES OF BIOLOGICAL AGING

Numerous molecular models have been proposed to explain the mechanisms of aging, there being about one theory per investigator in the field, with one not necessarily being an alternative to any of the others. The abundance of theories is an indication of the dearth of reliable data on aging.

Most theories of aging presume that a single mechanism is responsible for all the characteristic changes seen with aging. Moreover, most focus only on the derangements that occur at some target molecule. However, most ignore the possibility that aging may be the result of several independent events involving genetically programmed decay, random genetic changes, and environmental insults. If a unifying theory of such a complex process as aging is possible, it should account for aging in both replicative and post-mitotic cells and should differentiate between programmed senescence and that due to environmental damage to sensitive systems.

There is no simple way to catalog the various proposed theories. Here, in general, are those most often referred to.

Genetic Theories

1. Error theories The error theories of aging propose that senescence is related to the progressive accumulation of errors in macromolecules. In aging, the infidelities of DNA, RNA, and protein synthesis are now considered to be interconnected. The possibility of a dramatic acceleration of error frequency was suggested by Orgel (*20*) in 1963 in his "error catastrophe" theory. Because cellular metabolism, cellular and tissue interactions, and most life functions depend on the quality of proteins, errors in these macromolecules would eventually become great enough to impair function. The appeal of this theory was that it offered a simple translational explanation for aging and appeared to be testable.

The implications of this theory are particularly serious for cells that do not divide after they have differentiated, such as brain and muscle cells. If they function poorly, they die and are not replaced. The results are less serious for dividing cells, such as those of the liver or the lining of the gastrointestinal tract.

Evidence for the error catastrophe theory was supplied by Lewis and Holliday (*21*), who found that in cetain mutant strains of *Neurospora* senescence is accompanied by the synthesis of defective protein molecules, with a rapid increase in their production just before growth ceases. Holliday and Tarrant (*22*) showed that human diploid fibroblasts accumulate heat-labile enzymes during the final stages of their life-span in culture. However, Cristofalo (*23*) concluded that cells with errors serious enough to compromise their survival are overgrown by healthy cells so that the overall life-span of the population is not affected. Current modifications of this theory suppose that the rate of expression of such damage may be altered by several processes, including the repair capacity of the cell.

2. Somatic mutations The basic assumption of this hypothesis is that, just as spontaneous mutations occur in germ-cell lines, so they may also occur in somatic cells. Szilard (*24*) proposed that random events called aging hits occur with a constant probability per unit time throughout life. Because mutations cause some change in cell and tissue function, a sufficient number of cells carrying such mutations affect tissue or organ function. More often than not, functional capacity declines. If mutations are involved in senescence, then the efficiency of DNA repair mechanisms may also play a role.

Consistent with this theory is the increase in chromosomal breaks and aneuploidy with age. However, similar to the redundancy theory described next, the theory should predict that the life-span of a species is proportional to its DNA content. This proportionality is not borne out by data for species with large differences in life-span.

3. Redundancies Medvedev (*25*) suggested that aging is due to the loss of unique, nonrepeated, genetic information from the genome. The repetitions of some genes, the bulk of which are repressed, are postulated as being not only an evolutionary reserve, especially in cells of higher organisms, but also a reserve to reduce the rate of aging. Medvedev believes that different species' life-spans may be a function of the degree of repeated sequences. As mutations, and thus errors, accumulate in functioning genes, reserve sequences containing the same information take over until the redundancy of the system is exhausted, resulting in biological age changes. The differences in species life-spans are then thought to be a manifestation of the degree of gene repetition. Mutations in genes that are both unique and essential would be especially deleterious.

Nongenetic Theories

1. Immunological theories With aging the immune system tends to be less able to distinguish normal molecules from abnormal ones, and so abnormal cells may proliferate and autoimmune reactions may take place. As primarily advocated by Burnet (*26*), forbidden clones capable of a minor attack on tissues arise with greater frequency as age advances and such clones are themselves subject to partial or complete control that becomes less effective. Walford (*27*) suggested that aging results from long-term, minor histoincompatibility reactions in the cell population. In humans the frequency of autoantibodies in supposedly healthy older individuals increases remarkably. In C_3H mice and parabiotic hamsters, life has been shortened by an increase in low-grade histoincompatibility reactions.

2. Free-radical theory Free radicals are ubiquitous, short-lived, highly reactive chemicals produced during normal metabolic reactions. This theory postulates that free radicals combine with essential molecules, causing damage to DNA or other cellular structures, and that these reactions contribute to aging and age-associated diseases. Abnormal or uncontrolled free-radical reactions have been considered an important source of cellular damage in a variety of pathological processes. Dietary changes, such as the addition of vitamin E, designed to minimize free-radical reactions have been shown to increase the life-span of WI-38 cells grown in culture and enhance humoral and cell-mediated immune response. Studies in mice have also shown that administration of free-radical quenchers results in *increased* life-span.

3. Cross-linking theory Aging has been postulated to be caused by molecules becoming irreversibly immobilized with age as a result of strong cross-linking bonds. Changes in the characteristics of molecular cross-linking of substances have a profound effect on physiological function. For example, cross-linking of collagen, which is 25 per cent of total body protein, could affect the flow of nutrients and waste products from cells. These, in turn, are thought to produce age changes.

CONCLUSION

Old age is inevitable but need not be debilitating. Identifying and understanding the underlying cause or causes of senescence would be beneficial for intervening in—and slowing—the aging process, thus allowing for a longer period of well-being during a person's life with a relatively quick denouement.

REFERENCES

1. A. Heron and S. Chown, *Age and Function.* Little Brown, Boston, 1967.
2. B. L. Strehler and A. S. Mildvan, General theory of mortality and aging, *Science* **132:**14 (1960).
3. A. Leaf, Unusual longevity: The common denominators, *Hosp. Practice* **8:**75 (1973).
4. F. L. DeBusk, The Hutchison-Gilford progeria syndrome, *J. Ped.* **80:**697 (1972).
5. E. A. Cockayne, Dwarfism with retinal atrophy and deafness, *Arch. Dis. Child.* **11:**1 (1936).
6. D. Soffer, H. W. Grotsky, I. Rapin, and K. Suzuki, Cockayne syndrome: Unusual pathological findings and review of the literature, *Ann. Neurol.* **6:**340 (1979).
7. C. J. Epstein, G. M. Martin, A. L. Schultz, and A. G. Motulsky, Werner's syndrome: A review of its symptomatology, natural history, pathological features, genetics and relationship to the natural aging process, *Medicine* **45:**177 (1966).
8. U.S. Department of Health, Education, and Welfare, Development of the Rodent as a Model System of Aging, D. C. Gibson (ed). Publication NIH 72-121, Washington, D.C., Books I and II.
9. L. Hayflick, The limited in vitro lifetime of human diploid cell strains. *Exp. Cell. Res.* **37:**614 (1965).
10. G. M. Martin, Cellular aging. *Am. J. Pathol.* **89:**484 (1977).

11. D. R. Hollingsworth, J. W. Hollingsworth, S. Bogitch, and R. J. Keehn, Neuro-muscular tests of ageing in Hiroshima subjects, *J. Gerontol.* **24:**276 (1969).
12. F. Bourliere, C. DeBray, J. Hellemans, and J. Poitrenaud, L'ulcère gastro-duodénal du sujet âgé: Etude physiologique et psychologique, *Sem. Hop. Paris* **41:**391 (1965).
13. F. Clement, L'activite physique ralentit-elle le declin des capacites intellectuelles? Etude d'un groupe de vieux cyclistes particulièrement actifs physiquement, *Rev. Franç. Géront.* **7:**379 (1961).
14. A. Comfort, *The Biology of Aging,* 3rd ed. Elsevier North Holland, New York, 1979.
15. R. R. Hyde, Inheritance of the length of life in *Drosophila ampelophila, Indiana Acad. Sci. Rept. for 1913,* p. 113.
16. J. S. Siegel, Demographic Aspects of Aging and the Older Population in the United States. Current Population Reports, Special Studies, Series P-23, No. 59, GPO, Washington, D.C., 1976.
17. L. Hayflick, Genetic disparities of senescence, in *Biocultural Aspects of Disease* (H. Rothschid, ed.). Academic Press, New York, 1981.
18. R. Pearl and R. de W. Pearl, *The Ancestry of the Long-Lived.* H. Milford, London, 1934.
19. W. T. Brown, Human mutations affecting aging: A review, *Mech. Ageing Develop.* **9:**325 (1979).
20. L. E. Orgel, The maintenance of the accuracy of protein synthesis and its relevance to aging, *Proc. Natl. Acad. Sci. USA* **49:**517 (1963).
21. C. M. Lewis and R. Holliday, Mistranslation and ageing in *Neurospora, Nature* **228:**877 (1970).
22. R. Holliday and G. M. Tarrant, Altered enzymes in aging human fibroblasts, *Nature* **238:**26 (1972).
23. V. J. Cristofalo, Animal cell cultures as a model system for the study of aging, *Adv. Gerontol. Res.* **4:45 (1972).**
24. L. Szilard, On the nature of the aging process, *Proc. Natl. Acad. Sci. USA,* **45:**30 (1959).
25. Z. A. Medvedev, Repetition of molecular-genetic information as a possible role of infidelity of transfer of information on the accumulation of age changes in differentiated cells, in *Mechanisms of Ageing and Development.* Elsevier Sequoia SA, Lausanne, 1980.
26. M. Burnet, Somatic mutation and chronic disease, *Br. Med. J.* **1:**338 (1965).
27. R. L. Walford, *Immunologic Theory of Aging.* Munksgaard, Copenhagen, 1969.
28. F. Bourliere, Ecology of human senescence, in *Textbook of Geriatric Medicine and Gerontology* (J. C. Brocklehurst, ed.) Churchill Livingstone, Edinburgh, 1978.
29. N. W. Shock, Physiological and chronological age, in *Aging—Its Chemistry* (A. A. Dietz, ed.). American Association for Clinical Chemistry, Washington, D.C., 1979.
30. M. Rockstein, J. A. Chesky, and M. L. Sussman, Comparative biology and evolution of aging, in *Handbook of the Biology of Aging* (C. E. Finch and L. Hayflick, eds.) Van Nostrand Reinhold, New York, 1977.

2 Clinical Aspects of Physical Aging

Fred Allison Jr.

If clinicians are to recognize risk factors for senility, they must know the changes involved in the normal aging process. They must recognize that the aging process varies with cell type, organ system, and individual organism. Because of this variation, the function of one organ system may fail to match the performance of other systems in the same aging person.

From a practical viewpoint, aging probably begins at the time of physical maturation. Thus, aging presumably starts earlier for females than for males. In some ethnic groups, aging may begin earlier than in others. Genetic makeup is thought to be largely responsible for the rate of aging. Because of these variables, which may be unpredictable, physicians often must determine whether a physical change is due to aging or to disease.

SIGNS OF NORMAL AGING

Here the physical aspects of normal aging are reviewed briefly by organ system.

Skin and Nails

The most obvious and easily recognizable changes of aging occur in the integument. As a result of exposure to sunlight, extremes of temperature, and other physical stresses, the skin may be the first organ system to show the changes characteristic of aging. These alterations reflect subtle yet definite microscopic and biochemical events that lead to a decrease in the number of elastic fibers, to a fragmentation and reduction of collagen tissue, and to diminution of supporting ground substances (*1*). Associated with the aging of supporting tissue are concurrent changes in the pigment-producing cells of the skin, i.e., the melanocytes. Their number decreases, and they begin to loose the capacity to produce pigment, whereby the skin gradually and progressively loses color. Loss of skin pigment allows underlying blood vessels to show through, with the result that, even though the number of blood vessels per unit of skin may be reduced, subcutaneous vascular channels are more visible. There is a decrease in subcutaneous fat, especially of the fat padding over the bony prominences. This loss of fat increases the possibility of decubitus ulcer formation, especially in the invalided elderly. As the skin becomes thinner, an age-related loss of sweat and sebaceous glands results in wrinkling, greater dryness, and enhanced fragility. Wrinkling of the skin is most prominent in areas of the body exposed to the elements, i.e., about the eyes, face, and upper extremities. The loss of sweat and sebaceous glands often leads to difficulty in regulating body temperature, which in turn may lead to heat stroke.

Many benign, proliferative changes emerge as skin ages. First are the acrochordons (skin tags), most often found on exposed skin, such as the dorsum of the hands and around the upper eyelids. Cherry angiomata, benign proliferative formations of capillaries, found on the upper abdomen and thorax, become increasingly obvious with each passing decade after age 30. Of other proliferative changes of the skin, the seborrheic keratoses are particularly common in scalp areas and can be confused with actinic malignant lesions. Another proliferative lesion, sebaceous hyperplasia, most often occurs in those areas where sebaceous glands are plentiful, i.e., the axilla and groin, and resembles to some extent the sebaceous keratoses.

Especially bothersome from a cosmetic point of view are the freckles, or lentigo, that proliferate with aging, more commonly on exposed areas of the face and extremities. Senile purpura, encountered most often over the extremities, follows minor trauma and results from extravasation of small amounts of blood under the skin. These are sometimes referred to as "liver spots."

With aging, the fingernails and toenails may show trophic changes, with a reduced rate of growth, longitudinal ridging, and, in some instances, increased thickness in response to trauma.

Hair

Changes of hair color and growth are recognized as being among the early signs of aging and reflect a slowing of the metabolic activity of cells at the base of hair follicles. Specifically, the capacity of melanocytes to produce the pigment necessary for hair coloration decreases and the number of these cells gradually declines. Premature graying, often a familial trait, may begin as early as age 20 in persons having this genetic makeup. By age 50, however, about 50 per cent of the body hair becomes gray. Graying usually appears first at the temples and then becomes apparent gradually in ensuing years over the vertex of the head. Graying over the rest of the body may not be nearly as noticeable and may not appear until years later, particularly for the hair of the eyebrows, chest, axillae, and pubic area.

Balding, clearly a result of hair follicle failure, is one of the most commonly encountered events of aging, particularly in men. For persons having a strong family trait of balding, loss of hair bitemporally and over the vertex may be seen in men as early as age 20. About 60 per cent of white men have some degree of temporal hair loss by age 50. Progressive loss of hair over the vertex of the head, or coronal balding, follows bitemporal loss. Unfortunately, little information is available regarding the frequency and rate of balding in nonwhite races (*1*). However, about 65 per cent of women have extreme bitemporal balding by age 70; and 20 per cent of women in this age group have significant loss of hair over the vertex of the head.

Over the remainder of the body, metabolism and growth of hair vary, depending on family and genetic makeup. It is important to keep in mind that the amount of hair on the trunk may increase up to the fourth decade in both men and women. As women grow older, their loss of pubic hair exceeds that of men; by age 70, about 5 per cent of women have little or no pubic hair. Similarly, women loose axillary hair more rapidly than do men of the same age. In about 40 per cent of women, facial hair increases progressively, particularly after menopause, so that by age 55 growth of dark hair on the upper lip, chin, and cheeks may be noticeable. This distressing cosmetic problem often requires medical counseling. Both sexes seem to lose hair progressively on the arms and legs after age 60, unrelated to vascular integrity.

Eyes

As a consequence of the reduction of supportive connective and elastic tissue content on the dermis, particularly about the face, age-related skin changes around the eyes are often prominent. Sagging of the eyelids may be noted, with development of extra skin folds in both the upper and lower lids. Beneath the eyes this sagging takes the form of bags that may lead to partial eversion of the lids of such proportion that the person needs plastic repair. Some consider arcus senilis, a ring of white pigment at the cornea's outer edge and often seen by age 60 or 70, to be normal. When found at an earlier age, arcus senilis may reflect underlying abnormality of carbohydrate and lipoprotein metabolism accompanying diabetes mellitus or accelerated atherosclerosis.

Of particular importance are changes that take place in the lens with aging. A gradual loss of ability of the lens to increase in thickness, as required for accommodation to near vision, is recognized as presbyopia and is an almost invariable development by age 45 to 50. Clouding and opacification of the lens, on the other hand, with formation of cataracts, occur with increasing frequency after the sixth or seventh decade of life but are not necessarily an invariable consequence of aging; it is possible that some persons may live to advanced years and never form cataracts.

Many senior persons have a diminution in visual acuity, with reduction in the ability to discriminate detail. This diminution apparently results from a gradual "dropping out" of the neuronal elements of the retina. Retinal degeneration, with sloughing of the surface into the vitreous, is usually secondary to vascular insufficiency or inflammatory processes; these are abnormal changes and materially interfere with visual acuity. Thickening of the vascular walls invariably occurs with aging with the result that the arteries appear more opaque, lose their red color, and look like a copper wire when viewed through the ophthalmoscope. Increased compression of venous channels crossing under retinal arteries almost always results. The hydrostatic pressure of the intraocular environment should remain normal throughout life; nonetheless, a variety of degenerative changes associated with aging may frequently lead to increased pressure and the emergence of glaucoma.

Ear

With normal aging, auditory integrity should be well maintained into the sixth and seventh decades. Impairment of hearing may be accelerated or accentuated by previous pathological processes that damaged the auditory apparatus. Nevertheless, even without such traumatic events, the gradual decline in hearing acuity with advanced age varies considerably. Subtle yet definite thickening of the eardrum, a slow loss of resolution capacity of the ossicles of the middle ear, and age-related degenerative changes of the eighth nerve all impair hearing in the elderly. Excessive exposure to an environment contaminated by noise may accelerate hearing loss. Although some of these changes are clearly of genetic origin, others seem to be sporadic and unpredictable.

Senile deafness, or presbycusis, is most commonly first recognized by the loss of ability to detect high-frequency sounds. The ability to perceive and identify sounds is reduced concurrent with a fall-off in ability to discriminate and localize precisely the origin of sounds. Eventually, these events cause a modest-to-moderate compromise in the elderly person's ability to communicate with others and may insidiously produce a degree of isolation that causes a serious loss of contact with environment, the emergence of deepening depression, and eventually the loss of ability to function. For this reason, regular monitoring of auditory capability in the elderly is essential, not only to confront but also minimize as much as possible an easily correctable disability.

For many elderly persons, the simple problem of wax accumulation in the external auditory canal may impair hearing severely. This problem is easily rectified with simple instructions that show patients how to clean their ears regularly.

With advancing years, the vestibular apparatus of the inner ear also begins to lose its ability to maintain postural equilibrium. Sudden changes of position may then result in unsteadiness and cause the affected person to fall. Increasingly apparent after the seventh and eighth decades of life, this problem must not be confused with cerebral circulatory changes in the form of atherosclerosis, cardiac arrhythmias, or embolic transient ischemic attacks, which simulate closely the disequilibrium of vestibular dysfunction.

Mouth and Nasopharynx

The elderly may seek help for loss of gustatory pleasures brought about by failure of the senses of taste and smell. Deprivation of these subtle yet finite sensory supports, along with decreased saliva flow, has a ruinous effect on appetite and causes a poor intake of essential foods, reflected by loss in weight and physical strength. The importance of this loss must be appreciated if aging persons are to maintain adequate nutrition.

For patients past the age of 70, especially those partially debilitated, reduction in the cough reflex may increase the risk of aspiration. Because aspiration inevitably leads to lower respiratory tract infection, proper precautions must be taken to protect the airway in elderly persons known to have physical or neurological problems. Age-associated changes in the vocal cords cause an increased voice pitch along with loss of the spoken voice volume.

With improved prophylaxis coupled with preventive education by the dental profession, it is not unusual today to encounter people in the seventh and eighth decades with well-preserved gums and permanent teeth. Early care of dental caries, proper and regular hygiene, dietary conservatism, and aggressive care of the gingival margins—coupled with early recognition of mechanical problems of mastication—help ensure preservation of teeth well into old age. Osteoporosis, a common finding in the elderly, may result in weakened bony support of the mandible and maxilla, with loosening of the teeth and eventual loss of permanent teeth.

Pulmonary System

After age 20, one's pulmonary function begins to decline progressively, presumably as a result of aging alone. This decline is caused by a loss of elastic tissue found in the lungs, chest wall, and diaphragm, tissue that is responsible for the recoil mechanism in breathing. Other gradual degenerative changes of connective tissue in the thoracic wall and lungs tend to limit or restrict the capacity to change volume. As a consequence of these events determined by age, residual volume gradually but progressively increases, reflected by a fall-off in total ventilatory capacity. A simultaneous but age-related reduction in diffusion capacity at the alveolus level limits oxygen exchange but imposes little or no restriction on the movement of carbon dioxide. Consequently, although there is no evidence of

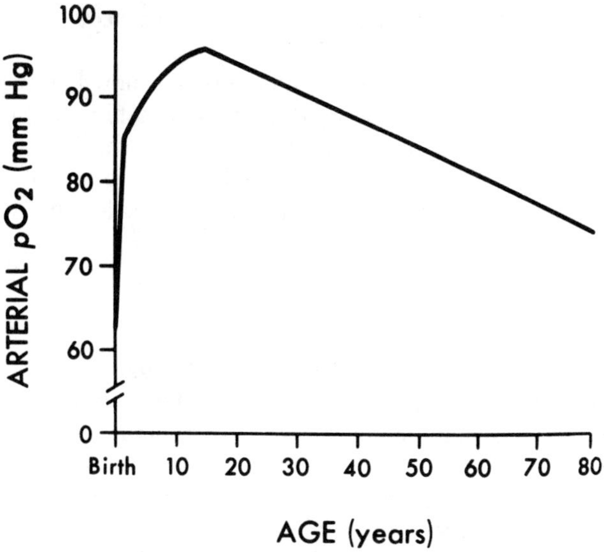

Figure 2-1. Effect of age on partial pressure of disssolved oxygen in arterial blood.

age-related carbon dioxide retention per se, a distinct age-linked effect on the partial pressure of dissolved oxygen in arterial blood can be demonstrated (Figure 2-1). The appropriate values for partial pressure of the oxygen in arterial blood corrected for age can be calculated easily according to the formula $pO_2 = 100.1 - 0.323 \times \text{age}$ (*2*). These subtle yet distinct ventilatory happenings must be understood if physicians are to interpret correctly the reduction in exercise tolerance and in laboratory results for blood gas determination encountered in patients of advanced age.

Cardiovascular System

After pathological conditions have been excluded, there can be identified distinct age-related changes that have a significant negative influence on cardiac function. Three fundamental events deserve emphasis. First, a gradual decrease in ventricular stroke volume reduces cardiac output. Second, increased peripheral resistance results in a gradual rise in systolic blood pressure, usually without an accompanying elevation in diastolic pressure. Third, these two events together limit the ability of aging persons to respond to exercise or stress. Expressed as limited cardiac reserve, this response limitation restricts their ability to mount a vigorous circulatory adjustment to stress (*3*). With advanced age, myocardial amyloid deposition becomes increasingly evident and may become a critical factor in reducing cardiac reserve. Whether amyloid represents a normal aging process or the end result of injury is not at all clear. All these changes lead to increased congestive heart failure.

It is not known whether physical conditioning, now highly popularized in the Western world and supported by many rehabilitation-minded physicians, preserves function or delays aging of the cardiovascular system. Physical exercise in moderation has substantial beneficial effects for many persons because it enhances a sense of well-being and vigorous health.

Kidney

As we age, it appears that both the total renal mass and the number of functioning nephrons decline. Whether this effect is purely age-related or a reflection of vascular changes and past inflammatory reactions that cause sclerosis and fibrosis of nephron units is unclear. Whatever the cause, there is a measurable reduction in glomerular filtration rate that seems to be independent of intrinsic or pre-existing renal disease but coincides with chronological age. Average age differences in physiological function among normal men aged 30 to 90 years are graphically portrayed in Figure 2-2 (*4*). Blood urea nitrogen (BUN) and creatinine levels are maintained within physiological ranges in healthy patients well up into the eighth and ninth decades. The reduced glomerular filtration rate does, nevertheless, compromise the capacity of older persons to sustain adequate renal function under conditions of stress (*5*). Thus, renal insuffi-

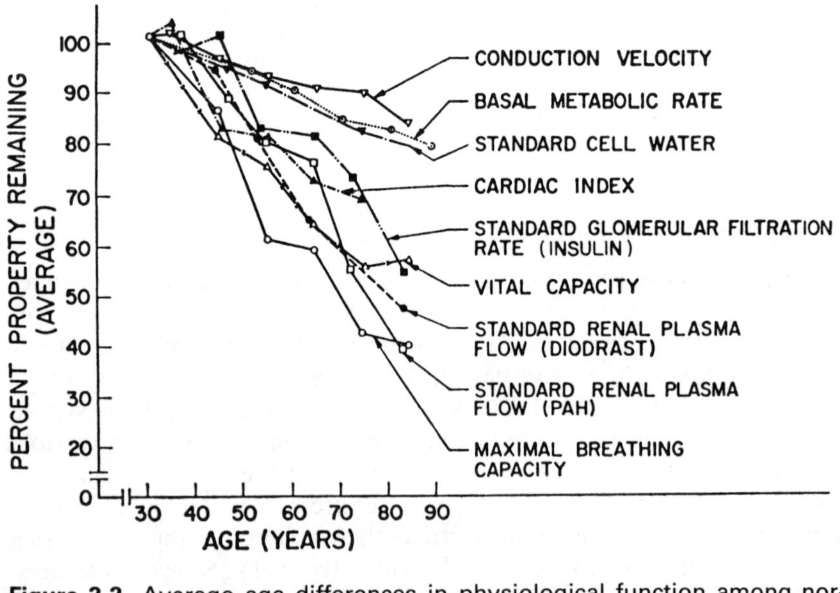

Figure 2-2. Average age differences in physiological function among normal men aged 30 to 90 years.

ciency may be encountered in the elderly after mild-to-moderate stress that is well tolerated by middle-aged patients.

Renin production by juxtaglomerular cells has been found to diminish with aging, as reflected in the release of aldosterone from the adrenal gland; this is an important step in the homeostatic maintenance of sodium, potassium, and magnesium metabolism in humans (*6*). Thus, when all factors are considered, elderly patients do not adjust well to sudden alterations in free water. For example, restriction of water intake may result in acute and serious elevations in the serum BUN/creatinine ratio. Conversely, sudden increases in water load with an expansion of plasma volume may cause life-threatening electrolyte abnormalities from excessive hemodilution, such as hyponatremia. As noted in Chapter 10, these changes also lead to drug toxicities when the kidney is the major route of excretion.

Endocrine System

Current evidence confirms that the hypophyseal-pituitary-thyroid feedback mechanism functions well throughout life. Specifically, levels of thyroid stimulating hormone (TSH) remain normal into old age and result in physiological levels of circulating thyroid hormone. There is, however, an age-related decline in peripheral or end-organ utilization of thyroid hormone. From this fact one may presume that the levels of thyrotropin-releasing hormone (TRH) from the hypothalamus are also adequate. This maintenance of TRH level persists even though the pituitary may be less responsive in its release of TSH on stimulation with exogenous TRH, but the physiological significance of this fact is unknown (*7*).

According to current evidence, adequate to slightly elevated levels of parathyroid hormone are found in later life (*8*). Calcitonin levels decline with age in both women and men. Calcium metabolism, as regulated by these two endocrine mediators, remains unaltered, although after age 60 intestinal absorption of calcium is reduced. With aging, demineralization of bone in the form of osteoporosis represents a major clinical problem not directly related to parathormone and calcitonin production (*9*).

Only minor age-related alterations in function of the pituitary-adrenal axis have been identified. Specifically, glucocorticoid metabolism, regulated by adrenocorticotropic hormone, remains at normal levels and is unmodified throughout life. The capacity to respond to stressful situations is well preserved so that absolute or relative adrenal insufficiency is not a problem associated with aging. Although aldosterone production is also maintained at normal levels in the elderly, it is important to know that adrenal gland responsiveness for release of extra aldosterone in response to stress is suboptimal. This limitation seems to be tied directly to an age-related decline in renin production by the kidney (*10*).

Of considerable interest to physicians in the field of geriatrics is gonadal integrity and function. This problem has been extensively studied, and the following facts seem secure. First, women after menopause have substantially less estrogen production from their involuted ovaries. Because their ovarian function has declined, the levels of follicle-stimulating hormone (FSH) and luteinizing hormone (LH) production by the pituitary gland are considerably elevated in venous blood samples. These high LH and FSH values fluctuate widely over 24-hour periods. Although the cause of cutaneous flushing, or hot flashes, a common problem in post-menopausal women, has not been proved, one is tempted to speculate that it relates in some way to the wide swing in levels of these hormones (*11*).

In healthy men over 65, increased LH levels in venous blood are thought to relate directly to a decreased responsiveness of testicular Leydig cells in releasing testosterone. Cutaneous flushing may be found in older men, but to a lesser extent than in women. From a practical point of view, blood levels of testosterone remain within the range of normal throughout life in response to the elevated LH production, and so the availability of androgen, for metabolic or other needs, is not reduced greatly (*12*).

Sexual drive in both elderly men and elderly women may remain intact but at a reduced intensity relative to that of younger persons. Libido commonly remains a strong force for women up until the time of menopause, whereas it declines gradually in men after they reach the middle years. For this reason, it is not unusual for patients in the eighth decade to have pertinent questions regarding this function and to remain sexually active. Atrophic epithelial vaginal changes with drying of surfaces, found in post-menopausal women, often cause mechanical problems and discomfort in sexual intercourse. Applying agents to lubricate surfaces and maintain pliability easily corrects this difficulty.

Release of the pituitary antidiuretic hormone (ADH) remains within normal ranges throughout life, although increased production in response to stress has been documented. As a consequence of an "inappropriate" secretion of ADH, the body's retention of an excess of water out of proportion to salt may lead to symptomatic and clinically significant hyponatremia (*13*).

Not much is known about the secretion of growth hormone or the somatomedins in elderly patients, although there is convincing evidence that pituitary response decreases in the presence of stress (*14*). In elderly women, prolactin production has been found to be below normal in response to reduced estrogen levels; in older men, these levels have yet to be documented clearly (*15*).

Fasting blood sugar levels are unchanged in healthy elderly persons. However, an intolerance to a glucose load has been documented as resulting from two possible mechanisms. First, the sensitivity of peripheral tissue to insulin is clearly reduced. This reduction may reflect an age-related alteration in insulin receptors (*16*). Second, in response to a glucose challenge, a decreased production of insulin by the pancreatic beta cells has been found by some observers, although many others have found a normal reaction (*17*). As a consequence of these subtle alterations, higher-than-normal serum glucose values may be detected after stress or a glucose challenge. Thus, elevated glucose levels should not be mistaken or misinterpreted as a clue for incipient or clinical diabetes mellitus. Rather, the values should be remeasured under ideal conditions to quantify precisely the dimensions of the disorder. Relevant to this question is the fact that glucagon produced by pancreatic alpha cells is apparently unchanged during aging (*18*).

Musculoskeletal System

Substantial and significant alterations are found in the bony skeleton as the human body ages. Primarily, a gradual reduction in total bone mass, osteoporosis, occurs with advancing age, more so in women than in men. Unquestionably, osteoporosis is accentuated in menopausal women. The mechanism responsible for osteoporosis is not known, although stabilization or slowing of the process may be brought about by addition to the diet of supplemental calcium, vitamin D, and fluoride. Supplemental estrogen may be of value to women with osteoporosis. Unfortunately, the potential alleged carcinogenic effects of estrogen administration have limited the advisability of its use for management of osteoporosis (*19*).

A well-known and direct result of osteoporosis is easily identified in the elderly by a gradual decrease or shortening of body stature in both men and women. Similarly, a loss in mechanical strength of bone increases the chance that minor injury will lead to a fracture. As noted previously, a serious consequence of osteoporosis of the mandible and maxilla leads to weakened support of, loosening, and eventual loss of the teeth. Such loss may also result in severe dietary modification, which in turn causes nutritional imbalances that accelerate and intensify other age-related problems.

With the decline in skeletal support is found a parallel loss of body striated muscle mass, even though physical activity continues. As a consequence, fatigue sets in more easily and a gradual reduction in physical strength limits the ability of elderly humans to carry out essential physical functions.

CONCLUSION

All these age-related changes result in a reduction in muscle, organ, and skeletal mass that is accompanied by an increase in body fat of about 35 per cent (*20*). At the same time, a gradual shrinking of plasma volume by as much as 8 per cent is accompanied by a decrease in body water of about 17 per cent, with an overall diminution of extracellular fluid volume of about 40 per cent. Thus the human body, as it ages, undergoes many changes that become evident in appearance, posture, and behavior.

REFERENCES

1. M.I.D. Hanna and A. L. MacMillan, Aging and the skin, in *Textbook of Geriatric Medicine and Gerontology* (J. C. Brockelhurst and C. Livingston, eds.), 2nd edn. New York, 1978.
2. J. F. Murray, Respiration, in *Pathologic Physiology: The Biologic Principles of Disease* (L. H. Smith Jr. and S. D. Thier, eds.). Saunders, Philadelphia, 1981.
3. N. O. Fowler, Circulatory changes with aging, in *Cardiac Diagnosis and Treatment* (N. O. Fowler, ed.), 3rd edn. Harper & Row, Hagerstown, Md., 1980.
4. N. W. Shock, in *Proceedings of Seminars* (F. S. Jeffers, ed.). Council on Gerontology, Duke University, Durham, N.C., 1962, p. 123.
5. J. W. Rowe, R. Andres, J. D. Tobin, A. H. Norris, and N. W. Shock, The effect of age on creatinine clearance in men: Cross sectional and longitudinal study, *J. Gerontol.* **31:**155 (1976).
6. J. W. Rowe, N. W. Shock, and R. A. DeFronzo, The influence of age on the renal response to water deprevation in man, *Nephron* **17:**270 (1976).
7. T. Olsen, P. Laurberg, and J. Weeks, Low serum triiodothyronine and high serum reverse triiodothyronine in old age: An effect of disease not age. *J. Clin. Endocrinol. Metab.* **47:**1111 (1978).
8. P. S. Wiske, S. Epstein, N. H. Bell, S. F. Queener, J. Edmonson, and C. C. Johnston Jr, Increases in immunoreactive parathyroid hormone with age, *N. Engl. J. Med.* **300:**1419 (1979).
9. L. J. Deftos, M. H. Weisman, G. W. Williams, D. B. Karpf, A. M. Frumar, B. J. Davidson, J. G. Parthemore, and H. L. Judd, Influence of age and sex on plasma calcitonin in human beings, *N. Engl. J. Med.* **302:**1351 (1980).
10. R. H. Noth, M. N. Lassman, S. Y. Tau, A. Fernandez-Cruz Jr, and P. J. Mulrow, Age and the renin-aldosterone system, *Arch. Int. Med.* **137:**1414 (1977).
11. S.S.C. Yen, C. C. Tsai, F. Naftolin, G. Vaudenberg, and L. Ajabor, Pulsatile patterns of gonadotropin release in subjects with and without ovarian function, *J. Clin. Endocrin. Metab.* **34:**671 (1972).
12. S. M. Harman, and P. D. Tsitouras, Reproductive hormones in aging men: I. Measurement of sex steroids, basal luteinizing hormone, and Leydig cell response to human chronic gonadotropin, *J. Clin. Endocrinol. Metab.* **51:**35 (1980).
13. J. H. Helderman, R. E. Vestal, J. W. Rowe, J. D. Tobin, R. Andres, and G. L. Robertson, The response of arginine vasopressin to intravenous ethanol and hypertonic saline in man: The impact of aging. *J. Gerontol.* **33:**39 (1978).
14. E. J. Sachar, G. Mushrush, M. Perlow, E. D. Weitzman, and J. Sassin, Growth hormone response to L-dopa in depressed patients, *Science* **178:**1304 (1972).
15. M Vekemaus and C. Robyn, Influence of age on serum prolactin levels in women and men, *Br. Med. J.* **4:**738 (1975).
16. R. A. DeFronzo, Glucose intolerance and aging: Evidence for tissue insensitivity to insulin, *Diabetes* **28:**1095 (1979).
17. D. K. Anderson, D. Elahi, J. C. Brown, J. D. Tobin, and R. Andres, Oral glucose augmentation of insulin secretion, *J. Clin. Invest.* **62:**152 (1978).
18. D. Berger, R. C. Crowther, J. C. Floyd, S. Pek, and S. F. Fajans, Effect of

age on fasting plasma levels of pancreatic hormones in man, *J. Clin. Endocrinol. Metab.* **47:**1183 (1978).

19. B. L. Riggs, E. Seeman, S. F. Hodgson, D. R. Taves, and W. M. O'Fallon, Effect of the fluoride/calcium regimen on vertebral fracture occurrence in postmenopausal osteoporosis, *N. Engl. J. Med.* **306:**446 (1982).
20. P. P. Lamy and R. V. Vestal, Drug prescribing for the elderly, in *The Geriatric Patient* (W. Reichel, ed.). H. P. Publishing, New York, 1978.

3 Neurobehavioral Changes in the Aged

F. William Black and Richard M. Paddison

Various terms have been used to refer to neurobehavioral disorders, including the recent American Psychiatric Association adoption of "organic brain syndromes" to mean a constellation of psychological and behavioral symptoms without regard to specific cause and "organic brain disorders" to refer to those alterations in behavior resulting from specific neurological origins (*1–3*). The essential point to consider here is that there is no unitary disorder, whether it be "organic" or "neurobehavioral," but rather a wide range of clinical disorders. They vary in their clinical manifestations and prognoses, depending on the nature of the cause, area of the brain affected, duration, and numerous other factors. The term "neurobehavioral" will be used in this chapter, as it stresses both the neurological origins of these disorders and their variable behavioral manifestations.

As one would expect, the aged are the group most highly at risk for the development of neurobehavioral disorders. Neuronal depletion results in greater susceptibility of the remaining brain tissue to a variety of adverse influences. Pfeiffer (*4*) has characterized this state as follows: "The healthy older brain is like a man walking along the edge of a cliff; he remains quite safe and intact in the absence of any disturbing influence." Unfortunately, the vulnerable brain of the aged person is subject to a range of disrupting factors.

RISK FACTORS IN THE AGED

As the body ages, organ function decreases. Because the brain is a high-energy-exchange organ, it depends on the integrity of the multiple organ systems that support somatic homeostasis. Any interference with brain homeostasis results in behavioral changes that can be seen in many forms, the most severe of which are known by such common terms as dementia, delirium, chronic brain syndrome, organic brain dysfunction, senile dementia, and Alzheimer's disease (*5*).

Though some have held the belief that a gradual decline in cognitive function ending in dementia is a natural consequence of the physiological deterioration associated with aging, studies have shown that this is not so. Although some cognitive functions, especially memory, psychomotor speed, and conceptual shifting, are more vulnerable than others to the effects of aging, there is little evidence that general cognitive functioning naturally declines with increasing age, even to the eighth decade (*6*). Clinically significant neurobehavioral changes are not typically the result of normal aging. This seems to hold for emotional as well as intellectual changes (*7*).

The aged patient is susceptible to a variety of insults that may result in neurobehavioral change. Toxic or substrate-reducing influences (e.g., stroke, tumor) slowly erode the reserve capacity of the aged brain, which has already undergone neuronal depletion as part of the normal aging process (*4,8,9*). In addition to physiological factors, the aged person is less resistant to the psychological stress of emotional or social change.

It is important to document those cases in which neurobehavioral disorders may be treatable. Table 3-1 summarizes data from various studies (*10–13*) and provides anterospective evaluations of consecutive hospital admissions of persons with severe mental dysfunction. The major point is that 70 to 82 per cent of patients with brain dysfunction can be categor-

Table 3-1. Cases of Treatable and Untreatable Dementing Illnesses from Three Published Sources

Dementia Evaluation	Freemon (*10*)	Marsden and Harrison (*11*)	Smith et al. (*12*)
Definable but untreatable			
Multi-infarct dementia	5	8	12
Alcoholic	4	6	17
Huntington's chorea	4	3	2
Other	3	10	7
Total	16 (27%)[a]	27 (29%)	38 (38%)
Treatable			
Normal-pressure hydrocephalus	7	5	7
Chronic drug toxicity	5	2	—
Resectable mass lesions	2	3	—
Depression	1	8	11
Other	3	1	—
Total	18 (30%)	19 (20%)	18 (18%)
Unknown disease	26 (43%)	48 (51%)	54 (54%)
Total of all three categories	60	94	100

[a]Percent of total of all three categories.

ized as having untreatable conditions or unknown disorders, whereas 18 to 30 per cent of persons admitted, studied carefully and given a satisfactory diagnosis, have a treatable disorder. Thus, no matter how gloomy predictions may be about the patient with brain dysfunction, the best diagnostic efforts should be extended to rescue those with treatable illness from the spectrum of patients with often confusing and idiosyncratic organic diagnoses (*14, 15*).

Physiological Insult

More than 100 conditions and disease states have been shown to result in changes in neurobehavioral status (*8, 9, 15–17*). Such changes may present either as an acute confusional state or as a dementia. Cerebral vascular disease is, of course, a prime cause of physiological dysfunction in the aged. Polypharmacy and self-medication are all too frequent in the aged population. (The important question of polypharmacy is considered in detail in Chapter 10.) Changes in cerebral blood flow have also been implicated in those patients with neurobehavioral disorders (*18*). Whether these changes are primary or secondary phenomena is not yet certain.

Trauma is not an uncommon cause of behavior change in the elderly. Although it can frequently be diagnosed by history, some patients present with vague histories of seemingly minor trauma yet show major neurobehavioral changes. A CT scan revealing a subdural hematoma arising from the stretched bridging veins is but one example of the vulnerable aged brain being unable to accommodate to an insult that would be relatively trivial in a younger person. Thus, the aged brain is vulnerable to a wide range of physiological insults, many of which are seemingly relatively minor yet are sufficient to upset the balance of the tenuously compensated elderly patient.

Psychological Insult

Just as the physiology of the aged brain is susceptible to external or internal insult, the emotional status of many elderly patients is such that psychological stress, social changes, and environmental confusion may precipitate dramatic neurobehavioral changes. The "coronary care syndrome" or the acutely confused elderly grandparent who must be returned from a trip to Europe are examples of such susceptibility. The presence of pre-existing functional disturbance (e.g., depression) only increases the possibility of neurobehavioral change, whether this change is provoked by psychological or physiological stress. The emotional reactions of either anxiety or depression may well result in personality disintegration, which causes a clinical picture of dementia or confusion that is more severe than what could be explained on the basis of structural brain impairment alone (*15*).

The aged patient, then, must be considered at risk from a host of both physiological and psychological stresses. Metaphorically poised on the brink of the cliff, the aged person can be pushed over the edge and a major neurobehavioral change precipitated by a wide range of factors, many of which would not be considered particularly stressful in the younger person.

NEUROBEHAVIORAL CHANGES IN THE AGED

The more common changes in behavior that are known to have organic causes are here divided into four major subgroups: (1) reversible organic brain syndromes, (2) dementia related to other diseases, (3) irreversible organic brain syndromes, and (4) neurobehavioral changes due to focal brain disease. This classification scheme, though differing from that used in the *DSM* (*3*), has been chosen because of its utility in patient evaluation and treatment.

A point that must be re-emphasized in discussing neurobehavioral disorders is that they are not a unitary organic brain syndrome but a spectrum of disorders, most of which have their own clinical presentations and pathological origins. There are, however, clusters of symptoms that do tend to correspond to rather specific groups of disorders, a fact that aids in both diagnosis and management. The differentiation of disorders is important because of several factors: (1) the causes of neurobehavioral changes frequently differ; (2) some neurobehavioral changes are treatable and reversible (e.g., acute confusional states) or are treatable toward preventing further deterioration (e.g., infection); and (3) prognoses differ depending on the particular disorder, resulting in different patient management programs (*2*).

Reversible Organic Brain Syndromes

An acute confusional state is a rapidly progressive, but reversible, change in behavior that is characterized by a clouding of consciousness, lack of coherence in thought, and difficulty with attention and concentration (*2*).

Although no single definition can encompass every aspect of the syndromes, the essential features are

1. Acute onset, usually hours to days
2. Clouding of consciousness, with fluctuations being common
3. Impaired attention
4. Disordered perception in all spheres
5. Disorientation to time, person, and place
6. Fluctuations in mental status

These syndromes usually, but not universally, have an organic cause, and most, but not all, cases are reversible (*8,9*). Therefore, the term "acute confusional state" is preferable when considering manifested behavior in reversible organic brain syndromes. Failure to diagnose the condition and to treat the patient appropriately may result in his or her deterioration to the point of death. Patient management includes (a) control of the abnormal behavior and (b) identification and correction of the underlying medical problem. Environmental structuring and the use of appropriate medication to sedate the patient, especially at night, are important considerations.

Irreversible Organic Brain Syndromes

A number of neurological processes result in irreversible organic brain syndromes (dementia). Dementia, a behavioral and descriptive term, refers to a group of brain disorders in which the patient has suffered a progressive deterioration of intellectual and adaptive functions (*19*). Use of the term "dementia" presumes knowledge that the patient at one time functioned more adequately. This presumption often poses a problem, especially during a first office visit in which no historical information is provided by anyone other than the patient. Dementia and the impaired cognition associated with the acute confusional states should be differentiated. Although some writers propose that patients with clouded intellect due to confusion be classified as demented, separating those patients whose primary symptoms are confusion and delirium from those whose primary clinical manifestation is dementia seems more appropriate. Therefore, the patient with lethargy and confusion due to an electrolyte imbalance would be considered to have an acute confusional state, whereas the patient who has a gradual deterioration of cognitive function secondary to normal-pressure hydrocephalus has a dementia related to a known neurological disease (see below).

Roth (*20*) and others have reported that between 15 and 35 per cent of persons over age 65 have significant mental disorders, with 5 to 6 per cent of the total having dementia. Other estimates of the incidence of dementia in patients over 65 vary from 40 per cent to 58 per cent (*21*). Organic brain disease (largely dementia) accounts for the almost all mental hospital admissions for patients over age 75. Katzman (*21*) has termed dementia a "malignant" disease that may be the fourth or fifth most common cause of death in the United States.

Although it has both varied causes and varied clinical presentations, dementia has this cardinal feature: progressive, usually unrelenting, deterioration of cognitive, adaptive, and emotional functions. The traditional distinction between Alzheimer's (or presenile) dementia occurring before age 65 and senile dementia appearing after age 65 is now less commonly accepted because the pathology, presentation, and clinical course have been found to be more alike than different for the two. The primary dementia syndrome is associated with a posterior atrophic process in most cases. The deterioration is gradual, progressing from the initial presentation of mild changes in cognition to significant dysfunction of all neurological functions and ultimate death. Although many patients show severe atrophic changes on CT scan, some do not. The converse is also true; some patients with severe atrophic CT scan changes carry out day-to-day activities relatively well. Accordingly, the diagnosis should be a clinical one, especially early in the course, with neurodiagnostic test results used only as collaborative evidence.

An ongoing controversy concerns the clinical separability of Alzheimer's and Pick's dementias. Although each disorder has a spectrum of clinical manifestations that may make initial differentiation difficult, the preliminary symptoms are typically distinct and usually recognizable with careful evaluation. Pick's dementia is secondary to a primary frontal atrophy: affected patients classically present with changes in personality and behavior before any change in cognition or neurological status is noted. Patients' disinhibition and social transgressions often result in their referral for evaluation. As the disease progresses, more posterior areas of the brain become involved and the clinical features begin to mimic those of Alzheimer's. Clinically, the early differentiation is based on the initial symptoms—involving emotional and behavioral changes in Pick's dementia and cognitive deterioration in Alzheimer's. Statistics are also helpful in the differential diagnosis; the frequency of Alzheimer's dementia is reported to be from 50 to 100 times that of Pick's.

Multi-infarct dementia is a progressive syndrome that results from multiple small cerebral infarctions. Clinically, such patients may be differentiated from those with other forms of dementia by (a) the presence of a history of cerebral vascular disease, (b) a history of stepwise deterioration in function, (c) neurological signs that are more dramatic than the dementia itself, (d) the presence of a pseudobulbar state, and (e) better performance on memory tests than on other cognitive-function tests.

Virtually all of the neurological degenerative diseases, e.g. Huntington's chorea, Parkinson's diseases, progressive supranuclear palsy, and Creutzfeldt-Jacob disease, have intellectual and emotional deterioration as a primary or associated manifestation.

Dementia Related to Other Diseases

Although a wide spectrum of diseases may present with dementia as a primary or prominent feature (9, 17), most demented patients continue to have untreatable brain diseases, such as cerebral arteriosclerosis or Alzheimer's disease. Furthermore, even though the outlook for patients presenting with dementia remains rather poor, developing diagnostic and therapeutic measures may offer some benefit to 10 to 15 per cent of patients in whom appropriate medical or surgical treatment will either reverse or halt neurobehavioral deterioration (17). In the past 75 years, a number of dementing disorders have been recognized and can be treated—one no longer sees pellagrous dementia and only rarely sees dementia from pernicious anemia. Neurosyphilis, until 20 years ago a frequent cause of dementia, is almost never seen.

1. Normal-Pressure Hydrocephalus (NPH) This entity is characterized by abnormality of gait, incontinence, and impaired mentation. Gait disorder is usually the first symptom, although the onset of mental dysfunction may occur concurrently or, rarely, as the first symptom. Later in the course of the illness, the thought processes and motor functions become slow and urinary incontinence may develop. In conjunction with these symptoms, the cerebrospinal fluid (CSF) pressure is normal and significantly enlarged ventricles are seen on CT scan.

This syndrome, first defined by Hakim and Adams (22), occurs in two general groups of patients: adults of any age in whom a causative factor is known and those in whom the cause may not be known (23). The NPH of unknown cause occurs in about 5 to 6 per cent of all patients presenting with dementia and has a peak incidence from ages 55 to 64.

The pathogenesis of NPH appears to be fibrosis and thickening in the arachnoid of the basal cisterns with obstruction of CSF flow. The mechanism is not fully understood but is known to be triggered by increased intracranial pressure. This pressure, determined by the degree that CSF is displaced and the brain parenchyma compressed, is the gradient between intraventricular CSF pressure and venous pressure (effective CSF pressure). When effective CSF pressure is increased by any mechanism, fluid is shifted out of the parenchyma, causing alterations in the lipid and protein content of the brain. The periventricular region receives the greatest stress; as the area is compressed, the ventricles enlarge. Homeostatic mechanisms that may operate to restore normal spinal fluid pressure include opening of blocked pathways in the basal cisterns, a reduction of CSF pressure, or an increased rate of absorption.

Persons who have NPH may have an initial complaint of difficulty in walking steadily and may have recent memory loss. Neurological examination shows no focal abnormality, but balancing is difficult when the patient starts to stand or walk. The patient's steps are short, and the base is wide. Plantar responses are often extensor, and grasping reflexes may be present. Mental function may first show a recent-memory defect that becomes severe.

The diagnosis is confirmed by evidence of enlarged ventricles on CT scan, no clinical evidence of increased intracranial pressure, normal findings on routine skull x-rays, and normal CSF pressure. NPH should be differentiated from Alzheimer's disease, which usually shows cortical atrophy and enlarged ventricles on the CT scan.

Adult-onset NPH may be secondary to subarachnoid hemorrhage, trauma, meningitis, postoperative lesions, or, rarely, brain tumor.

Lumbar puncture with drainage of 25 ml or more of fluid may improve the patient's condition. The definitive treatment is surgical shunting either by ventricular peritoneal or ventricular venous shunt. Improvement may begin in 24 hours to one week. Shunting will not help a degenerative brain disorder such as Alzheimer's disease, senile dementia, or various dementing disorders.

2. Metabolic Disorders Chronic renal, hepatic, pulmonary, or cardiac disease can lead to symptoms that mimic dementia. Dementia may result from myxedema, hypoglycemia, or vitamin B12 or folate deficiency. Manic affect may result from hyperthyroidism, general paresis, or stimulant drugs, whereas depressed affect may result from hypothyroidism, hypocorticalism, or hypercalcemia. Sleep deprivation, psychological distress, sensory deprivation, or immobolization may exacerbate such symptoms.

3. Trauma-Induced Disorders In those persons whose brain is diminishing in size, the cortical bridging veins run a relatively longer, unprotected course. With relatively minor head acceleration or trauma, shearing forces may be generated, with resultant injury to these bridging veins. Venous oozing occurs and a collection of blood forms that, via osmotic and other influences, may slowly gather volume, resulting in clinical manifestations—subacute or chronic behavioral changes and possibly focal neurological symptoms later in the course of the disease. In elderly patients the greatest suspicion should be directed toward those who have recently acquired a behavioral disorder and who have waxing and waning of their level of awareness. Such phasic alterations of awareness should alert the physician to the possibility of a readily treatable disorder—the subdural hematoma. Diagnosis may be established via CT scan, isotope scan, or ultrasound scan for midline shift. However, if a high index of suspicion exists, the preferred and most accurate diagnostic test is a cerebral angiogram with an AP projection. Treatment is, of course, surgical drainage of the collection of fluid.

4. Drug-Induced Dementia About 72 per cent of persons aged 45 to 64 have at least one medically treated chronic physical illness, and about 33 per cent of that group have two or more. At age 65 and older, 86 per cent have at least one such illness and about 50 per cent have two or more. The incidence of psychiatric illness in late life is 100 times greater than that of persons 15 years of age or younger. The older person becomes a ready subject for the prescription of innumerable drugs to treat varied physical illnesses. Many drugs have side effects or interactions that can lead to production of delirium or an organic confusional state (*24*).

The adverse effects of drugs are numerous, but several agents can specifically cause the CNS changes of encephalopathy, extrapyramidal syndromes, and myelopathy. Encephalopathy has been associated with antibiotics, such as penicillin, chloramphenicol, cycloserine, isoniazid, gentamycin, and griseofulvin. Cardiac glycocides can produce toxic manifestations in the elderly. Autonomic agents, including atropine, diphenhydramine, ergotamine, methysergide, L-dopa, ephedrine, and methylphenidate, can cause behavioral change. The antiserotonin drugs, such as methysergide (Sansert) and cyproheptadine (Periactin), can cause euphoria, hallucinations, and psychotic episodes. The psychotherapeutic drugs, including phenothiazines, tricyclic antidepressants, lithium, butyrophenones, and benzodiazepines, can all produce severe nervous system and and behavioral alterations. L-dopa and combinations of L-dopa and carbidopa (Sinemet) can produce severe mental symptoms, especially depression. Prolonged use of L-dopa products may end in a dementia that includes associated hallucinatory and illusionary experiences. Unknown is whether this dementia is specifically drug-induced, the result of aging, or a combination of the two.

GI tract motility and absorbtion, slow cerebral blood flow, and impaired renal and hepatic function can all add to the risks of drug utilization in the elderly.

5. Pseudodementia Resulting from Depression (25) Persons affected by social problems of the aged often withdraw; they may become uninterested, fail to eat, have impaired sleep patterns, seem so apathetic that they are called "senile" or "dotty" and may become hostile and act indifferently (pseudodementia). Pseudodementia must be considered in the differential diagnosis of all patients presenting with impaired cognitive functioning. Although pseudodementia is classically described as a feature of depression, it has also been noted in association with conversion hysteria and several other psychiatric conditions. Although differentiation may be difficult at first contact with a severely disordered patient, the careful examiner may be able to distinguish between the two conditions in almost all cases. Some of the many important differential points are

1. The patient with depressive illness often has a life history of cyclic emotional problems.
2. Acute psychotic depression or other reactive depressions usually have a recognizable antecedent precipitating cause.
3. In depression, the emotional change (usually blunting of affect and interest) precedes the cognitive (usually memory) change, whereas the opposite is typically true in dementia.
4. The depressed patient frequently has disturbed sleep, crying spells, self-deprecation, and other behavioral signs, whereas the demented patient is usually more apathetic.
5. Mental status testing of the depressed patient reveals good constructions and, with some encouragement, evidence of adequate new learning ability and abstraction.
6. Neuropsychological testing of the depressed patient reveals normal nonverbal skills, with errors primarily noted in memory, reasoning, and tasks related to psychomotor speed and sustained attention.
7. Perhaps most important, the depressed patient responds to stimulation and encouragement; the demented patient cannot.
8. In most cases, functional behavioral changes have an onset before age 40; initial behavioral complaints in the patient over age 40 should alert the clinician to the possibility of organic changes.

It must be understood that many patients will have overlapping problems. The primarily depressed patient can also develop a dementia, and similarly many demented patients can show significant degrees of depression. In many cases, treatment of the depressive component (or other functional component) of the demented patient will result in improved functioning, at least for a time. A careful mental status assessment may separate the depressed pseudodemented patients from those with dementia.

Neurobehavioral Changes Due to Focal Brain Disease

Thus far, the information here has concerned relatively generalized disorders secondary to diffuse brain disease. In contrast, the focal syndromes are manifestations of a type of lesion different from those seen in the acute confusional states or dementias. Focal syndromes are relatively discrete changes in behavior due to localized cerebral lesions, such as an infarct, tumor, or abscess. Aphasias, apraxias, amnesias, and other relatively specific behavioral changes are associated with damage or dysfunction of particular areas of the brain (*2, 26, 27*).

NEUROBEHAVIORAL EVALUATION OF THE AGED PERSON

In many cases, the behavioral assessment shows evidence of organic brain disease long before the appearance of neurological abnormalities. Thus, certain types of patients should routinely receive mental status examinations, including the following:

1. Elderly patients who present, or are presented by their families, with histories of recent behavior change.
2. Patients having documented brain disease.
3. Patients of any age, but especially the elderly, in whom a brain lesion is suspected by virtue of a changed medical course, a change in behavior, or recent trauma.
4. Patients in whom the diagnosis of neurological disease is equivocal.
5. Patients presenting with a history of psychiatric disturbance, especially when symptoms appear rather acutely in an aged person having a history of otherwise normal emotional and behavioral functioning. Organic changes often present initially with emotional or behavioral changes, especially in cases of frontal lobe disease. Accordingly, they frequently present first to the family physician as a functional disorder.
6. Patients who present with vague physical or behavioral complaints that are impossible to substantiate or quantify by standard medical techniques. Such problems typically include those of memory and attention, a deterioration of interest in family, work, or life, and elusive physical complaints that cannot be clearly ascribed to an organic cause. In such cases, the physician should be alert to the possibility of

organic brain disease. Often the differential diagnosis is difficult and involves consideration of brain functions or other medical and functional implications.

Brief Screening Mental Status Examination Several clinically and empirically derived "mini-exams" have been developed for office and bedside use. The primary advantages of such examinations are their brevity; utility in broadly differentiating organic, functional, and combined subgroups; and reasonable objectivity and reliability. Even a brief examination should encompass a sufficient variety of cognitive and emotional factors to assure that an adequate overview of the patient's functioning is obtained. Among the critical areas that should be evaluated are (1) appearance and behavior, (2) orientation, (3) language functions, (4) constructions, (5) mood, (6) memory, and (7) general intellect. Because of this need for evaluation of a behavioral spectrum, "single factor" tests (e.g., Bender Gestalt designs) to assess the possibility of brain dysfunction are more misleading than they are clinically useful.

The mini-examination will suffice for the acutely confused patient and for screening, whereas patients with dementias and more focal neurobehavioral disorders require a more comprehensive evaluation.

The Comprehensive Mental Status Examination The advantages of this examination are that it is systematic, based on hierachial principles of neurobehavioral function, and comprehensive. Although this form of the mental status examination is considerably more comprehensive than the screening examinations, in the hands of an experienced examiner it can be completed rapidly (15 to 25 minutes) and yields valuable data otherwise unavailable in the work-up of the patient with a neurobehavioral disorder.

The mental status examination is outlined in Table 3-2.

A patient with a known nonterminal brain lesion should be evaluated neuropsychologically as part of planning the rehabilitation program. Data regarding the effect of brain dysfunction on cognitive function, emotional status, general behavior, and social adjustment are critical for overall prognosis.

Neuropsychological Evaluations

Briefly, the neuropsychological evaluation is an objective, comprehensive assessment of a wide range of cognitive, adaptive, emotional, and related behaviors that reflect the adequacy (or inadequacy) of the patient's cortical functioning. It differs from the mental status examination in that it is more extensive and typically includes tests and procedures that have been well standardized on samples of normal and brain-damaged subjects. The use of standardized measures enables the evaluator to compare the patient's performance with that of normative groups. In addition, the ade-

Table 3-2. Key Elements of the Mental Status Examination

- Patient information
- Patient's level of consciousness
- Behavioral observations
- Attention
  - Observation
  - Digit repetition
  - Random letter or "A" test for vigilance
- Language
  - Description of the patient's spontaneous speech
  - Comprehension
    - Patient's response to sequential pointing commands
    - Patient's response to yes-no questions
  - Repetition of sentences of increasing length and complexity
  - Naming of colors, objects, and body parts and word finding
  - Reading, writing, and calculations
- Memory
  - Immediate recall
  - Orientation to person, place, and time
  - Remote memory
    - Personal information
    - Knowledge of basic historical facts
  - New learning ability
    - Ability to retain four unrelated words for varying times
    - Verbal story read to the patient and then immediately recalled
    - Paired associate learning
    - Visual memory (hidden subjects)
- Constructional ability
  - Drawings to command
  - Reproduction drawings
  - Block designs
- Higher cognitive functions
  - Fund of general information
  - Proverb interpretation
  - Verbal similarities
  - Calculations
- Related cortical functions
  - Ideomotor apraxia
  - Right-left orientation
  - Finger agnosia
  - Presence of denial and neglect
  - Frontal lobe functions—alternating sequences (written and hand movements)

quacy of the patient's functioning in a variety of different areas can be readily contrasted. Because of the wide range of performance assessed and the depth to which they are evaluated, the neuropsychological evaluation is better able to detect subtle deficits early in the course of a disease than is the mental status examination (*2,28*). The neuropsychological evaluation has several advantages over most currently available neurodiagnostic techniques. It is a noninvasive procedure and accordingly has no risk of mortality or morbidity.

CONCLUSION

Two factors make neurobehavioral changes particularly worthy of the physician's attention: they are extremely common in medical practice, posing difficult diagnostic and management problems, and their causes are at times treatable. Familiarity with the neurobehavioral disorders and a careful evaluation of the behavioral as well as the mental status of the patient presenting with alterations in emotions or behavior result in appropriate diagnosis, treatment when indicated, and proper planning for patient management. Such awareness also eliminates the referral of patients having abnormal behavior due to organic brain syndromes to mental health facilities, which are less likely to assess properly the medical and neurological component of the patient's problem. Use of well-constructed mental status examinations and the resources of the neuropsychologist when indicated lead to early diagnosis.

Some senile brain changes seem to occur in all of us. However, in that vast wasteland of senescence, senility, organic brain syndromes, and dementia, we may find 20 to 30 per cent of older persons have treatable disorders.

REFERENCES

1. D. F. Benson, preface in R. L. Strub, and F. W. Black, *The Organic Brain Syndromes.* Davis, Philadelphia, 1981.
2. R. L. Strub, and F. W. Black, *The Organic Brain Syndromes.* Davis, Philadelphia, 1981.
3. American Psychiatric Association Task Force, *Diagnostic and Statistical Manual of Mental Disorders DSM/III.* American Psychiatric Association, Washington, D.C., 1980.
4. E. Pfeiffer, Clinical manifestations of senile dementia, in *Senile Dementia: A Biomedical Approach* (K. Nandy, ed.) Elsevier North-Holland, New York, 1978.
5. C. E. Wells (ed.), *Dementia,* 2nd edn. Davis, Philadelphia, 1977, p. 284.
6. A. L. Benton, P. J. Eslinger, and A. R. Damasio, Normative observations on neuropsychological test performance in old age. *J. Clin. Neuropsychol.* **3**:33 (1981).
7. R. D. Savage, Intellect and personality in the aged, in *Aging and Dementia* (W. L. Smith and M. Kinsbourne, eds.) Spectrum, Jamaica, N.Y., 1977.
8. A.J. Levenson (ed.), *Neuropsychiatric Side-Effects of Drugs in the Elderly.* Raven Press, New York, 1979.
9. A. J. Leven and R. C. Hall (eds.), *Neuropsychiatric Manifestations of Physical Disease in the Elderly.* Raven Press, New York, 1981.
10. F. R. Freemon, Evaluation of patients with progressive intellectual deterioration, *Arch. Neurol.* **33**:658 (1976).
11. C. D. Marsden and M.J.G. Harrison, Outcome of investigation of patients with presenile dementia, *Br. Med. J.* **1**:50 (1972).
12. J. S. Smith, L. G. Kiloh, G. S. Ratnavale, and D. A. Grant, The investigation of dementia: The results of 100 consecutive admissions, *Med. J. Australia* **2**:403 (1976).

13. Editorial: The investigation of dementia, *Med. J. Australia* **2:**397 (1976).
14. M. F. Folstein, S. E. Folstein, and P. R. McHugh, "Mini-mental state": A practical method for grading the cognitive state of patients for the clinician. *J. Psychiatr. Res.* **12:**189 (1975).
15. H. S. Wang, Dementia in old age, in *Dementia* (C. E. Wells, ed.). Davis, Philadelphia, 1977.
16. D. R. Crapper-McLachlan and U. DeBoni, Etiologic factors in senile dementia of the Alzheimer type, in *Aging of the Brain and Dementia* (L. Amaducci, A. N. Davison, and P. Antuono, eds.). Raven Press, New York, 1980.
17. G. R. Haase, Diseases presenting as dementia, in *Dementia* (C. E. Wells, ed.). Davis, Philadelphia, 1977.
18. L. Gustafson and J. Risberg, Regional blood flow related to psychiatric symptoms in dementia with onset in the presenile period. *Acta Psychiatr. Scand.* **50:**516 (1974).
19. C. E. Wells (ed.), *Dementia.* Davis, Philadelphia, 1977.
20. M. Roth, Aging of the brain and dementia: An overview, in *Aging of the Brain and Dementia* (L. Amaducci, A. N. Davison, and P. Antuono, eds.). Raven Press, New York, 1980.
21. R. Katzman, The prevalence and malignancy of Alzheimer's disease. *Arch. Neurol.* **32:**217 (1976).
22. S. Hakim, and R. D. Adams, The special clinical problem of symptomatic hydrocephalus with normal cerebrospinal fluid pressure: Observations on cerebrospinal fluid dynamics. *J. Neurolog. Sci.* **2:**307 (1965).
23. R. G. Ojemann, Normal pressure hydrocephalus in *Current Surgical Management of Neurologic Disease* (C. B. Wilson, and J. T. Hoff, eds.). Churchill Livingston, New York, 1980.
24. A. J. Levenson (ed.), Neuropsychiatric Side-Effects of Drugs in the Elderly, in *Aging,* vol. 9. Raven Press, New York, 1979.
25. V. T. Sherr, Benjamin Franklin and geropsychiatry: Vignettes for the bicentennial year, *J. Am. Geriatr. Soc.* **24:**447 (1976).
26. D. F. Benson, *Aphasia, Alexia and Agraphia.* Churchill Livingston, New York, 1979.
27. H. Hecaen, and M. Albert, *Human Neuropsychology.* Wiley, New York, 1978.
28. R. L. Strub, and F. W. Black, *The Mental Status Examination of Neurology.* Davis, Philadelphia, 1977.

4 Pathophysiology of Aging

Kenneth R. Brizzee

Over two decades ago, Strehler (*1*) proposed that any age-associated change, to be considered part of the basic aging process, should be (a) universal (b) intrinsic (c) progressive and (d) deleterious. Medawar (*2*) suggested that senescence is of at least twofold origin. One set of factors, which he considered to be innate, is developmental. Strehler referred to these as "determinate processes." The other set, comprising the cumulative effects of injurious influences, is environmental. Risk factors for senility fall into the latter category, which includes infection, disease, stress, radiation, trauma, toxins, temperature extremes, and tumor-producing agents. Such factors undoubtedly exert a significant influence on the intrinsic process of aging but do not conform to Strehler's essential criteria for this process.

This chapter describes the major structural alterations in the mammalian brain that have been consistently demonstrated to occur during aging. These structural changes, most of which we consider to be the visible manifestation of the determinative or innate factors, appear to form a substrate upon which risk factors of various types may impinge to alter both the severity and the rate of aging. The sociomedical advances that have lengthened the average human lifespan in developed countries since the turn of the century (*3*) have resulted mainly from the amelioration of such risk factors.

GROSS STRUCTURAL CHANGES

A common gross alteration in the human brain observed during aging is a widening, and apparent deepening, of sulci, together with a decrease in width and mass of gyri, apparently due in large part to a reduction in the mass of the white matter in the centrum semiovale as well as to a reduction in cell number and neuropil (*4*) (Figure 4-1). Although such changes

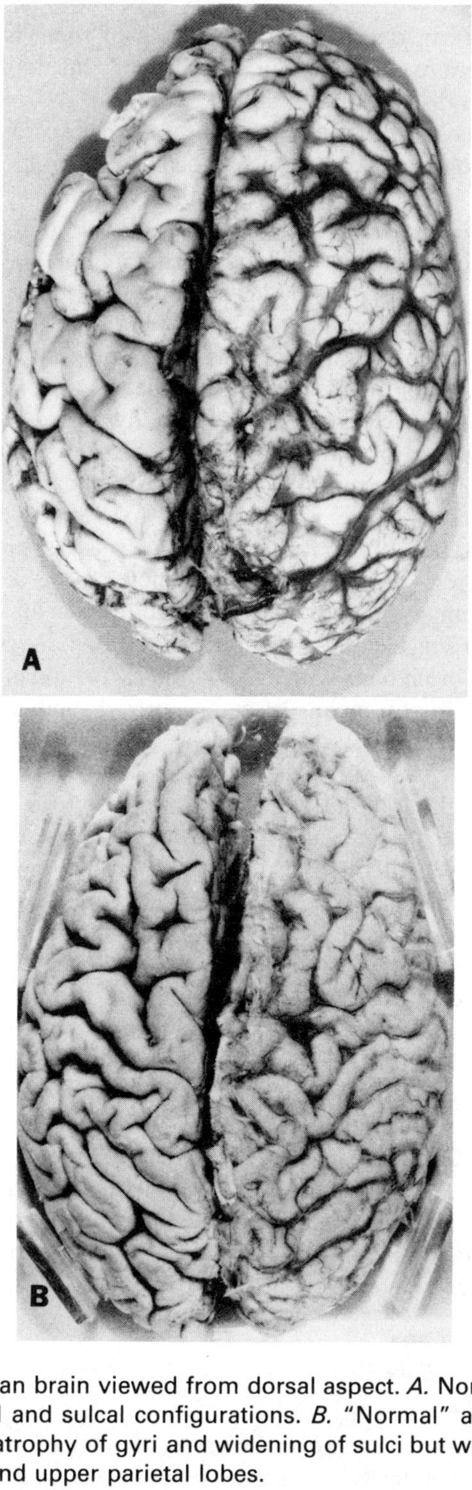

Figure 4-1. Human brain viewed from dorsal aspect. *A.* Normal adult showing normal gyral and sulcal configurations. *B.* "Normal" aged brain showing generalized atrophy of gyri and widening of sulci but with severe alterations in frontal and upper parietal lobes.

may be moderate in degree, some evidence of them is found in a high percentage of brains of aged human patients, including those without histories of brain disease or dementia.

Recently it was shown that brain volume, expressed as a percentage of cranial cavity volume, decreases significantly in nondemented patients over 60 years of age (*5*). In another recent quantitative study of cerebral atrophy in old age and senile dementia, the ratio of brain volume to cranial capacity was noted to decline with age so that a total of about 5 per cent of brain volume is lost in advanced old age in control (nondemented) patients (*6*). Dementia patients younger than 80 years of age generally showed excessive brain atrophy relative to controls. In some cases the deficit was as much as 18 per cent of the mean control value. However, the ratio of brain volume to cranial capacity in dementia patients over age 80 did not differ significantly from that of controls of the same age.

In a large group of hospital patients considered representative of the population at large, the mean brain weight for men decreased from 1449 grams in subjects 20 to 30 years of age to 1344 grams in subjects 70 to 80 years of age (*7*). The regression of EEG frequency in senescence followed the general trend of many growth curves, including that for brain weight (*8*). This observation suggests the possibility of a broad direct relationship between the loss in brain mass with age and the regression in EEG frequency.

Barron et al. (*9*), by means of computerized tomography (CT), measured changes in ventricular volume with age and showed a progressive increase from the first through the sixth decades and an even larger increase in the eight and ninth decades. In a more recent CT study (*10*), a significant increase in ventricular size with age was observed and a significant enlargement of sulci was also seen in human subjects. Those investigators reported no apparent relationship between measures of brain mass and mental status. Similarly, no significant relationships existed between measures of mental function and sulcal score (obtained from the sum of the widths of the four largest sulci scanned in the upper three CT sections). Furthermore, there was no significant correlation between ventricular and sulcal measures. Drechsler (*11*) recognized the possibility that the slowing of cerebral activity, which he observed in a long series of EEG studies in young and aged human subjects, may relate to senile atrophy of the CNS. By means of a new CT method combined with previously used CT techniques in 43 outpatients, each having a presumptive diagnosis of senile dementia of the Alzheimer's type (*12*), the physical measurement of the third ventricle was noted to be the single most powerful linear correlate of cognitive impairment.

MICROSCOPIC CHANGES

Neuron Nucleus

Some investigators have observed increased pallor of nuclei in aged neurons. A loss of regularity of nuclear outline and an absence of a sharp demarcation between nucleus and cytoplasm of some cerebral cortical neurons have also been found in aged rhesus monkeys. Nuclear inclusions and nuclear invaginations in neurons appear to be more numerous in aged than in young adult rats (Figure 4-2).

A reduction of nuclear volume with age was observed in the chinchilla by Cammermeyer (*13*), and similar changes have been described recently by Lin et al. (*14*) in several hypothalamic areas in the rat.

Neuron Perikaryon

In the perikaryon of some large pyramidal neurons in the motor cortex of aged rhesus monkeys, basophilia was reduced and Nissl substance apparently depleted. Other investigators have observed similar changes in various species (*13*). Some of these workers have emphasized that the depletion of Nissl material appears to coincide with an increase in lipofuscin in the perikarya of the same neurons and have suggested a causal relationship between the two phenomena.

Using optimal stereologic methods, Haug (*15*) recently showed that the total visual cortex (area 17) in human brains does not diminish in volume,

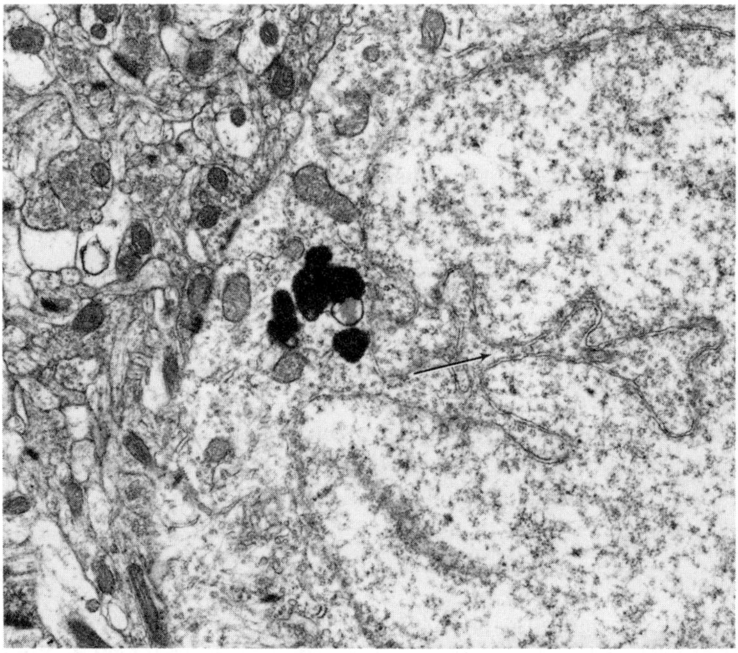

Figure 4-2. Electron micrograph of a neuron nucleus, showing an extensive invagination (*arrow*) in the caudatus-putamen of a 29-month-old Fischer 344 rat (x 27 000).

but neuron size (presumably soma volume) in all classes does decrease moderately. In parietal area 7, a decrease in tissue volume was noted, but the decrease in neuron size was less than that in area 17. In premotor area 6, a continuous decrease in volume of cortical neurons was observed during life. The neurons of area 11 showed a distinct size decrease only after age 65. Haug emphasized that the aging processes in the human brain differ considerably from region to region. He suggested that those cortical areas that are most active begin aging later than those areas that are less active throughout life.

Ultrastructural studies in neurons of the lateral vestibular nucleus in rats revealed a sparse pattern of rough surface endoplasmic reticulum (RER) relative to that in young adult rats. Hinds and McNelly (*16*) noted a threefold increase in the volume of cisternae of RER per mitral cell in the rat olfactory bulb from 3 to 27 months postnatally and a halving from 27 to 30 months.

Hinds and McNelly also observed a linear increase in the volume of Golgi complex cisternae per mitral cell in the rat olfactory bulb throughout the period from the third to the twenty-seventh month, and no evidence of a decrease was seen from the twenty-seventh to the thirtieth month. Others have observed similar Golgi vesicle dilation in the lateral vestibular nucleus of 18-month-old rats.

In mitochondria, a loss in the outer unit membrane accompanied by vesiculation of cristae and formation of multivesicular bodies has been observed in older mice. Disintegration of the single unit membrane of the vesicular bodies resulted in residual masses of vesicular material. Hinds and McNelly (*16*) showed that the volume of mitochondria per mitral cell in the rat olfactory bulb increased from the third to the twenty-seventh month, but they observed a considerable decrease in that volume from the twenty-seventh to the thirtieth month.

Melanin

That pigment melanin appears in the perikarya of neurons of the substantia nigra and locus ceruleus at birth and increases linearly until middle age has been reported. In old age, however, the pigment content of these structures actually decreases, possibly due to the selective atrophy of the most highly pigmented neurons rather than as a result of a general pigment loss from all such cells.

Lipofuscin

In electron micrographs, the lipofuscin granules have a granular, electron-dense component and a vacuolar or vesicular electron-lucent component. The entire granule, made up of a varying number of such components, is ensheathed in a single limiting membrane. Figure 4-3 shows an electron micrograph of lipofuscin granules in the cytoplasm of a neuron from the

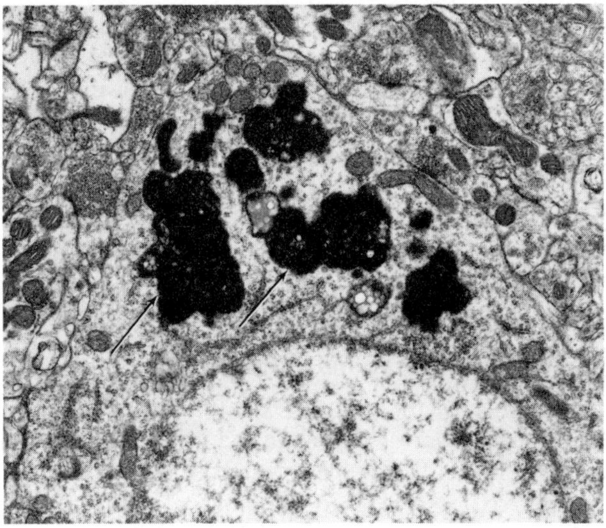

Figure 4-3. Electron micrograph of a portion of the perikaryon of a neuron in the caudatus-putamen of a Fischer 344 rat, showing an extensive accumulation of lipofuscin granules (*arrows*) (x 27 000).

nucleus caudatus-putamen of an aged Fischer 344 rat. Glees and Hasen (*17*) recognized six patterns of lipofuscin deposition: homogeneous, finely granular, vacuolated, lamellated (banded), coarsely granular, and compound or heterogeneous. These patterns correspond to those we observed in the rat and rhesus monkey.

Quantitative histological studies on regional differences in the accumulation of lipofuscin in the rhesus monkey revealed that the neurons of the inferior olivary nucleus accumulated the greatest amount of the pigment, whereas the neurons of the medial nucleus of the superior olive accumulated the least (*18*). The same study found that the accumulation of lipofuscin in glial cells differed decidedly from region to region. Lipofuscin was especially abundant in the glia cells adjacent to the Purkinje neurons of the cerebellum and in glia adjacent to the neurons in the medial nucleus of the superior olive. The low pigment content in the neurons of these structures, in contrast to the large amount in the adjacent glia cells, suggests that these glial elements may be directly involved in removing lipofuscin from the neurons.

Several authors have reported that the amount of lipofuscin in the perikarya of neurons decreases after the chronic administration of the hydrochloride of the dimethylaminoethyl ester of parachlorophenoxyacetate (Helfergin, centrophenoxine, meclophenoxate, Lucidril). Nandy (*19*) reported that the behavioral performance of old rats in reversal learning situations improved significantly after chronic daily treatment with centrophenoxine for periods up to 12 weeks.

The functional significance of lipofuscin is unknown. Some investigators have suggested that the pigment mass may damage the neuron by distorting and disturbing the cell geometry, crowding out other organelles, altering or blocking diffusion and transport pathways, and generally decreasing the neuron's metabolic efficiency. The accumulation of large amounts of pigment, especially at dendritic branching points, by interfering with protoplasmic transport to cell processes, might result in degeneration and loss or distortion of the cell process with age of the type described by Scheibel and Scheibel (*20*).

Axonal Changes and Alterations in the Neuropil

In the pyramidal tract of the aged C57BL/10 mouse, significant decreases were noted in the number of mitochondria in the axons and in the number of neurofilaments and a significant increase was seen in the number of microtubules per axon from 8 to 26 months of age. Samorajski (*21*) reported an age-related decrease in the total number of myelinated fibers per nerve in the posterior tibial nerve in C57BL/10 mice, with a fairly uniform loss across all caliber of fibers. However, the size of the individual nerves increased with age, as did the mean axon diameter of individual fibers and the proportion of connective tissue between fibers in the older nerves. Ultrastructural studies showed an increase in mean axon circumference of myelinated fibers between three and eight months and of unmyelinated fibers between eight and twenty-six months. Mitochondrial concentration in myelinated fibers also decreased between eight and twenty-six months of age. In the posterior tibial nerve, no change was observed in concentration of filaments and microtubules or in blood vessels or myelin sheath thickness with increasing age.

In humans, Toghi et al. (*22*) reported that the average small myelinated fiber density in the sural nerve decreased gradually with age after the second decade. The mean number of fibers for each square millimeter cross-sectional area for the eighth decade was 74 per cent of that for the second decade. The large myelinated fiber density in the ninth decade was only 54 per cent of that in the third decade. These results seem to show that the ratio of small to large myelinated fiber density increases with age. In the sural nerve studies of Toghi et al., the nuclear density (mainly Schwann cells and fibroblasts) increased gradually from the second to the eighth decade.

A comparative study of peripheral motor nerve conduction in nondemented and demented elderly humans showed that maximum forearm conduction velocity in the median nerve was significantly lower in demented than in control patients (*23*). In nondemented psychiatric patients, conduction velocity and wrist latency values were comparable with published normal values.

On the other hand, LaFratta and Canestrari (*24*), testing the medial nerves of male patients, reported a significant decline in values of both sensory and motor nerve conduction velocity with increasing age. However, statistically valid relationships between alterations in nerve fibers and functional decrements remain to be demonstrated.

Alterations in Dendrites

In CNS tissue stained with the rapid Golgi method, the first age-related changes in dendrites in the mouse lower brain stem and spinal cord appear as irregular swellings and "lumpiness" of cell bodies and initial portions of dendrites. These changes are followed by increasing nodularization of the dendrite tree and apparent loss of spines and postsynaptic specializations normally seen in the young adult (*20*). In the hypothalamus, the cytoarchitecture becomes progressively disrupted, paralleled by deterioration and loss of dendrite surface. Those who investigated the changes suggested that such alterations in the hypothalamic dendritic tree contribute to the physiological phenomena associated with the decline in the brain-gonadal functions in old persons.

Morphometric studies on age changes in cerebral cortical dendrites in rats showed a decrease in dendritic diameters and a decrease in the number of dendritic spines per unit length of dendrites. That some dendrites appeared aspinous was also noted. The density of basal dendritic arborizations in the auditory cortex of aged rats was reported to be greatly decreased, but the extent of the dendritic arborizations did not change. In neurons of the human cerebral cortex, distortion and loss of dendritic processes with age have been reported.

Hasan and Glees (*25*) reported an increase in the incidence of dendritic profiles and dendrodendritic contacts without intervening glial fibers in aged rats. Those authors suggested that such data may have important implications for explaining observed decremental changes in the integration of complex motor skills and decreased responsiveness of motor pathways that occur in senescence.

In Buell and Coleman's study (*26*) of dendritic changes in the human parahippocampal gyrus, the dendritic trees were found to be more extensive in elderly persons (average age 79.6 years) than in younger adults (average age 51.2). Most of the difference was due to increases in the number and average length of terminal segments of the dendritic tree. In senile dementia (average age 76.0 years) dendritic trees were less extensive in elderly brains than in adult brains, largely because the former group's terminal segments were fewer and shorter. However, cells with shrunken dendritic trees were found in all brains. Buell and Coleman interpreted their data as suggesting a model of aging in the CNS in which one population of neurons dies and regresses and the other survives and grows. They were of the opinion that the latter appeared to be the dominant neuron population in aging without dementia.

Synaptic Alterations

Ultrastructural studies of rhesus monkey cerebral cortex have revealed that the number of synaptic vesicles decreases with age but synaptic clefts are well preserved. In the rat hippocampus, axosomatic synapses were observed less frequently in old than in young animals.

A decreased number of cortical synapses in the superior frontal gyrus in aged human brains (Figure 4-4) and in the molecular layer of the dentate gyrus in aged rats was found in several ultrastructural studies (*27*). Drechsler (*11*) suggested that the short latencies he observed in the first component of somatosensory evoked potentials (SEP) (median nerve stimulation) and visual evoked potentials (VEP) (light flashes) indicate that they are transmitted "through paucisynaptic pathways to the specific cortical response area." He noted that the SEP and VEP have prolonged latencies of all components in aged as compared with young adult subjects, and he maintained that the long latencies of the late components support the hypothesis that these are evoked through polysynaptic pathways. He postulated that the quantitatively different prolongations of the different components of the evoked potentials probably relate to age-dependent changes of the synaptic transmitter mechanism. It seems reasonable to assume that such alterations in evoked potentials in the cerebral cortex might be caused by losses of synapses with age.

In the rat cerebellar glomeruli, a significant decrease in surface density

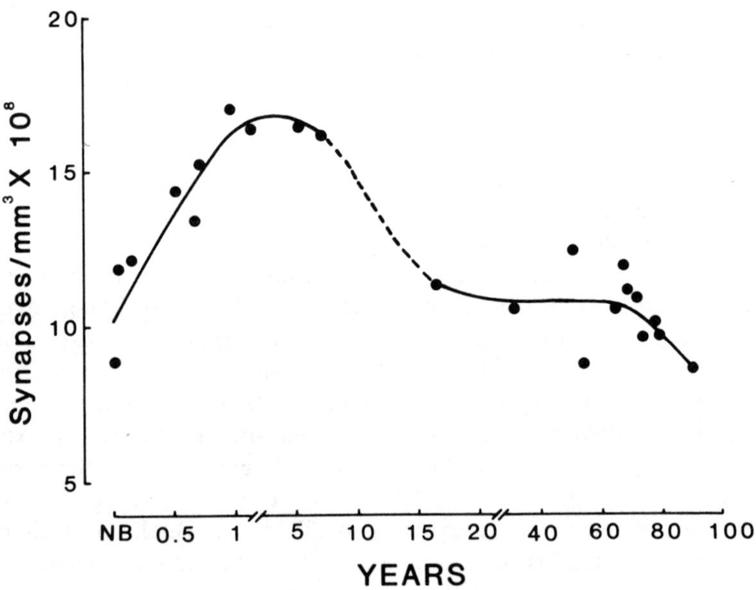

Figure 4-4. Life-span changes in density of synapses in human frontal cortex. From Huttenlocker (*27*).

of synaptic contact zones per unit area, in total length of the synaptic contact zones per unit area, and in numerical density of synapses was observed in aged animals. Fredarri and Giuli (*28*) regarded the age-dependent decrease in synaptic parameters observed in the cerebellar glomerulus as a morphological basis for the known decline in the integration of complex motor activities by the cerebellum. They suggested that any deterioration of the contact zones between nerve elements may influence the processing of the information coming from the periphery, necessary for complete motor coordination.

Neurofibrillary Changes, Amyloid and Senile Plaques

Although neurofibrillary tangles are characteristic of the cytological changes in the brain in Alzheimer's disease, they are also found in fewer numbers in the course of normal aging. They occur preponderantly in the frontal and temporal cerebral cortex and hippocampus but may occasionally be found in the mesencephalon and rostral rhombencephalon.

Neurofibrillary tangles shown in light microscope preparations consist of compact clusters of neurofibrils in neuron perikarya or dendrites and axon synaptic terminals, resulting in abnormal intraneuronal configurations. They exhibit birefringence in polarized light and are argyrophilic. As shown in electron micrographs, the neurofibrillary material consists of masses of modified microtubules. These measure 200 to 220 Å in diameter, as compared with about 240 Å for normal microtubules. A large proportion of such tubules appear crescentric rather than circular in outline when cut transverse to their long axis. In the human brain, they exhibit periodic constrictions every 800 Å and are actually in the form of paired helical filaments. In a single aged rhesus monkey brain, similar structures have been observed and with the periodic constrictions occurring at intervals of about 500 Å (*29*).

A recent quantitative study of cerebral atrophy in old age and senile dementia showed that the incidence of neurofibrillary tangles in the hippocampal gyrus was greater in most demented patients than in controls and was unaffected by the age of the subjects (*6*). On the other hand, senile plaque formation was said to be unrelated to clinical status and showed some tendency to increase with age. The investigators concluded that disease processes, rather than exaggerated age change, underlie primary neuronal dementia of the Alzheimer type.

Amyloid has been observed in animal and human brains both in "normal" aging and in age-related pathological conditions, such as Alzheimer's disease. In the CNS, amyloid commonly occurs in blood vessels and senile plaques. The "classical" plaque consists of a central core of amyloid surrounded by degenerating neuronal processes and reactive cells. Data from recent ultrastructural studies on the genesis of senile plaques indicate that degenerating neuronal processes are the most important source of these structures. In hospital patients without evidence of dementia, the incidence of plaques was small in middle-aged patients but increased notably in older subjects.

NEURON LOSS

Ellis (*30*) reported a negative correlation between age and number of Purkinje cells per equivalent unit area of cerebellar tissue, and most later reports on cell population changes in cerebral and cerebellar cortex have generally supported the concept of a loss of neurons with age. However, data from studies on age changes in certain structures of the brain in some species or strains of subprimate mammals suggest that neuron loss with age, at least in some regions of the brain, may be less severe in certain strains or species than in humans or perhaps nonhuman primates.

One widely quoted study on age changes in neuron number in human cerebral cortex is that of Brody (*31*), who reported that the greatest neuron loss was found in the superior temporal and precentral gyri, area striata, and postcentral gyrus, in decreasing order. All cell layers were affected, with the greatest loss occurring in the external and internal granular layers. Tomlinson and Henderson (*32*) reported a significant decrease in numbers of neurons measuring between 27 and 31 micrometers in longest horizontal chord in brains from nondemented human subjects from about 15 to over 90 years of age. As Drechsler (*11*) pointed out, the analysis, differentiation, and synthesis of the continuous influx of information by the cortex is possible only by its selective limitation to specific cortical structures via selective cortical inhibition. In aging human subjects, Drechsler observed a spread of the somatosensory-evoked response over the whole hemisphere. He suggested that this phenomenon probably relates to a progressive decrease of inhibitory processes during aging. Cerebral "neuron fallout" with age, together with age-related alterations in dendrites, might contribute to a disruption of the normal balance of the processes of excitation and inhibition, thus contributing to the functionally debilitating spread of the somatosensory cortical response over the whole hemisphere.

In the study on Long-Evans rats, we (*33*) observed that, although the neuron packing density did not decrease with age, the glial packing density in the old animals increased significantly. Other workers have also reported increases in glial numbers with age in specific CNS structures.

In a recent quantitative study of 90 normal human subjects (42 female, 48 male), counts of cerebellar Purkinje cells showed a mean reduction of 2.5 per cent per decade, or 25 per cent during 100 years (*34*). The data indicate that the reduction in the Purkinje cell population first became apparent on curvilinear graphs at about the sixtieth year. In another study, atrophy of all three laminae in the human cerebellar cortex with severe loss of Purkinje cells was observed in aged subjects (*35*).

Studies in our laboratory revealed a significant decrease in the number of neurons in the lamina pyramidale of the CA-1 zone of the hippocampus in 29-month-old, as compared with 11-month-old, Fischer rats (*36*). Lipofuscin content in the neuron perikarya increased greatly in the old animals and correlated significantly with the decrease in the number of neurons with age.

In a quantitative study of age changes in neuron populations in the human hippocampus, including counts of all neuron nucleoli in the ventrolateral quadrant (*37*), the best linear regression lines comparing nerve cell density and age showed a negative correlation for nondemented patients. The mean neuron densities did not differ significantly for the right and left sides of the brain, and neuron density in these tissues was reported to decrease 27 per cent in the 50-year period between ages 45 and 95.

A significant decrease in cell packing density in the amygdala of behaviorally normal aged, as compared with young and middle-aged adult, human subjects has been described by Herzog and Kemper (*38*). No statistically significant change in volume of individual divisions between the two age groups was found, however. On the other hand, all divisions of the amygdala in brains from aged demented subjects underwent a statistically significant decrease in cell packing density in comparison with either the young or the aged normal group.

The data available to date give no indication of an increase in glial packing density in the hippocampus of the aged rat or in human subjects. However, astroglial hypertrophy and increased oligodendroglial satellitosis are prominent features of the hippocampus in the aged rat.

A significant decrease in the neuronal populations of the human substantia nigra and the locus ceruleus suggests the possibility of a dysfunction of central monoaminergic systems in aged persons. Tomlinson and associates (*39*) reported that the mean count of neurons in the locus ceruleus was significantly less in brains obtained from patients with senile dementia of the Alzheimer type (SDAT) than in normal aged subjects. There was also some evidence that the more severe cases of SDAT, in terms of neocortical plaque formation, had the greatest loss of locus ceruleus neurons.

A loss of both small and large neurons with age, together with a decrease in volume, has been reported in the human putamen (*40*) (Figure 4-5). Recent studies in our laboratory revealed a significant decrease in the neuron packing density in the ventrolateral region of the caudatus-putamen in 25-month-old, as compared with 5-month-old, Fischer 344 rats (*41*). A significant increase in the glial packing density in the older animals was seen in the same tissues.

That the volume of the human brain's ventral cochlear nucleus decreases with age has been reported, but the total number of neurons in this nucleus does not decrease. In the spiral ganglion of the cochlea of the rat, the number of neurons (both type I and type II) decreased by 14 per cent from the age of 1 or 2 months to 23 months and by 20 per cent at 27 to 29 months. In animals of 33 to 34 months of age, the mean neuron loss was 28

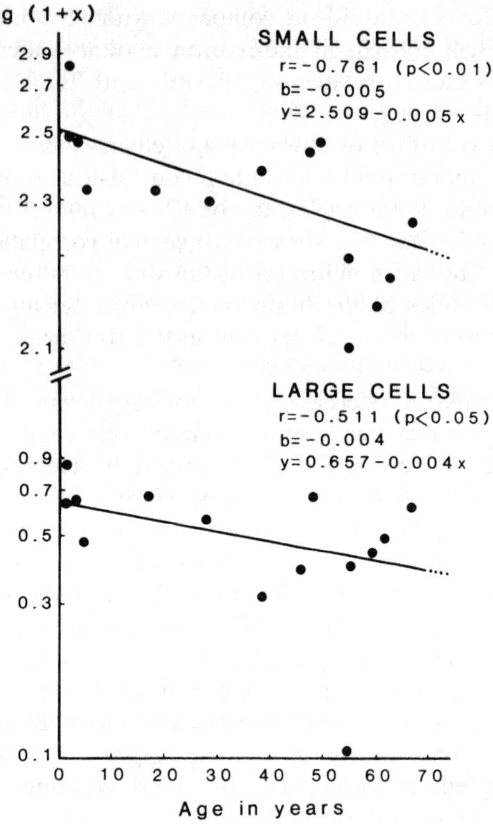

Figure 4-5. Linear regression lines illustrating the decrease of small and large cells with age in the human putamen. From Bugiani et al. (*40*).

and 33 per cent, respectively. In human subjects, primary degeneration of the first-order cochlear neurons is the pathological basis of the *neural type* of presbycusis. In this condition, which is much more prevalent in aged than in young patients, there is a loss of speech discrimination that is more severe than the hearing loss for pure tone frequencies (*42*).

As in the case of the ventral cochlear nucleus, the human trochlear and abducens nuclei show no loss in neurons in advanced age. Some earlier studies in the human inferior olivary nucleus also revealed no changes in the total neuron number with age. However, more recent investigations by Sandoz and Meier-Ruge (*43*) indicated a significant decrease in number of neurons in this nucleus in aged humans. The discrepancy in results between these studies remains to be resolved.

Maleci in 1936 (*44*) reported finding the total number of neurons in the facial nucleus in humans decreased slightly with age. However, a more recent study showed no influence of age on the number of cells in the facial nucleus in the cat, dog, or human.

In a series of 47 spinal cords from human subjects between 13 and 95 years of age, no loss of motor neurons was evident in lumbosacral segments up to 60 years of age. Above 60 years of age, however, several cases showed motor neuron counts of only 50 per cent of that in early adult life or middle age (Figure 4-6). Such cell loss appeared to be uniform throughout all segments and was unaccompanied by any other striking morphological change (*45*).

Alterations in Glial Cells

In ultrastructural studies on age changes in glia cells, oligodendroglial satellitosis, binucleated cells, fusion of oligodendroglia, and invagination of oligodendroglial nuclear membranes with pronounced marginal condensation of nuclear chromatin have been observed in the hippocampus of rats. No changes in astrocytes were observed, but many lipid vacuoles were seen in microglia.

In the nuclei of Bergman astrocytes in the chinchilla cerebellum, nuclear membranes were commonly found to be indented and invaginated, with the tip of each invagination ending near a nucleolus. Deep pink periodic acid-Schiff-stained bodies of various configurations (irregular rods, bars, spheres, or faceted bodies) were observed in astrocyte nuclei (*13*).

In the olfactory bulb of aged human subjects, degenerative changes in astrocytes have been reported. In these elements, a homogenization of the soma and gradual loss of processes were observed, resulting in a round, homogeneous, dark-stained body with no resemblance to a cell.

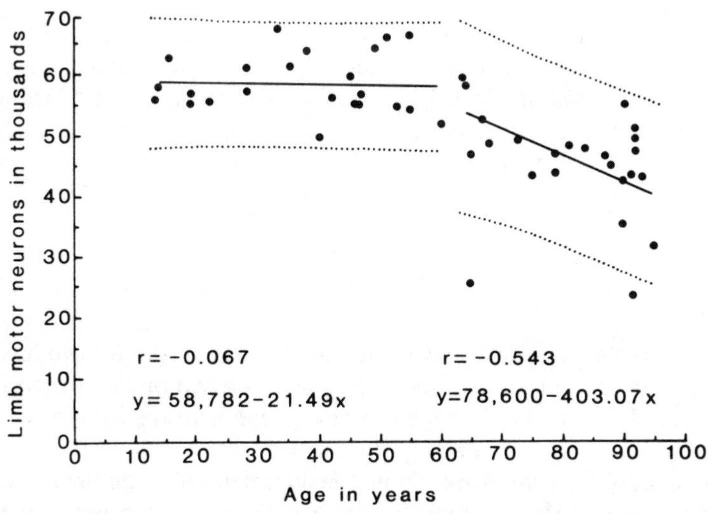

Figure 4-6. Numbers of limb motor neurons in the human lumbosacral cord in 47 subjects from 13 to 95 years of age. From Tomlinson and Irving (*45*).

Table 4-1. Results of stereologic studies on vascular changes with age in human cerebral cortex

Stereologic parameters	Precentral gyrus, age-dependent differences	
	Young	Aged
Diameter, μm	6.73	7.21
Projected area, %	2.32	2.97
Specific surface area, μ^{-1}	0.129	0.120
Mean linear distances, μm	451	373
Length/unit cortex volume, cm/mm^3	20.65	24.05

Source: Hunziker et al. (*47*).

Alterations in Blood Vessels

Investigations on vascular effects of aging in the human hippocampus showed that the diameter of both capillaries and arterioles increases with age (*46*). The density of capillaries decreased, whereas that of the arterioles increased significantly. The authors suggested that the capillary changes may indicate a reduced exchange potential accompanying aging. In the same study the overall capillary diameters and densities in brains of persons with Alzheimer's disease did not differ from those of age-matched controls. However, those hippocampal zones showing the greatest severity of, or increment in, nerve cell lesions were found to correspond to those having the largest increase in capillary density. This finding was interpreted as suggesting a direct association between neuronal susceptibility to Alzheimer's changes and the degree of regional blood supply.

Hunziker and associates (*47*) reported that capillary specific surface area and mean linear distances decreased in the human neocortex of young adults as compared with elderly subjects, whereas capillary volume and diameter and capillary length/unit cortex volume increased (Table 4-1).

Burns et al. (*48*) reported attenuation of capillary walls and declining numbers of endothelial mitochondria per capillary profile with increasing age in the frontal and occipital cortices of the pigtail monkey (*Macaca nemestrina*).

COMMENT

Although the motor and sensory manifestations of the infirmities of age are familiar to everyone, statistically valid correlations of structural and functional decrements with age are few. Some investigators (*8*) have suggested that, if the number of brain cells decreases with age, signal strength would be reduced. Noise level might also be increased in a relative sense if the number of nerve cells and synapses available for progressive refinement of the signals received is reduced. Similar functional deficits might occur if the functional integrity of a significant proportion of the nerve cells is reduced through age changes such as the reported reduction in RNA content, loss of dendrites, and loss or alterations of dendritic spines and synapses.

These data and thinning of the cortex may also help to explain the long aftereffects seen in EEG studies on aged subjects (*49*). As Timiras (*8*) pointed out, such aftereffects tend to blur subsequent signals, with the degree of interference depending on the intensity of the aftereffect in relation to that of the primary cortical activity resulting from the signals actually present. This single phenomenon, possibly resulting from neuron fallout and/or alterations in residual neurons, may explain the increased time necessary for aged persons to perform simple tasks.

As to the question of whether arousal is reduced with age, galvanic skin-response and skin-conductance tests tend to be lower in aged subjects. EEG studies, on the other hand, suggest higher arousal levels (*50*). Our own studies in the Fischer 344 rat showed that pain-elicited aggression, considered to be a measure of behavioral arousal, declined significantly in animals 29 months of age (*36*). In the same animals, a significant loss of neurons occurred in the CA zone of the hippocampus in the aged as compared with 11-month-old rats. Whether these phenomena are causally related remains to be determined.

The severe and relatively selective degeneration in the amygdala in senile dementia as compared with behaviorally normal aged subjects is believed to strengthen the notion that the amygdala, which is considered to play a major role in emotion, motivation, and memory, may be involved in the pathogenesis of deficits in these functions in senile dementia.

That the velocity of conduction in some human nerves decreases with age has been known for many years. Norris et al. (*51*) stated that the observed reduction in conduction velocity could not be attributed to nerve fiber degeneration. They suggested that alterations in nerve metabolism associated with membrane permeability and/or other transfer changes might be the most suitable explanation for changes in conduction velocity.

REFERENCES

1. B. L. Strehler, Origin and comparison of the effects of time and high-energy radiations on living systems, *Quart. Rev. Biol.* **34:**117 (1959).
2. P. B. Medawar, *An Unsolved Problem of Biology*. Lewis, London, 1951.
3. J. F. Fries, Aging, natural death, and the compression of morbidity, *N. Engl. J. Med.* **303:**130 (1980).
4. V. F. Shefer, Hippocampal pathology as a possible factor in the pathogenesis of senile dementias, *Neurosci. Behav. Physiol.* **8:**236 (1977).
5. P.J.M. Davis and E. A. Wright, A new method for measuring cranial cavity volume and its application to the assessment of cerebral atrophy at autopsy, *Neuropath. Appl. Neurobiol.* **3:**341 (1977).
6. B. M. Hubbard and J. M. Anderson, A quantitative study of cerebral atrophy in old age and senile dementia, *J. Neurol. Sci.* **50:**135 (1981).

7. A. S. Dekaban and D. Sadowsky, Changes in brain weights during the span of human life: Relation to brain weights of (body heights and body weights). *Ann. Neurol.* **4**:345 (1978).
8. P. S. Timiras, *Developmental Physiology and Aging.* Macmillan, New York, 1972.
9. A. S. Barron, L. Jacobs, and W. R. Kinkel, Changes in the size of normal lateral ventricles during aging determined by computerized tomography, *Neurology* **26**:1011 (1976).
10. C. P. Hughes and M. Gado, Computed tomography and aging of the brain, *Radiology* **139**:391 (1981).
11. F. Drechsler, Quantitative analysis of neurophysiological processes of the aging CNS. *J. Neurol.* **218**:197 (1978).
12. M. J. deLeon, S. H. Ferris, A. E. George, B. Reisberg, I. I. Kricheff, and S. Gershon, Computed tomography evaluations of brain-behavior relationships in senile dementia of the Alzheimer's type, *Neurobiol. Aging* **1**:69 (1980).
13. J. Cammermeyer, Cytological manifestations of aging in rabbit and chinchilla brains. *J. Geront.* **18**:41 (1963).
14. K. H. Lin, Y. M. Peng, and M. T. Peng, Changes in nuclear volume of rat hypothalamic neurons in old age, *Neuroendocrinology* **21**:247 (1976).
15. H. Haug, Quantitative results on normal aging of the human cortex, *Proceedings of the 2nd International Ernst Reuter Symposium on Brain Aging.* Berlin, July 1981.
16. J. W. Hinds and N. A. McNelly, Aging in the rat olfactory bulb: Quantitative changes in mitral cell organelles and somato-dendritic synapses. *J. Comp. Neurol.* **184**:811 (1979).
17. P. Glees and M. Hasen, Lipofuscin in neuronal aging and disease, *Norm. Pathol. Anat. (Stuttgart)* **32**:1 (1976).
18. K. R. Brizzee, J. M. Ordy, and B. Kaack, Early appearance and regional differences in intraneuronal and extraneuronal lipofuscin accumulation with age in the brain of a nonhuman primate, *J. Geront.* **29**:366 (1974).
19. K. Nandy, Lipofuscinogenesis in mice early treated with centrophenoxine, *Mech. Ageing Develop.* **8**:131 (1978).
20. M. E. Scheibel and A. B. Scheibel, Structural changes in the aging brain, *Aging,* vol. 1 (H. Brody, D. Harman, and J. M. Ordy, eds.). Raven Press, New York, 1975.
21. T. Samorajski, Age differences in the morphology of posterior tibial nerves of mice, *J. Comp. Neurol.* **157**:439 (1974).
22. H. Toghi, H. Tsukagoshi and Y. Toyokura, Quantitative changes with age in normal sural nerves, *Acta Neuropath. (Berlin)* **38**:213 (1977).
23. R. Levy and E. W. Poole, Peripheral motor nerve conduction in elderly demented and nondemented psychiatric patients, *J. Neurol. Neurosurg. Psychiat.* **29**:362 (1966).
24. C. W. LaFratta and R. E. Canestrari, A comparison of sensory and motor nerve conduction velocities as related to age, *Arch. Phys. Med. Rehabil.* **47**:286 (1966).
25. M. Hasan and P. Glees, Ultrastructural changes in hippocampal neurons, synapses and neuroglia, *Exp. Gerontol.* **8**:75 (1973).
26. S. J. Buell and P. D. Coleman, Dendritic growth in the aged human brain and failure of growth in senile dementia, *Science* **206**:854 (1979).

27. P. R. Huttenlocher, Synaptic density in human frontal cortex: Developmental changes and effects of aging, *Brain Res.* **163:**195 (1979).
28. C. B. Fredarri and C. Giuli, A quantitative morphometric study of synapses of rat cerebellar glomeruli during aging, *Mech. Ageing Develop.* **12:**127 (1980).
29. H. M. Wisniewski, B. Ghetti, and R. D. Terry, Neuritic (senile) plaques and filamentous changes in aged rhesus monkeys, *J. Neuropath. Exp. Neurol.* **32:**566 (1973).
30. R. S. Ellis, Norms for some structural changes in the human cerebellum from birth to old age, *J. Comp. Neurol.* **32:**1 (1920–21).
31. H. Brody, Organization of the cerebral cortex: III. A study of aging in the human cerebral cortex, *J. Comp. Neurol.* **102:**511 (1955).
32. B. E. Tomlinson and G. Henderson, Some quantitative cerebral findings in normal and demented old people, in *Neurobiology of Aging* (R. D. Terry and S. Gershon, eds.). Raven Press, New York, 1976.
33. K. Brizzee, N. Sherwood and P. Timiras, A comparison of cell populations at various depth levels in cerebral cortex of young adult and aged Long-Evans rats. *J. Geront.* **23:**289 (1968).
34. J.A.N. Corsellis, Some observations on the Purjinke cell population and on brain volume in human aging, in *Neurobiology of Aging* (R. D. Terry and S. Gershon, eds.). Raven Press, New York, 1976.
35. E. Tarnowski-Dziduszko, Morphological picture of the cerebellum in the course of the aging process, *Neuropathol. Pol.* **11:**199 (1973).
36. K. R. Brizzee and J. M. Ordy, Age pigments, cell loss and hippocampal function, *Mech. Ageing Develop.* **9:**143 (1978).
37. M. J. Ball, Neuronal loss, neurofibrillary tangles and granulovacuolar degeneration in the hippocampus with ageing and dementia: A quantitative study, *Acta Neuropath.* **37:**111 (1977).
38. A. G. Herzog and T. L. Kemper, Amygdaloid changes in aging and dementia, *Arch. Neurol.* **37:**625 (1980).
39. B. E. Tomlinson, D. Irving, and G. Blessed, Cell loss in the locus coeruleus in senile dementia of Alzheimer's type, *J. Neurol. Sci.* **49:**419 (1981).
40. O. Bugiani, S. Salvarani, F. Perdelli, G. L. Mancardi, and A. Leonardi, Nerve cell loss with aging in the putamen, *Europ. Neurol.* **17:**286 (1978).
41. K. R. Brizee, T. Samorajski, R. C. Smith, and D. L. Brizzee, The effect of age and chronic neuroleptic drug treatment on cell populations in the neostriatum of Fischer 344 rats, in *Aging 17, Brain Neurotransmitters and Receptors in Aging and Age-Related Disorders* (S. Enna, T. Samorajski, and B. Beer, eds.). Raven Press, New York, 1981.
42. R. R. Gacek, Degenerative hearing loss in aging, in *Neurological and Sensory Disorders in the Elderly* (W. S. Fields, ed.). Year Book, Chicago, 1975.
43. P. Sandoz and W. Meier-Ruge, Age-related loss of nerve cells from the human inferior olive, and unchanged volume of its gray matter, *IRCS J. Med. Sci.* **5:**376 (1977).
44. O. Maleci, Sul rapporto numbricotra le cellule dei nuclei di origine e la fibre di nervi motori encefalici dell'uomo, con osservazioni differenze qualitative delle fibre, *Arch. Ital. Anat. Embriol.* **35:**559 (1936).
45. B.E. Tomlinson and D. Irving, The numbers of limb motor neurons in the human lumbosacral cord throughout life, *J. Neurol. Sci.* **34:**213 (1977).

46. M. A. Bell and M. J. Ball, Morphometric comparisons of hippocampal microvasculature in ageing and demented people: Diameters and densities, *Acta Neuropathol. (Berlin)* **53:**299 (1981).
47. O. Hunziker, S. Abdel, and U. Schulz, The aging human cerebral cortex: A stereological characterization of changes in the capillary net, *Gerontology* **24:**27 (1978).
48. E. M. Burns, T. W. Kruckeberg, L. E. Comerford, and M.B.T. Buschmann, Thinning of capillary walls and declining numbers of endothelial mitochondria in the cerebral cortex of the aging primate, Macaca nemestrina, *J. Geront.* **64:**642 (1979).
49. M. C. Diamond, R. E. Johnson, and C. A. Ingham, Morphological changes in the young adult and aging rat cerebral cortex, hippocampus and diencephalon, *Behav. Biol.* **14:**163 (1975).
50. A. C. Mundy-Castle, Central excitability in the aged, *Aging Around the World: Medical and Clinical Aspects of Aging,* vol. 4 (H. T. Blumenthal, ed.). Columbia University Press, New York, 1962.
51. A. H. Norris, N. W. Shock, and I. H. Wagman, Age changes in the maximum conduction velocity of motor fibers of human ulnar nerves, *J. Appl. Physiol.* **5:**589 (1952).

5 Risk Factors for Senile Dementia

Jacob A. Brody and Lon R. White

In the study of senile dementia epidemiologists have tried, thus far unsuccessfully, to discern patterns that would distinguish the afflicted minority from the general population. An important preliminary question is, How does senile dementia differ from Alzheimer's disease? This chapter considers the conditions associated with neuropathological changes described in Alzheimer's disease, which includes both senile and presenile forms. Of greatest interest are the former. For convenience and perhaps from some sense of conviction (see below), we keep the two forms separate. Because much more is known about the senile form, the bulk of this chapter deals with those entities generally embraced by the term "senile dementia, Alzheimer's type" (SDAT). Some overlap will be obvious.

Having made this semantic demarcation, the next issue is whether SDAT is a disease or merely one form of normal aging. Considering SDAT to be a disease is convenient and potentially useful because, even if it is not a disease (a difficult word to define), it certainly involves a specialized pattern of degeneration. Thus, although SDAT shares elements with normal aging, there must be factors that cause it to appear and be recognizable in some persons and not in others.

The issue of whether Alzheimer's disease is one entity with two forms—presenile and senile—cannot yet be resolved. Some argue that the early and late forms involve the same changes, both clinically and pathologically, but at different ages, and thus should be considered one entity. Others, including ourselves, consider it premature to combine the two entities because we lack rigorous data indicating that the pathogenesis and natural history of the early form are identical with those of the senile form. Furthermore, etiological research is better served if the entities are considered as separate. If one is caused by factor X and the other is not, we could miss the critical association by case dilution; if both are caused by factor X, it will be manifest in both groups.

A critical gap in the data pertains to the age-specific incidence of the presenile and senile forms. If the distribution is bimodal, with an early peak followed by a trough and then a steady rise, and if the clinical or epidemiological patterns differ in the earlier and later forms, separate causes are implied.

EPIDEMIOLOGY

Epidemiologists do not need a fixed and final diagnosis to ply their trade. Within the present state of knowledge, therefore, deciding whether SDAT is a clinical or pathological diagnosis is not a critical issue as long as specialists generally agree about the terms. The more germane problem is suggested by a quotation from Roth (*1*): "The most significant challenge of all is that presented by the contrast between ordinary senescence and Alzheimer's and other forms of dementia." How do we treat the entity that Kral (*2*) refers to as benign senescent forgetfulness? Perhaps epidemiologists will be able to determine whether this entity is simple normal aging or indeed a part of the natural history of SDAT.

It is clear that the incidence and prevalence of dementia increase with age and that the problem is one of enormous magnitude both economically and in terms of lost human potential and disrupted lives. Even though a limited proportion of the people afflicted with this condition are actually institutionalized, approximately half of the institutionalized elderly in the United States appear to be cognitively disabled (*3*).

In almost all series, regardless of the criteria used, we find that among those who are clinically diagnosed as having a senile dementia, from 50 to 65 per cent will have SDAT-like neuropathological changes (*4*). Although malignant and nonmalignant forms are recognized, a general conformity of data—derived from neuropathology studies, population surveys, and, to some extent, regional institutional surveys—suggests that diagnosticians are probably discussing the same entities.

The magnitude of the problem and clues to pathogenesis are described and sought by epidemiologists through comparisons of incidence, prevalence, and mortality among groups of individuals categorized according to a characteristic or an exposure. Each of these indices of disease frequency has its own set of methodological problems. Mortality data are generally not useful in dementia research because of great underreporting. Determination of incidence is especially difficult and expensive because it requires that a large population be under surveillance for a period after a baseline evaluation, in order to determine who becomes demented during the period of observation. Cross-sectional studies of prevalence are the least expensive and have provided most of the information on the epidemiology of this condition. The validity of prevalence estimates depends on several factors relating to the identification of all or nearly all cases in the population. Approaches that depend on recognition of dementia during conventional medical contacts are of unacceptably limited utility because of the many cultural, social, and behavioral factors that might produce inaccuracies and spurious differences. For example, the person who lives with her or his family in a sheltered environment is certainly much less likely to come to medical attention than one who does not. Another difficulty is that the degree of impairment often varies, with persons slipping into and out of states of impaired cognitive functioning (*5*). This variability may lead to underdiagnosis or to ambiguous diagnosis. Varying educational and language backgrounds also influence the expression and/or recognition of cognitive disability (*6*). Among the several problems that interfere with comparing rates of dementia reported in various studies, probably the most perplexing is that of differing diagnostic criteria.

Estimates of the incidence of dementia have been few and of uncertain comparability. Among the residents of Rochester, Minnesota, over 29 years of age, Kokmen and Schoenberg (*7*) reported an annual incidence of 110 new cases per 100 000. Their figures were based on fixed and rather restrictive criteria applied to persons whose condition had been recognized and documented by physicians in medical facilities in that area during a five-year period. In a study done in Sweden, Akesson (*8*) estimated the annual incidence of "senile psychosis" among persons aged 60 and older as 380 per 100 000. His estimate for the incidence of dementia due to "severe arteriosclerotic psychosis" was 520 per 100 000 in the same population.

No data suggest that trends exist or that rates have changed over time. Descriptions compatible with the clinical features of SDAT exist in the literature from earliest writings. Obviously, with the increasing number of persons surviving to late age, the absolute number of cases is increasing rapidly. The possibility that changes in reported mortality and prevalence of dementia might actually reflect a changing incidence within a single community was considered by Gruenberg (*9*) with reference to a study carried out in southern Sweden between 1947 and 1957. His conclusion was that improvements in medical treatment had increased the duration of illness (and thereby the point prevalence) but that these did not indicate a true increase in incidence. It seems generally accepted that the frequency of dementia in the elderly is, in fact, fairly constant over time and over large geographic areas.

Estimates of the prevalence of dementia from population studies in northern Europe have ranged from 3.9 per cent to 21.6 per cent (severe dementia, 1.3 to 6.2 per cent; mild impairment 2.6 to 15.4 per cent) among the elderly (*10–16*). A recent study conducted in Copiah County in rural Mississippi resulted in an estimate of 1 per cent for severe dementia among county residents aged 40 and older, climbing to a 7 per cent prevalence among residents aged 80 or older (B. S. Schoenberg, personal communication). These figures reflect stringent criteria and the inclusion of only severe cases. In Akesson's study, the age-specific prevalence of severe dementia at age 80 and above was 4.8 per cent (*8*). Less restrictive criteria resulted in higher age-specific prevalence figures, such as 12.6 per cent (*15*) and 22 per cent (*13*) among persons age 80 or older. In general, the increase in age-specific prevalence between the ages of 60 and 80 appears to be 10- to 20-fold, exceeding 20 per cent by 80 to 85 years. That these figures are probably underestimates of the true prevalence is also generally agreed.

Unanswered questions involve the age-specific rates from the presenile through the oldest age groups. SDAT rates probably continue to increase with age. Many neurological diseases begin later in life but then diminish. This diminution is certainly true of amyotrophic lateral sclerosis and multiple sclerosis. Even Parkinson's disease seems to decline after the eightieth or eighty-fifth year (*17*). Some pathological observations among extremely old persons suggest a decrease in the presence of Alzheimer's associated neuropathological changes (*18*). Autopsy studies in extremely old persons, are, of course, subject to considerable bias because a person who dies having a diagnostic problem is much more likely to undergo autopsy than someone having only general senile mental changes.

Clinicians are aware that the initial signs and symptoms of SDAT vary widely and encompass a variety of entities and causes. SDAT probably has a life-shortening effect. Available studies, however, have not found this effect consistently. More frequently, age, male sex, and poor general physical condition at the time of diagnosis of SDAT are associated more strongly with early death. Thus the question arises as to whether or not SDAT itself is a fatal condition.

Clinicians tend to agree that more women than men have SDAT. However, EEG findings over time suggest that fast-wave activity is better preserved in women than in men (*19*). The likelihood is great that clinicians see more female patients because women far outnumber men in the older, more susceptible age groups. Furthermore, elderly women are much more likely to be widowed and living alone than elderly men and hence would require institutionalization in the absence of social supports. In the United States among persons over age 65, there are about 5.5 million women and only 1.6 million men living alone or with nonrelatives. That a true sex difference has been documented is unlikely from the information available, although such a difference may exist (*20*).

Among the Chamorro people of Guam and the other Mariana Islands is a focus of dementia resembling presenile Alzheimer's disease associated with extrapyramidal features (*21*) (see Chapter 6). No other known focus or geographic localization by country, latitude, urban-rural status, or other common factor has yet been defined. No one would suggest that this topic has been addressed systematically, but wherever old people are studied, senile dementia has been reported.

What has been said for geographic distribution can also be said for race: no patterns have been detected. Throughout the United States between 1950 and 1965 a high proportion of SDAT patients were institutionalized. Since epidemiologists and other health researchers have for many years been interested in different rates of and reasons for institutionalization, it seems reasonable to expect that a race differential would have been reported if it actually existed. Longevity and cardiovascular disease patterns among black and white elderly Americans do differ substantially. The apparent absence of differences in age-specific dementia rates suggests that the factors determining risk for dementia are probably dissimilar from the major factors responsible for racial differences in cardiovascular morbidity and mortality. This line of reasoning focuses attention away from life-style, obesity, smoking, stress, diet, medical care, and the like and toward genetic, early-life, and late-life characteristics and exposures.

There is no suggestion in the literature concerning clusters of cases with common exposure or occupations. One exception to this is among prizefighters, who develop a syndrome that shares much with Alzheimer's disease. Thus, trauma (at least that of the severity to which prizefighters are exposed) joins Guam in providing a deviation from the absolutely random pattern of observed dementia.

Although medical and psychiatric histories have not been reported to relate to the likelihood of developing SDAT, an association of SDAT with lower social status has been reported (*6*). The significance of the association with social status is uncertain, however, since individuals with fewer social supports would likely be more heavily represented in institutions. Furthermore, most test batteries would tend to discriminate against people with less education. Again, these points are raised not to claim that socioeconomic variables are not related to SDAT but to emphasize that convincing evidence of a causal association is lacking.

In short, SDAT presents no comfortable epidemiological pattern. It is perhaps the only disease in which no acceptable pattern that would aid epidemiological thinking is even suggested.

PATHOLOGY AND NEUROCHEMISTRY

Epidemiologists look to pathology and neurochemistry for facts, and facts are plentiful although not definitive. Yet to be determined, for example, are those factors that are causally sufficient or necessary for SDAT. A cluster of changes associated with normal aging exists, but those changes also characterize the predominant findings in Alzheimer's disease (see Chapter 4). These include the neurofibrillary tangles in the form of paired helical filaments, senile plaques, granulovacuolar bodies, and Hirano bodies (*4*). In addition, congophilic angiopathy is frequently observed, and evidence is increasing that the dendritic arbor disintegrates. Considerable data have been accumulated about the anatomic patterns of these findings and their intensity.

Chlorine acetyltransferase (CAT) is similarly depressed with age but more so with SDAT (*22*). Gerontologists are gradually learning about enzyme levels that normally increase or decrease with age, and frequently those that decline are observed at still lower levels among patients with SDAT. This enzyme level difference for both groups seems to be true for norepinephrine and dopamine. Most attention, however, seems to be focused on the functioning of the cholinergic system.

It has been postulated that a combination of the neuropathological alterations described above somehow reaches a threshold beyond which clinical SDAT proceeds. A similar argument should be made for decreases in CAT levels. In the many studies of brains of persons dying in a state of senile dementia, about 50 per cent have the above-mentioned neuropathological changes. About 20 per cent do not have these changes but have severe atherosclerosis. The significance of this group remains unclear because SDAT is not a vascular disease. In another 15 per cent or so, both Alzheimer-like changes and atherosclerotic changes occur, and in about 10 per cent there are other specific causes for the demented state. In a final 5 to 10 per cent, no distinctive disease characteristics are encountered (*4*). Contrariwise, in at least 10 per cent of the elderly population without mental illness the changes usually ascribed to Alzheimer's disease occur at a frequency sufficient to overlap that usually encountered in SDAT. Thus persons without senile dementia can have the neuropathological changes associated with Alzheimer's disease, and patients with senile dementia can have histologically normal brains. This nonspecificity implies that we cannot yet associate pathological lesions with symptoms.

Some investigators have tried to correlate the degree of dementia before death with the concentration of neurofibrillary tangles and senile plaques. Some evidence seems to show the two are correlated, albeit loosely. Although the correlation has not been reported among non-Guamanian patients with dementia, Hirano et al. (*23*) did find that the number of neurofibrillary tangles diminishes with progression of disease. Whether senile plaques similarly diminish with age and severity is not clear.

This observation makes the attempt to correlate clinical with neuropathological findings an elusive undertaking. Part of the problem involves deciding whether cell loss occurs in SDAT patients to a greater degree than in control patients of the same age. This question is currently a matter of dispute (*4*). If cell loss occurs, then it too would be one of the critical neuropathological findings. Here, however, only the appearance of abnormal cells and particles is of concern. It is doubtful that all areas (hippocampus?) have been surveyed adequately enough to allow us to state definitively the numbers of cells or concentrations of cells with lesions.

We want to emphasize further that, although Alzheimer-like structural changes are observable, the chemical abnormalities deserve considerable attention. The logic of the importance of a chemical lesion is supported by Busse and Wang's study (*5*), in which the clinical course was not steadily progressive but regularly involved remissions and exacerbations. Furthermore, clinical improvement is common in patients at certain times of the day and for rather surprisingly long periods. Conversely, clinical status often declines after a minor illness or following a geographic move.

These rapid swings are more likely to be chemically than anatomically mediated. Lazarus notwithstanding, dead cells do not come back to life. One should recall that in Parkinson's disease, patients who have been practically immobile for years are able to move normally for a short time after intense emotional stimulation. Part of the chemical lesion in Parkinson's disease is now understood and amenable to treatment with L-dopa. Optimism is high in some quarters that an analogy exists with SDAT and the cholinergic system and that clinical improvement may result from flooding the nervous system with choline percursors (lecithin).

THE CORRELATION SCRAMBLE

Some of the recent directions in SDAT investigations are considered next.

Data from aluminum studies in cats, tissue culture, and neurons containing neurofibrillary tangles confirm a higher affinity for aluminum in specific tissues in SDAT (*24*). The significance is far from clear, however, because persons exposed to high levels of aluminum, such as aluminum workers and patients on renal dialysis, do not necessarily develop neurofibrillary tangles or SDAT. Perhaps aluminum is an indicator of some metabolic process, one involving the parathyroid and metallic ions, that is either causally or passively associated with SDAT.

Genetic influences have been considered with regard to presenile and senile forms of Alzheimer's diseases (*25*). Most of the early clinical studies showed varied patterns compatible with (a) no genetic influence, (b) a relationship between presenile dementia and SDAT in the same families, and (c) mathematical models that could be interpreted as autosomal dominant inheritance with incomplete penetrance or with age-dependent penetrance, implying that if the person lived long enough eventually penetrance would be complete. The possibility of polygenic factors has also been dicussed. Data necessary to sustain autosomal dominant inheritance with incomplete penetrance or polygenic inheritance are virtually impossible to obtain and certainly unavailable at present. In the Guam form of dementia, which occurs at an extraordinary high rate, no Mendelian pattern of inheritance has emerged. One extremely rare form of familial Alzheimer's disease in which many of the cases have onset in the presenile age range has been well documented (*26*).

Recent studies of families of autopsied patients with Alzheimer's disease of presenile and senile forms encountered an elevated frequency of Down's syndrome. The association is much stronger when the Alzheimer's disease appeared in its presenile form (*27*). Several groups are studying Down's syndrome to detect whether the association can be sustained, starting with patients having that syndrome and determining rates of SDAT among family members. Studies are also under way to detect whether Alzheimer's disease occurs more frequently in the offspring of elderly parents. That Alzheimer's disease could be late-onset Down's syndrome has been suggested. The chromosomal dislocations encountered in Down's syndrome are not seen in Alzheimer's disease, but impetus to conduct these studies is provided by the observation that most Down's syndrome patients who survive into adulthood develop neurofibrillary tangles that are indistinguishable from those found in Alzheimer's disease. Chromosomal studies among familial and nonfamilial Alzheimer's disease (presenile and senile forms) have given inconsistent results. The most persistent finding is of aneuploidy in Alzheimer's disease (*28*). Aneuploidy is, of course, a difficult finding to interpret, particularly if results are not consistent from patient to patient and laboratory to laboratory. When chromosomes are prepared for study, perhaps the most common artifact is apparent aneuploidy resulting from the loss of a chromosome during the extensive manipulation.

Recent histocompatibility typing data were summarized from about 60 patients, including nearly equal numbers having SDAT and the presenile form of Alzheimer's disease. Data for the two groups did not differ. HLA type B^7 was significantly increased in all Alzheimer's disease. Previous reports of positive associations with other HLA types were not sustained. Nonetheless, workers in the field have the impression that some associations are likely. Homozygosity of HLA types increases with age. Most intriguing is a suggestion of a $B^7 - CW^3$ haplotype being greatly increased among Alzheimer's patients of all ages when compared with the frequency in the general population (*29*). More will surely be heard concerning HLA typing and senile dementia. It is worth noting that the types apparently associated with Alzheimer's disease are not found in Down's syndrome.

The possibility that SDAT is caused by an unconventional ("slow") virus cannot be dismissed. Studies among Guamanians with dementia were coupled with the original kuru studies in the first primate experiments. Thus far, the Guam extract has been negative when studied by the techniques used to transmit kuru and several human slow-virus diseases of the central nervous system. In the late 1960s, extracted material from several unusual patients with familial Alzheimer's disease produced a spongiform degeneration in chimpanzees indistinguishable from the neuropathology encountered with inoculations from kuru brains. Numerous attempts to reproduce these transmissions from the original material and from many other patients with familial and nonfamilial dementias of the presenile and senile forms have been negative to date (*30*). The early observations, thus, are essentially uncorroborated by the scientists who did the original work, and today the virus studies must be considered negative.

Many causes of immunopathology among SDAT patients have been suggested. A brain-specific antibody and some immunoglobulins identified in senile plaques have been reported. Attempts to correlate immunoglobulin levels with disease or test performances have, on occasion, given positive or "suggestive" results. Eisdorfer and associates (*31*) summed up the data nicely: "In the aggregrate, there appears to be a nagging relationship between components of the immunoglobulin system and certain aspects of cognitive performance." Yet another provocative observation is an association of Alzheimer's disease, both presenile and senile, with haptoglobin gene Hp^1. This gene is also reported to be associated with an excess risk of leukemia and a less efficient general immune responsiveness. In Down's syndrome a diminished immune responsiveness and excess risk of leukemia are also suggested. Haptoglobin type distribution in Down's syndrome, however, is apparently normal (*32*).

"CONCERNING HUMAN UNDERSTANDING" AND THE EPIDEMIOLOGICAL METHOD

With a topic as difficult as SDAT, one must evoke faith in strict technique and proceed according to the rules with a logical, and at times tedious, dedication. The impediments to direct acquisition of information are all too clear from the numerous examples of positive and less-than-positive data and suggestions given earlier in this chapter. Because we are hampered by lack of useful definitions, epidemiologists will have to obtain functional definitions that are testable in populations. Of primary need is a series of viable clinical and psychometric instruments. These must include instruments that can be used for field testing, others that can be used in hospitals and clinical settings, and still others that are useful for following up patients over time. Until scales with high degrees of correlation with outcomes are found, progress will be slight. Another need is for a rough rating score, such as that referred to as the Kurtzke Scale for multiple sclerosis, which quantifies severity of a range of clinical signs and symptoms.

We suggest that these efforts go on in many populations with many different instruments and types of patients. Of course, communication between investigators is necessary, but the most important factor is for enough investigators to keep working until there begin to emerge epidemiological patterns that suggest the cause of senile dementia—or at least the direction laboratory studies should take.

Perhaps during this challenging and lengthy evolutionary phase, a pathologist or immunologist or chemist will get lucky and shortcut all our efforts. We do, however, profess to the prejudice that the hippocampus is harder to get to than a well-studied series of populations.

What can be sadder than an epidemiologist investigating a disease that has no pattern? We must take heart from Hume's discussion of miracles in his essay "Concerning Human Understanding?": "That no testimony is sufficient to establish a miracle, unless the testimony be such a kind that its falsehood would be more miraculous than the fact which it endeavors to establish." It is clearly more miraculous that there be no pattern than that the evidence thus far accumulated—suggesting the absence of a pattern—is incomplete and incorrect.

REFERENCES

1. M. Roth, Diagnosis of senile and related forms of dementia, in *Aging,* vol. 7: *Alzheimer's Disease: Senile Dementia and Related Disorders* (R. Katzman, R. D. Terry, and K. L. Bick, eds.). Raven Press, New York, 1978.
2. V. A. Kral, Benign senescent forgetfulness, in *Aging,* vol. 7: *Alzheimer's Disease: Senile Dementia and Related Disorders* (R. Katzman, R. D. Terry, and K. L. Bick, eds.). Raven Press, New York, 1978.
3. *National Nursing Home Survey: United States 1973–1974.* GPO, Washington, D.C., 1977.
4. R. D. Terry, Aging, senile dementia, and Alzheimer's disease in *Aging,* vol. 7: *Alzheimer's Disease: Senile Dementia and Related Disorders* (R. Katzman, R. D. Terry, and K. L. Bick, eds.). Raven Press, New York, 1978.
5. E. W. Busse and H. S. Wang, Multiple factors contributing to dementia in old age, in *Psychiatry II* (R. DelaFuenta and M. H. Weisman, eds.). American Elsevier, New York, 1973.
6. B. J. Gurland, The borderlands of dementia: The influence of sociocultural characteristics on rates of dementia occurring in the Senium, in *Clinical Aspects of Alzheimer's Disease and Senile Dementia* (N. E. Miller and G. D. Cohen, eds.) Raven Press, New York, 1981.
7. E. Kokmen and B. S. Schoenberg, Epidemiological patterns and clinical features of dementia in a defined U.S. population (abstract), *Ann. Neurol.* **8:**116 (1980).
8. H. O. Akesson, A population study of senile and arteriosclerotic psychoses, *Human Hered.* **19:**546 (1969).
9. E. M. Gruenberg, Epidemiology of senile dementia, in *Neurological Epidemiology: Principles and Clinical Applications* (B. S. Schoenberg, ed.). Raven Press, New York, 1978.
10. T. R. Bollerup, Prevalence of mental illness among 70-year-olds domiciled in nine Copenhagen suburbs: The Glostrup survey, *Acta. Psychiat. Scand.* **51:**327 (1975).
11. G. A. Broe, A. J. Akhtar, G. R. Andrews, F. I. Caird, A.J.J. Gilmore, and W. J. McLennan, Neurological disorders in the elderly at home, *J. Neurol. Neurosurg. Psychiat.* **39:**362 (1972).
12. E. Essen-Moller, H. Larsson, C. Uddenberg, and G. White, Individual traits and morbidity of a Swedish rural population, *Acta Psychiat. Neurol. Scand.,* suppl. 100, 1956.
13. D.W.K. Kay, K. Bergmann, E. M. Foster, A. A. McKechnie, and M. Roth, Mental illness and hospital in the elderly: A random sample followed up, *Comp. Psychiat.* **11:**26 (1970).
14. D.W.K. Kay, P. Beamish, and M. Roth, Old age mental disorders in Newcastle upon Tyne: I. A study of prevalence, *Br. J. Psychiat.* **110:**146 (1964).
15. J. Nielson, Geronto-psychiatric period-prevalence investigation in a geographically delimited population, *Acta Psychiat. Scand.* **38:**307 (1963).
16. E.J.R. Primrose, *Psychological Illness. A Community Study.* Charles C Thomas, Springfield, Ill., 1962.
17. L. T. Kurland, J. F. Kurtzke, I. D. Goldberg, N. W. Choi, and G. Williams, Parkinsonism, in *Epidemiology of Neurologic And Sense Organ Disorders,* (L. T. Kurland, J. F. Kurtzke, and I. D. Goldberg, eds.). Vital and Health Statistics Monographs, APHA, Harvard University Press, Cambridge, Mass., 1973.

18. N. S. Peress, W. C. Kane, and S. M. Aronson, Central nervous system findings in a tenth decade autopsy population, in *Neuro-biological Aspects of Maturation and Aging* (D. H. Ford, ed.). Elsevier, Amsterdam, 1973.
19. E. W. Busse and W. D. Obrist, Significance of focal electroencephalographic changes in the elderly, *Postgrad. Med.* **34:**179 (1963).
20. J. A. Mortimer, L. M. Schuman, and L. R. French, Epidemiology of dementing illness, in *The Epidemiology of Dementia* (J. A. Mortimer and L. M. Schumann, eds.). Oxford University Press, New York, 1981.
21. J. A. Brody, J. M. Stanhope, and L. T. Kurland, Patterns of amyotrophic lateral sclerosis and parkinsonism-dementia of Guam, in *Topics on Tropical Neurology* (R. W. Hornabrook, ed.). Contemporary Neurology Series, Davis, Philadelphia, 1975.
22. E. G. McGeer, Aging and neurotransmitter metabolism in the human brain, in *Aging,* vol. 7, *Alzheimer's Disease: Senile Dementia and Related Disorders* (R. Katzman, R. D. Terry, and K. L. Bick, eds.). Raven Press, New York, 1978.
23. A. Hirano, N. Malamud, T. S. Elizan, and L. T. Kurland, Amyotrophic lateral sclerosis and parkinsonism-dementia complex on Guam, *Arch. Neurol.* **15:**35 (1966).
24. D. R. Crapper, S. Karlik, and U. DeBoni, Aluminum and other metals in senile (Alzheimer's) dementia, in *Aging,* vol. 7, *Alzheimer's Disease: Senile Dementia and Related Disorders* (R. Katzman, R. D. Terry, and K. L. Bick, eds.). Raven Press, New York, 1978.
25. J. A. Mortimer, Epidemiologic aspects of Alzheimer's disease, in *The Aging Nervous System* (G. J. Maletta and F. J. Pirozzolo, eds.). Praeger, New York, 1980.
26. J. Goudsmit, B. J. White, L. R. Weitkamp, B.J.B. Keats, C. H. Morrow, and D. C. Gajdusek, Familial Alzheimer's disease in two kindreds of the same geographic and ethnic origin: A clinical and genetic study, *J. Neurol. Sci.* **49:**79 (1981).
27. L. L. Heston and A. R. Mastri, The genetics of Alzheimer's disease: Associations with hematologic malignancy and Down's syndrome, *Arch. Gen. Psychiat.* **34:**976 (1977).
28. B. E. Ward, R. H. Cook, A. Robinson, and J. H. Austin, Increased aneuploidy in Alzheimer disease, *Am. J. Med. Genetics* **3:**137 (1979).
29. R. L. Walford and S. E. Hodge, HLA distribution in Alzheimer's disease, in *Histocompatibility Testing* (P. I. Peresaki, ed.). UCLA Tissue Typing Lab, Los Angeles, 1980.
30. J. Goudsmit, C. H. Marrow, D. M. Asher, R. T. Yanagihara, C. L. Masters, C. J. Gibbs Jr., and D. C. Gajdusek, Evidence for and against the transmittability of Alzheimer's disease, *Neurology* **30:**945 (1980).
31. C. Eisdorfer, D. Cohen, and C. E. Buckley III, Serum immunoglobulins and cognition in the impaired elderly, in *Aging,* vol. 7, *Alzheimer's Disease: Senile Dementia and Related Disorders* (R. Katzman, R. D. Terry, and K. L. Bick, eds.). Raven Press, New York, 1978.
32. F. C. Stam and W. Op den Velde, Haptoglobin types in Alzheimer's disease and senile dementia, in *Aging,* vol. 7, *Alzheimer's Disease: Senile Dementia and Related Disorders,* (R. Katzman, R. D. Terry, and K. L. Bick, eds.). Raven Press, New York, 1978.

6 Pacific Cultures: A Paradigm for the Study of Late-Onset Neurological Disorders

Ralph M. Garruto and D. Carleton Gajdusek

The cross-cultural study of senescence and of the biology of aging in diverse human populations remains an important challenge to modern medicine. The impact of sociocultural, genetic, and environmental factors varies from one society to another, thereby modifying the biological characteristics of aging populations.

Brizzee (*1*) and Tomlinson (*2*) underline the conceptual distinction between normative aging and the pathological and physiological changes associated with late-onset disorders. Among the influences on the lifespan of an individual or population are genetics, nutrition, activity patterns, environmental conditions, and behavioral patterns. These same factors are associated with the physiological and pathological changes observed in many late-onset disorders.

In recent years, there has been a specific effort to document patterns of aging and increased longevity in non-Western cultures. In tropical Africa, forest pigmies, Kalahari bushmen, West African agricultural groups, and East African pastoralists have been studied. Farther to the east, the biology of Indian and Asiatic populations has been studied, as has that of the diverse Pacific islanders, which include Melanesians, Micronesians, and Polynesians. On the American continents, Eskimo and Amerindians, including the pastoral populations of the Andes, have been studied. This effort led to the highly publicized discovery, documentation, controversy, and eventual refutation of extreme longevity in three populations relatively free of late-onset disorders: the Vilcabamba in southern Ecuador, the Hunzas of Pakistan, and the Georgians of the Soviet Union (*3,4*).

In contrast, a number of populations have unusual concentrations of disease in older age groups. Perhaps the best illustrations of such concentrations are a number of chronic degenerative diseases of the central nervous system occurring in six geographic isolates in the Pacific: kuru among the Fore people of the eastern highlands of Papua New Guinea,

Viliuisk encephalitis among the Iakut people of the Soviet Union, the newly discovered neurological complex occurring among the Australian aborigines living on Groote Eylandt and adjacent Arnhem Land, and the three high-incidence foci of amyotrophic lateral sclerosis and parkinsonism syndromes found among the Chamorros of the Mariana Islands, the Auyu and Jakai people of West New Guinea, and the people from the Kii Peninsula of Honshu Island, Japan (*5–13*) (Figure 6-1). Such hyperendemic foci of disease in geographic isolates offer a unique opportunity for solving etiological and epidemiological problems of widespread medical significance. As "natural experiments," they are generally uncomplicated by the changing cultural, genetic, and environmental conditions that often mask or complicate the analysis of major medical problems and inquiry in larger, genetically open, cosmopolitan communities. Such foci are important not only to the study of pathobiological aging but also to the study of general senescence among diverse human groups.

Here we limit our remarks to the three high-incidence foci of amyotrophic lateral sclerosis and parkinsonism syndromes in the western Pacific. After describing the ecology and natural history of these disorders within each focus, we compare their epidemiological, clinical, and neuropathological features to identify risk factors that may be related to their causes.

FOCI OF AMYOTROPHIC LATERAL SCLEROSIS AND PARKINSONISM SYNDROMES IN THE WESTERN PACIFIC

During the past 30 years, unusually high-incidence foci of amyotrophic lateral sclerosis (ALS) and parkinsonism syndromes have been recognized in, and later investigated among, geographic isolates in the western Pacific. A disease of the motor neurons of the brain and spinal cord, ALS is characterized by muscle weakness, progressive atrophy of skeletal muscles, and paralysis. By comparison, parkinsonism is characterized by slowness of voluntary motor activity, muscular rigidity, tremor, and masked facies and, in these foci, is often accompanied by progressive mental deterioration. Both disorders are late-onset, uniformly fatal, and of unknown origin. The hyperendemic foci of ALS and parkinsonism, all located in the western Pacific, represent natural experimental models of late-onset chronic degenerative disease that occur in different cultures in different ecological zones and among genetically divergent populations.

Kii Peninsula Focus

The first account of the high incidence of ALS in the Kii Peninsula of Honshu Island, Japan, was documented as early as 1911 (*14*). By 1925, Hirata (*15*) had confirmed Miura's earlier finding of a high incidence of ALS in the Kii Peninsula, specifically localized in the Mie and Wakayama prefectures. Later studies represented detailed analyses of the distribu-

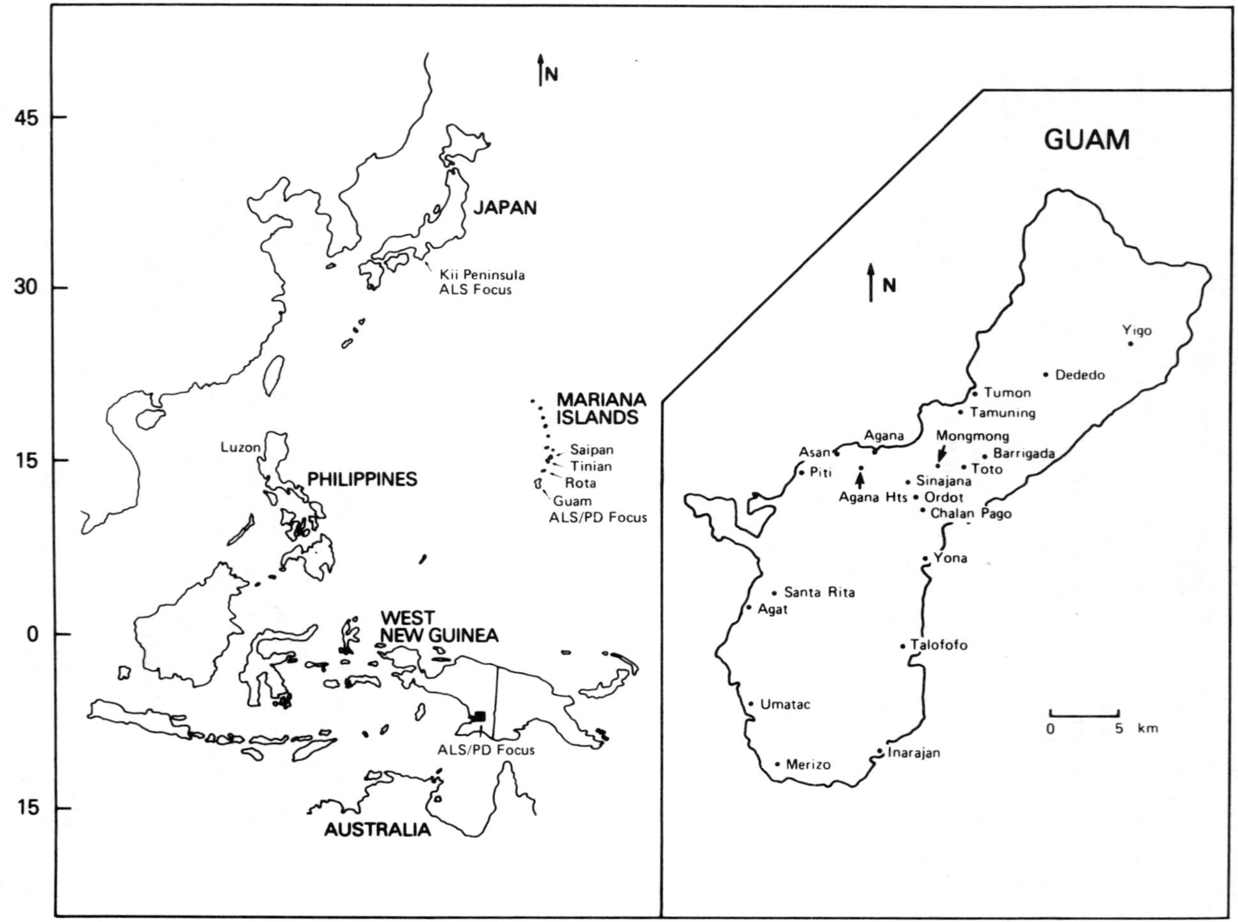

Figure 6-1. High-incidence foci of amyotrophic lateral sclerosis (ALS) and

tion of these cases within the affected prefectures. The earlier surveys relied solely on hospital records, and not until the systematic surveys of the early 1960s did the epidemiological patterns and geographic limits of the focus become well defined (*16,17*).

In the Kii Peninsula, two separate foci of ALS have been discovered thus far: the Kozagawa focus, with a population of 6200, and the Hobara focus, with a population of 2100. The foci are separated by about 200 kilometers, and both are located in remote, mountainous regions with farming and lumbering the main occupational activities (*17*). Kozagawa, with a larger population, has a male-to-female sex ratio for ALS of 2.5:1, an older age at onset, and a slightly longer duration of illness. The Hobara focus, although only one third the population of Kozagawa, has an incidence rate (55/100 000) four times that of Kozagawa and 100 times that of the whole of Japan. In Hobara, the familial occurrence of the disease reaches 70 per cent and the degree of consanguinity, based on first-cousin marriages, is 10 per cent. Additionally, the Hobara ALS focus is associated with several patients who have parkinsonism and/or dementia. In both regions, calcium and magnesium levels in water and soil are low, and in Kozagawa the soil and hair of cattle have high manganese content, in contrast to that found in nearby control villages that are without disease.

Neuropathologically, patients with ALS and parkinsonism in the Kii Peninsula focus show the interesting hallmark of Alzheimer's neurofibrillary tangles, so commonly seen in the Marianas focus (*17*). Clinical and epidemiological monitoring of the Kii population indicates that both disorders are in steady decline (*18*).

West New Guinea Focus

The most recent and most remote focus of ALS and parkinsonism to be systematically studied is that found among the Auyu and Jakai people living on the southern coastal plain of West New Guinea. This focus, first described by Gajdusek in 1963, has been intensively studied during the past seven years (*8,19*). Among a population of about 7000, there have been recorded 97 cases of ALS, 18 cases of parkinsonism, and 18 cases of a condition reminiscent of Landry-Guillan-Barre syndrome, which Gajdusek and Salazar (*19*) have termed poliomyeloradiculitis. The overall crude average annual incidence rate for ALS alone reaches 147/100 000, almost 150 times that of the U.S. mainland and the highest recorded level anywhere in the world. In selected villages, the prevalence rate exceeds 1300/100 000. The focus is geographically discrete, and after repeated surveys, neither ALS nor parkinsonism is found outside the focal region in the surrounding larger population.

The ecology of the region is that of a low coastal plain covered by tropical rain forest 100 to 200 kilometers inland from tidal swamplands. Villages are located near rivers, which are used as the major avenue of transportation. The Auyu people live a seminomadic subsistence-level life that includes producing sago flour (a staple carbohydrate source), fishing, food-gathering, and, only more recently, some horticultural activity. The Jakai people, on the other hand, are more sedentary.

In this focus, the male-to-female ratio for ALS is 1.8:1. The age at onset of disease is rather low, with a mean of 33 years and a duration of 3.5 years. Thirty-seven per cent of all ALS patients are younger than age 30. In several cases, mild-to-moderate parkinsonism features are observed. Except for a younger age at onset, the clinical picture is consistent with that of ALS worldwide (*19*).

Parkinsonism, found in association with the high incidence of ALS, was recognized during the second survey of the area about 12 years after the first report of ALS. In West New Guinea, parkinsonism occurs with or without dementia and is much less common than ALS. The male-to-female ratio is 3:1. The mean age at onset is 43, ten years later than that for ALS, and the mean duration of illness is six years. Clinically, the parkinsonism syndrome seen in this focus is strikingly similar to that reported in the Guam focus. No autopsy has as yet been done on any decedent who had either ALS or parkinsonism in this extremely isolated focus.

The third condition, poliomyeloradiculitis, has been recognized in the same area and in patients not suffering from ALS. The disease occurs in the same villages and even in the same households concurrently with ALS and parkinsonism. The mean age at onset (26 years) is the lowest for the three conditions, with 70 per cent of the affected persons being younger than age 30. The disease has an acute onset, is associated with physical exhaustion and stress, and rapidly progresses to weakness of all limbs. Fever and prostration are frequent, but headache is not. Paralysis progresses for several weeks or months, with the patient usually recovering three to six months thereafter. Repeated attacks are common. A relationship of poliomyeloradiculitis to ALS seems possible but is as yet unclear, and neither an infectious condition nor a deficiency syndrome, such as beri-beri or pellagra, has been ruled out.

Mariana Islands Focus

Of the three known foci of ALS and parkinsonism, none has been more closely monitored clinically, epidemiologically, and neuropathologically than that among the Chamorro people of Guam. During the past 30 years, intensive systematic studies on Guam have shown an initial incidence rate for ALS (locally referred to as *lytico*) 50 to 100 times higher than that of the continental United States (*11*). Ten years after the reported high incidence of ALS on Guam, a second uniformly fatal neurological disorder, parkinsonism-dementia (PD) (locally referred to as *bodig*), was clinically and neuropathologically described (*20,21*). Parkinsonism-dementia often occurs in association with the high incidence of ALS, often in the same sibship, and even together in the same patient.

Since the first systematic observations began more than 30 years ago, 765 patients from a mean Chamorro population base of about 40 000 have been clinically diagnosed as having either ALS or PD, and another 76 patients are currently suspected of having one or the other. All patients who develop disease are followed up throughout their clinical course, and more than 65 per cent have had neuropathological verification. Both disorders are late in onset and previously accounted for one in five deaths among Chamorros over age 25 (*22*).

Historically, the original ancestors of the native Chamorros are presumed to have migrated from Malaysia and the Philippine Islands as early as 2000 B.C. (*23*). Europeans first arrived on the island with Magellan in 1521. Under early Spanish rule, the population declined dramatically as a result of the Spanish-Chamorro Wars, severe typhoons, and disease. The declining native Chamorro population intermarried extensively, particularly with Filipinos and, to a much lesser extent, with Mexican and Spanish colonials (*24*).

Until recently, the population remained genetically stable, although its extensive early admixture modified the original gene pool such that "pure" Chamorros are unlikely to exist today. The current 1980 U.S. census of Guam lists the total population of the island at 106 000 (*25*). Of that total, we estimate that about 64 000 are native Chamorros, 20 000 Filipinos, and 22 000 Caucasians (mostly short-term military personnel and their dependents) and other ethnic groups. The main economic activity of the island was originally subsistence farming and fishing, but since 1950 Westernization and the development of a dollar economy have increased, mainly through the large U.S. military presence on the island.

The initial crude incidence rate for ALS was more than 50/100 000, with a similar frequency for PD (*26*). For ALS and PD, the original male-to-female ratios were 2:1 and almost 3:1 respectively; the mean ages at onset were 46 and 54 years, with durations between 4 and 4.5 years. Geographically, both conditions are found throughout the island but least prominently in the western part and in highest incidence among the more traditional communities in the volcanic southern end of the island. Both disorders are often familial, and it is not unusual to find the conditions spanning several generations in a family and, on occasion, manifesting themselves in the same person.

The disorders occur in high incidence not only among the Chamorro people of Guam but also among the Chamorros of Rota, just 70 kilometers north of Guam. Yet the Chamorro people of Tinian, Saipan, and the more northerly inhabited islands of Anatahan, Alamagan, Pagan, and Agrihan in the Mariana chain do not have an unusually high incidence of either disorder (*27*).

Additionally, our studies of ALS and PD in migrants have shown that Chamorro migrants to the U.S. mainland (*28*) have a fivefold increased risk of developing disease and that long-term Filipino migrants to Guam have a similar increased risk of developing disease (*29*). Both groups develop disease after about two decades' residence on Guam, either as children and adolescents (as with the Chamorro migrants) or as middle-aged adults (as with the Filipino migrants). In neither case has the disease reached the level of that currently observed among Chamorros on Guam. The small endogamous Carolinian migrant group and the much larger short-term Caucasian migrant population of American military personnel living on the island do not show any increased risk of developing disease (*30*).

Clinically, ALS on Guam is identical to the disease described by Charcot in 1884 (*31*) and of classical ALS found throughout the world today, except for its high, but not invariable, association neuropathologically with Alzheimer's neurofibrillary changes. The clinical and neuropathological features of PD include insidious onset of extrapyramidal symptoms, progressive organic mental changes, and the frequent development of motor neuron involvement in the sixth and seventh decades of life. Neuropathologically, PD almost invariably shows a characteristic presence and distribution of neurofibrillary tangles (NFTs) in the brain and spinal cord, without associated senile plaques, Lewy bodies, or spongiform change. Nonaffected Chamorro controls have also unexpectedly been found to develop NFTs at a relatively early age (*32,33*). Thus, ALS and parkinsonism patients on Guam and the Kii Peninsula show this intriguing tendency toward NFT formation. Yet recent reports indicate that the occurrence together of ALS, parkinsonism, and dementia, with or without associated NFTs, is not a rare event and that these conditions are found in various combinations in Western populations more often than had been previously recognized (*34,35*).

Our continued neuroepidemiological studies confirm that ALS and PD are rapidly disappearing from Guam and, in fact, from the entire Mariana Archipelago (*26,27,36*). The decline on Guam is most dramatic among males and among those from the traditional high-incidence southern end of the island, such that the male-to-female ratio for both disorders is now approaching unity. The proportional number of deaths from ALS and PD, compared with other causes in those older than age 25, has fallen dramatically from 20 to 6 per cent during the past 30 years. Increasing evidence suggests a cohort phenomenon involving exposure to selected environmental factors or traditional cultural practices on the island. Although we do not know the reason for the decline, its pattern is not unlike that of kuru, except that the sexual prevalence is reversed.

COMPARISON OF ALS AND PARKINSONISM SYNDROMES IN GUAM, THE KII PENINSULA, AND WEST NEW GUINEA

The identification of all three high-incidence, ethnically and geographically limited foci of chronic progressive motor neuron disease, located in the Pacific Basin and each associated with parkinsonism and presenile dementia, raises important questions concerning their interrelationships, risk factors, and common causes.

Table 6-1. Ecologic and Demographic Comparisons of High-Incidence Foci of ALS and PD

	Guam (ALS + PD)	Kii Peninsula (ALS)	West New Guinea (ALS + PD)
Location	13°N, 144°E	34°N,136°E	7°S, 139°E
Genetic history	Malay/Filipino/other	Mongoloid/Oriental	Australoid/Mongoloid
Population size	60 000	8300	7000
Ecological zone	Tropical, mountainous, southern zone	Temperate, mountainous	Tropical inland coastal plain
Economic activities	U.S. gov't, farming	Lumber, farming	Subsistence level; food gathering, fishing, horticulture

Table 6-1 shows the general ecologic and demographic profiles of the three foci. The West New Guinea focus is the most isolated, with a subsistence and food-gathering economic base, whereas the Kii Peninsula and Guam are less isolated and now on a dollar economy. West New Guinea and Guam are in tropical ecozones, whereas the Kii has a more temperate climate. Demographically, Guam has a native population base seven or eight times that of the other two foci and a genetic history different from that of either the Kii or the West New Guinea focus.

The elemental chemistry of garden soil and drinking water has identified similarities in trace and essential elements among the three foci. Table 6-2 shows a partial comparison of elements from the more than 50 we have identified in soil and 30 in drinking water from these foci. The elements selected for comparison are those currently under investigation for their

Table 6-2. Trace and Essential Elements in Water and Soil from High-Incidence Foci of ALS and PD[b]

	Al (ppm)	Ca (ppm)	Mg (ppm)	P (ppm)	Mn (ppm)
		Water			
Guam[a]	0.07	1.4	0.3	0.07	0.01
Kii Peninsula	—	0.3	0.3	—	1.7
West New Guinea	0.8	1.0	0.4	ND	0.01
Ilocos	0.01	79	8.8	0.05	0.01
United States	—	10–100	3–30	—	0.05
		Soil			
Guam[a]	50 000	3100	8500	680	1200
Kii Peninsula	85 000	1200	7100	1200	900
West New Guinea	42 000	1000	600	880	90
Ilocos	70 000	25 000	19 000	800	1500
United States	60 000	24 000	9200	420	560

[a]High-incidence southern area.
[b]Preliminary results based on partial data.

possible involvement in the pathogenesis of ALS and parkinsonism. An assessment of the elemental content of water clearly shows low levels of calcium and magnesium in all three foci relative to levels on the U.S. mainland. Similarly, soil samples from Guam, the Kii Peninsula, and West Guinea show an 8- to 25-fold decrease in calcium, with magnesium levels more equivalent to those of the U.S. mainland. Table 6-2 also includes a comparison of water and soil from the Ilocos region of the Philippine Islands, a potential high-incidence area for the disease. Values for calcium from the Ilocos region were equivalent to those of the U.S. mainland, rather than showing the low levels observed among the high-incidence ALS areas in Guam, the Kii Peninsula, and West New Guinea.

Epidemiologically, the incidence of ALS and parkinsonism is clearly decreasing both on Guam and in the Kii Peninsula, whereas it has remained unchanged in West New Guinea (Table 6-3). The decrease in incidence of both diseases on Guam has been most striking among males, particularly those living in the more traditional high-incidence southern region of the island (*26,27,36*). The mean age at onset of ALS and parkinsonism in West New Guinea patients is rather young, followed respectively by Guam and the Kii Peninsula. All three foci have a sizable proportion of affected persons living more than five years after onset. The family history for ALS varies significantly within each focus, ranging from 2 per cent in West New Guinea to 70 per cent in the Hobara region of the Kii Peninsula. Yet, except for the higher incidence and larger number of persons who survive more than five years, the overall characteristics in Table 6-3 suggest a closer resemblance between the Kii focus and classical ALS worldwide than between either of the other two foci.

Clinically, with the exception of earlier age at onset in Guam and West New Guinea, ALS patients from all three foci show the same overall

Table 6-3. Comparison of High-Incidence Foci of ALS and PD in the Western Pacific

		Guam		Kii Peninsula		West New Guinea	
	Classic ALS	ALS	PD	ALS Hobara	ALS Kozagawa	ALS	PD
Crude incidence	1.5	52	36	55	14	147	79
Sex ratio	1.5:1	2:1	2.8:1	1.8:1	2.5:1	1.8:1	3:1
Mean age at onset (years)	52	46	54	51	54	33	43
Age 30(%)	—	12	0	—	—	37	10
Mean age at death (years)	55	50	58	54	57	37	49
Mean duration (years)	2.5	4	4.4	2.6	3.2	3.5	6
5 Years (%)	8	34	24	28	28	27	60
Family history (%)	2	14	14	70	—	2	—
Trend in incidence	Stable	Decreasing		Decreasing		?Stable	

Note: This table is modified after Gajdusek and Salazar 1981 (*19*), and all data represent earlier figures rather than current figures for comparison.

Table 6-4. Comparison of Clinical and Pathological Features of ALS and PD

	Classic ALS	Guam ALS	Guam PD	Kii Peninsula ALS	West New Guinea ALS	West New Guinea PD
		Clinical Features (%)				
Extrapyramidal	1	4	100	+	5	100
Dementia	3	3	100	+	(5)	95
Bulbar signs	39	35	10	+	40	7
Motor neuron signs	100	100	46	100	100	60
		Pathological Features				
Neurofibrillary tangles	0	+	+	+	—	—
Amyloid plaques	0	0	0	0	—	—
Spongiform change	0	0	0	0	—	—

Source: Modified after Gajdusek and Salazar (*19*).

clinical features as those of patients with classical ALS described by Charcot, with an anamnestic history that indicates a similar mode of onset (Table 6-4). Additionally, in all three foci, dementia and extrapyramidal disease are also found singly or in combination with ALS.

Pathologically, NFTs have been observed in predilected areas of the brain and spinal cord of patients from Guam and the Kii Peninsula (Table 6-4) (*17,37*). Such tangles are a hallmark characteristic of ALS and PD cases on Guam but are also found among Chamorros who are neurologically normal (*32,33*). No decedents having ALS or parkinsonism-dementia have as yet been autopsied in the remote West New Guinea focus. Neither on Guam nor in the Kii Peninsula does one observe senile plaques or spongiform change associated with either ALS or parkinsonism. The observation of NFTs in neurons in tissues obtained from both foci suggests some common causative factor. If tangles are found to be primarily associated with ALS and parkinsonism in these foci, then those observed in nonaffected Chamorro controls may indicate incipient disease. However, the precise association between NFTs and ALS or parkinsonism is now obscure. The coexistence of these phenomena may actually represent only a spurious relationship or a secondary association at best. Without autopsies of ALS and parkinsonism patients in the critical West New Guinea focus and without further studies on the relationship between the tangles, ALS, and parkinsonism in general, we cannot easily predict functional or causal relationships.

RISK FACTORS AND SUSPECTED ETIOLOGIES IN FOCI OF HIGH-INCIDENCE ALS AND PARKINSONISM

A major consideration in assessing risk factors for ALS and parkinsonism has been the relative contribution of genetics and environment to these disorders. The extensive studies in the Kii Peninsula and particularly on

Guam initially suggested that the disorder was genetically autosomal dominant with variable or incomplete penetrance. There is clearly a familial and sporadic form of disease in all three foci, but no viable genetic pattern has been identified. In addition to a dominant theory with incomplete penetrance, hypotheses including a polygenetic form of inheritance, a genetic susceptibility, or a multifactorial threshold effect have been offered. Intensive genetic studies have included pedigree analyses, calculations of coefficients of inbreeding, development of prospective case-control registries, and the search for specific gene markers associated with either disorder (including HLA antigens at the A and B loci, red blood cell enzymes, haptoglobins, serum proteins, blood groups, immunoglobulin allotypes, and dermatoglyphic patterns). None has yielded a satisfactory genetic explanation (*17,38,39*).

The disappearance of ALS and parkinsonism on Guam and the Kii Peninsula, the known genetic diversity in the three foci, the extensive genetic studies with the lack of any clear genetic pattern for the disease, and the increased risk of developing disease among migrants to and from Guam suggest that environmental factors are involved in pathogenesis. However, efforts to transmit ALS and PD experimentally to primates and other laboratory animals have been unsuccessful (*40*), as has the search for a virus by cultivation of brain tissue in vitro, by inoculation of cell cultures, or by an attempt to find a viral protein, antigen, antibody, or nucleic acid in the tissues of patients (*41,42*).

No association of ALS and PD with plant and animal toxins has become evident thus far, despite extensive research on the cycad nut, cassava, and fish toxins on Guam (*43,44*). In the West New Guinea focus, we know that the population has only recently been exposed to a number of factors that are customarily associated with modern technology. Thus, with ALS and parkinsonism already present, the Auyu and Jakai had never had contact with most domestic animals (except dogs and pigs) or exposure to wild carnivores. Only plant species native to that region of the Pacific (which would exclude rice, corn, wheat, and other grains) were available. No exposure to such items as seafood, coffee, teas, cocoa, petrochemicals, paints, soaps, insecticides, fertilizers, manufactured medicines, textiles, and ceramics occurred (*19*).

However, deficiencies and excesses of certain trace and essential elements in soil and water are consistently found in all three foci (Table 6-2) (*45,46*). It has been postulated that abnormalities in the mineral environment are involved in ALS and PD (*47*). Yase (*48*) has proposed that chronic nutritional deficiencies of calcium and magnesium lead to abnormalities in mineral metabolism (secondary hyperparathyroidism), which, in the presence of excessive accumulations of certain divalent and trivalent cations, result in the deposition of these elements in motor neurons as hydroxyapatites, culminating eventually in cell destruction. Levels of metals such as aluminum that are not known to be toxic for normal persons may become toxic as a result of chronic calcium and magnesium deficiency. Alternately, abnormal calcium levels may disrupt the neuronal cytoskeleton and axoplasmic flow. Indeed, the clinical similarity between ALS and the neuromuscular syndromes of primary and secondary hyperparathyroidism, the occasional association of parathyroid diseases (particularly hypoparathyroidism) with extrapyramidal dysfunction and dementia, the unusually low levels of calcium in drinking water and garden soils from all three geographically limited foci, and the recent demonstrations of high concentrations of calcium, magnesium, aluminum, and manganese in brain and spinal cord tissue from patients with ALS and parkinsonism from Guam and the Kii Peninsula all suggest that disordered mineral metabolism may be involved in the pathogenesis of these diseases (*49–59*). Detailed studies of mineral metabolism, neuroendocrine function, and the quantitative and qualitative determinations of the mineral content of central nervous system tissue from patients with ALS and parkinsonism are now in progress.

The intriguing medical enigma of ALS and associated parkinsonism and dementia, and perhaps the aging process per se continues to unfold as these unique hyperendemic foci are studied. Such isolated Pacific foci represent a paradigm of natural experimental models for the elucidation of risk factors and the mechanisms for the origin and dissemination of disease to an extent not possible in larger, Westernized societies. The natural decline of ALS and parkinsonism on Guam and the Kii Peninsula continues, thus alleviating more than a century of burden from these populations that have suffered inordinately from their effects.

Acknowledgment

We thank Doreen Arion for her invaluable assistance in the comparative analysis, particularly with regard to the Kii Peninsula focus of ALS, and gratefully acknowledge the editorial assistance of Richard T. Yanagihara, Cathy Daum, and Diane Molchon.

REFERENCES

1. K. R. Brizzee, Age changes in relation to diseases of the nervous system, in *Neurobiology of Aging* (J. M. Ordy and K. R. Brizzee, eds.). Plenum Press, New York, 1975.
2. B. E. Tomlinson, Morphological brain changes in nondemented old people, in *Ageing of the Central Nervous System: Biological and Psychological Aspects* (H. H. Van Praag and A. F. Kalverboor, eds.). Bohn, Haarlem, the Netherlands, 1972.
3. A. Leaf, *Youth in Old Age.* McGraw-Hill, New York, 1975.
4. R. B. Mazess and S. H. Forman, Longevity and age exaggeration in Vilcabamba, Ecuador, *J. Gerontol.* **34:**94 (1979).
5. D. C. Gajdusek and V. Zigas, Degenerative disease of the central nervous system in New Guinea: The endemic occurrence of "kuru" in the native population, *N. Engl. J. Med.* **257:**974 (1957).

6. D. C. Gajdusek, Unconventional viruses and the origin and disappearance of kuru, in Les Prix Nobel en 1976. P. A. Norstedt, Stockholm, 1977.
7. P. A. Petrov, Viliuisk encephalitis in the Iakut Republic (U.S.S.R.), *Am. J. Trop. Med. Hyg.* **19:**146 (1970).
8. D. C. Gajdusek, Foci of motor neuron disease in high incidence in isolated populations of East Asia and the western Pacific, in *Advances in Neurology,* Vol. 36, Human Motor Neuron Diseases (L. P. Rowland, ed.). Raven Press, New York, 1982.
9. D. C. Gajdusek, E. Millard and D. Goldgaber, *Bibliography of Viliuisk Encephalomyelitis in the Iakut People of Siberia.* National Institutes of Health, Bethesda, Md., 1982.
10. L. G. Kiloh, A. K. Lethlean, G. Morgan, J. E. Cawte, and M. Harris, An endemic neurological disorder in tribal Australian aborigines, *J. Neurol. Neurosurg. Psych.* **43:**661 (1980).
11. L. T. Kurland and D. W. Mulder, Epidemiologic investigations of amyotrophic lateral sclerosis: I. Preliminary report on geographic distribution, with special reference to the Mariana Islands, including clinical and pathological observations, *Neurology (Minneap.)* **4:**355, 438 (1954).
12. K. Kimura, Y. Yase, Y. Higashi, S. Uno, K. Yamamoto, M. Iwasaki, I. Tsumoto, M. Sugiura, S. Yoshimura, H. Kawaguchi, K. Namikawa, J. Kumura, S. Iwamoto, I. Yamamoto, Y. Handa, M. Yata, Y. Yata, M. Kanzaki, S. Nakai, H. Utsunomiya, Study on amyotrophic lateral sclerosis: (I) Epidemiological, geomedical and genetic studies on amyotrophic lateral sclerosis and its allied diseases in Kii Peninsula, Japan, *Psychiat. Neurol. Japon.* **65:**31 (1963).
13. Y. Yase, N. Matsumoto, F. Yoshimasu and Y. Handa, Clinico-epidemiological studies in a new focus of motor neuron disease in Japan. *Neurol. India* **20** (suppl. IV):531 (1973).
14. K. Miura, Amyotrophische lateralsklerose unter dem bilde von sog: Bulbarparalyse, *Neurol. Japon.* **10:**366 (1911).
15. U. Hirata, Statistical observation of amyotrophic lateral sclerosis, *Neurol. Japon.* **25:**418 (1925).
16. K. Kimura, Studies of amyotrophic lateral sclerosis in the Kozagawa district in the Kii Peninsula, Japan, *Wakayama Med. Reports* **9:**177 (1965).
17. H. Shiraki and Y. Yase, Amyotrophic lateral sclerosis in Japan, in *Handbook of Clinical Neurology* (P. Vinken and G. W. Bruyn, eds.). Elsevier, New York, 1975.
18. Y. Uebayashi, Epidemiological investigation of motor neuron disease in the Kii Peninsula of Japan and on Guam: The significance of long survival cases, *Wakayama Med. Reports* **23:**13 (1980).
19. D. C. Gajdusek and A. Salazar, Amyotrophic lateral sclerosis and parkinsonian syndromes in high incidence among the Auyu and Jakai people of West New Guinea, *Neurology* **32:**107 (1982).
20. A. Hirano, L. T. Kurland, R. S. Krooth and S. Lessell, Parkinsonism-dementia complex, an endemic disease on the island of Guam: I. Clinical features, *Brain* **84:**642 (1961).
21. A. Hirano, N. Malamud and L. T. Kurland, Parkinsonism-dementia complex, an endemic disease on the island of Guam: II. Pathological features, *Brain* **84:**662 (1961).
22. J. A. Brody and L. T. Kurland, Amyotrophic lateral sclerosis and parkinson-

ism-dementia in Guam, in *Tropical Neurology,* (J. D. Spillane, ed.). Oxford University Press, New York, 1973.

23. A. Spoehr, Marianas prehistory: Archaelogical survey and excavations on Saipan, Tinian, and Rota, in Fieldiana, *Anthropology* **48,** Chicago Natural History Museum, 1957.
24. L. Thompson, *Guam and Its People.* Princeton University Press, Princeton, N.J., 1947.
25. U.S. Bureau of the Census: *Census of Population, General Population Characteristics.* GPO, Washington, D.C., 1980.
26. D. M. Reed and J. A. Brody, Amyotrophic lateral sclerosis and parkinsonism-dementia on Guam, 1945–1972: I. Descriptive epidemiology, *Am. J. Epidemiol.* **101:**287 (1975).
27. R. T. Yanagihara, R. M. Garruto and D. C. Gajdusek, Epidemiological surveillance of amyotrophic lateral sclerosis and parkinsonism-dementia in the Commonwealth of the Northern Mariana Islands, *Ann. Neurol.* **13:**79 (1983).
28. R. M. Garruto, D. C. Gajdusek and K.-M. Chen, Amyotrophic lateral sclerosis among Chamorro migrants from Guam, *Ann. Neurol.* **8:**612 (1980).
29. R. M. Garruto, D. C. Gajdusek and K. M. Chen, Amyotrophic lateral sclerosis and parkinsonism-dementia among Flipino migrants to Guam, *Ann. Neurol.* **10:**341 (1981).
30. J. A. Brody, A. H. Edgar and M. M. Gillespie, Amyotrophic lateral sclerosis: No increase among U.S. construction workers in Guam, *JAMA* **240:**551 (1978).
31. J. M. Charcot, De la sclerose laterale amyotrophique, *Progress Med.* **2:**325 (1874).
32. F. H. Anderson, E. P. Richardson, H. Okazaki and J. A. Brody, Neurofibrillary degeneration on Guam: Frequency in Chamorros and non-Chamorros with no known neurological disease, *Brain* **102:**65 (1979).
33. L. Chen, Neurofibrillary changes on Guam, *Arch. Neurol.* **38:**16 (1981).
34. A. J. Hudson, Amyotrophic lateral sclerosis and its association with dementia, parkinsonism and other neurological disorders: A review, *Brain* **104:**217 (1981).
35. H. Sroka, T. S. Elizan, M. D. Yahr, A. Burger and M. R. Mendoza, Organic mental syndrome and confusional states in Parkinson's disease, *Arch. Neurol.* **38:**339 (1981).
36. R. M. Garruto, D. C. Gajdusek, K.-M. Chen and C. J. Gibbs, Jr., Changing epidemiological and clinical characteristics of amyotrophic lateral sclerosis and parkinsonism-dementia in the Mariana Islands, in Abstracts of the Twelfth World Congress of Neurology, Kyoto, September 1981. International Congress Series No. 548, *Excerpta Medica,* Amsterdam, 1981.
37. N. Malamud, A. Hirano and L. Kurland, Pathoanatomic changes in amyotrophic lateral sclerosis on Guam: Special reference to the occurrence of neurofibrillary changes, *Arch. Neurol.* **5:**401 (1961).
38. R. M. Garruto, C. C. Plato, M. S. Schanfield, N. Myrianthopoulos, D. C. Gajdusek, Blood groups, immunoglobin allotypes and dermatoglyphic frequencies in patients with amyotrophic lateral sclerosis and parkinsonism-dementia of Guam, *Am.J.Med. Genet.,* **14:**289 (1983).
39. N. M. Blake, R. L. Kirk, S. R. Wilson, R. M. Garruto, D. C. Gajdusek, C. J. Gibbs, Jr. and P. Hoffman, Search for a red cell enzyme or serum

protein marker in amyotrophic lateral sclerosis and parkinsonism-dementia of Guam, *Am. J. Med. Genet.* **14**:299 (1983).
40. C. J. Gibbs, Jr. and D. C. Gajdusek, An update on long-term in vivo and in vitro studies designed to identify a virus as a cause of amyotrophic lateral sclerosis, parkinsonism-dementia and Parkinson disease, in *Advances in Neurology,* Vol. 36, Human Motor Neuron Diseases (L. P. Rowland, ed.). Raven Press, New York, 1982.
41. D. E. Kohne, C. J. Gibbs, Jr., L. White, S. M. Tracy, W. Meinke and R. A. Smith, Virus detection by nucleic acid hybridization: Examination of normal and ALS tissues for the presence of poliovirus. *J. Gen. Virol.* **56**:223 (1981).
42. M. V. Viola, J. C. Myers, K. L. Gann, C. J. Gibbs, Jr. and R. P. Roos, Failure to detect poliovirus genetic information in amyotrophic lateral sclerosis, *Ann. Neurol.* **5**:402 (1979).
43. L. T. Kurland, Geographic isolates: Their role in neuroepidemiology, in *Advances in Neurology,* Vol. 19 (B. S. Schoenberg, ed.). Raven Press, New York, 1978.
44. D. Reed, C. Plato, T. Elizan and L. T. Kurland, The amyotrophic lateral sclerosis/parkinsonism-dementia complex: A ten-year follow-up on Guam: Part I. Epidemiologic studies, *Am. J. Epidemiol.* **83**:54 (1966).
45. D. C. Gajdusek, R. M. Garruto and R. Yanagihara, Low levels of calcium and magnesium in drinking water and soil samples from the high incidence focus of amyotrophic lateral sclerosis and parkinsonism-dementia in West New Guinea, in *Abstracts of the Tenth International Congress on Tropical Medicine and Malaria,* Manila, November 1980.
46. D. C. Gajdusek, R. M. Garruto and A. M. Salazar, Ecology of high incidence foci of motor neuron disease in eastern Asia and the western Pacific and the frequent occurrence of other chronic degenerative neurological diseases in these foci, in *Abstracts of the Tenth International Congress on Tropical Medicine and Malaria,* Manila, November 1980.
47. R. T. Yanagihara, Heavy metals and essential minerals in motor neuron disease, in *Advances in Neurology,* Vol. 36, Human Motor Neuron Diseases (L. P. Rowland, ed.). Raven Press, New York, 1982.
48. Y. Yase, ALS in the Kii Peninsula: One possible etiological hypothesis, in *Amyotrophic Lateral Sclerosis,* (T. Tsubaki and Y. Toyokura, eds.). University of Tokyo Press, Tokyo, 1979.
49. L. E. Mallette, B. M. Patten and W. K. Engel, Neuromuscular disease in secondary hyperparathyroidism, *Ann. Intern. Med.* **82**:474 (1975).
50. B. M. Patten, J. P. Bilezekian, L. E. Mallette, A. Prince, W. K. Engel and G. Aurbach, Neuromuscular disease in primary hyperparathyroidism, *Ann. Intern. Med.* **80**:182 (1974).
51. F. Ikuta and T. Makifuchi, Distribution of aluminium in the spinal motor neurons of ALS, examined by wavelength dispersive x-ray microanalysis, in *Annual Report of the Research Committee of Motor Neuron Disease.* The Ministry of Health and Welfare of Japan, Tokyo, 1977.
52. H. M. Kurlander and B. M. Patten, Metals in spinal cord tissue of patients dying of motor neuron disease, *Ann. Neurol.* **6**:21 (1979).
53. D. P. Perl, D. C. Gajdusek, R. M. Garruto, R. T. Yanagihara and C. J. Gibbs, Jr., Intraneuronal aluminum accumulation in amyotrophic lateral sclerosis and parkinsonism-dementia of Guam, *Science* **217**:1053 (1982).
54. R. M. Garruto, R. Fukatsu, R. Yanagihara, D. C. Gajdusek, G. Hook and

C. Fiori, Imaging of aluminum and calcium in brain tissue from patients with amyotrophic lateral sclerosis and parkinsonism-dementia of Guam, in *Proceedings of the Conference on Aluminum Analysis in Biological Materials,* Charlottesville, Virginia, June 1983.

55. R. D. Traub, T. C. Rains, R. M. Garruto, D. C. Gajdusek, and C. J. Gibbs Jr., Brain destruction alone does not elevate brain aluminum, *Neurology* **31:**986 (1981).
56. R. Yanagihara, R. M. Garruto, D. C. Gajdusek, A. Tomita, Y. Konagaya, T. Uchikawa, K.-M. Chen, C. C. Plato, C. J. Gibbs, Jr. and I. Sobue, Calcium and vitamin D metabolism in Guamanian Chamorros with amyotrophic lateral sclerosis and parkinsonism-dementia, *Ann. Neurol.* **15:**42 (1984).
57. S. Nakagawa, S. Yoshida, C. Suematsu, E. Shimizu, T. Hirahata, T. Kumamoto, Y. Yase, K. Kawai and S. Iwata, The calcium-magnesium-deficient rat: A study on the distribution of calcium in the spinal cord using the electron probe microanalyser, *Experientia* **33:**1225 (1979).
58. Y. Yase, The role of aluminum in CNS degeneration with interaction of calcium, *Neurotoxicology* **1:**101 (1980).
59. F. Yoshimasu, M. Yasui, Y. Yase, S. Iwata, D. C. Gajdusek, C. J. Gibbs Jr., and K. M. Chen, Studies on amyotrophic lateral sclerosis by neutron activation analysis: 2. Comparative study of analytical results on Guam PD, Japanese ALS and Alzheimer disease cases, *Folio Psychiatrica Neurologica Japon.* **34:**75 (1980).

7 Mental Stimulation and Deprivation as Risk Factors in Senility

Fred B. Charatan

A question of theoretical and practical importance is whether sensory deprivation can contribute to, or even cause, dementia in the elderly. Dementia is precisely defined as a loss of intellectual abilities of sufficient severity to interfere with social or occupational functioning (*1*). The deficit is multifaceted and involves memory, judgment, abstract thought, and a variety of other higher cortical functions; changes in personality and behavior also occur. Although in the past the term "dementia" usually meant an irreversible process, current usage implies that dementia may be a progressive, static, or remitting condition. Busse and Blazer (*2*), using data from longitudinal studies, have shown that mild-to-moderate organic brain disease can undergo remissions and exacerbations during an extended period. Dementia, then, can be an episodic disease before becoming a chronic disorder. Thus, the underlying cause plus the availability and timely application of therapy may determine whether the dementia is reversible or not.

SENSORY DEPRIVATION

The term "sensory deprivation" came into general use in the 1950s after it was shown that volunteers under conditions of visual, auditory, and tactile deprivation reacted after a few days with increased suggestibility (*3*). Soon, what is now called the sensory deprivation state was described (*4*). It is characterized by anxiety, tension, impaired concentration, increased suggestibility, bodily illusions, somatic complaints, intense subjective emotional accompaniment, and vivid sensory imagery, usually visual and sometimes reaching hallucinatory intensity. When sensory input was reduced to as near zero as possible by immersing the subjects in a tank of water at body temperature and having them breathe through a blacked-out head mask, symptoms appeared earlier and more intensely. After normal sensory input was restored, the sensory deprivation state was relatively short-lived; nonetheless, prolonged solitary confinement was thought to be a factor in prison psychosis, in "brainwashing," and in the altered behavior first observed in U.S. prisoners during the Korean War.

SENSORY DEPRIVATION IN GERIATRIC PATIENTS

Sensory deprivation operates in a number of important ways in elderly patients residing in nursing homes, health-related facilities, and old-age homes (see Chapter 2).

Impairment of the Special Senses

Vision In normal aging, the size of the blind spot increases and the visual fields become progressively reduced. Dark adaptation takes longer. Common visual impairments include senile cataract, glaucoma, and senile macular degeneration, the latter condition being the greatest single cause of visual loss in the elderly. Furthermore, the high prevalence of cerebrovascular accident as single-hemisphere stroke in this population often results in hemianopia, blindness in half of the visual field.

Hearing Of the elderly population in nursing homes, 90 per cent have a hearing impairment (5). Patients with hearing aids frequently do not use them or neglect to replace dead batteries.

Taste and Smell Both of these senses deteriorate with age. Anosmia in the community elderly can result in asphyxiation, as happened with coal gas in one circumstance because the victim was unable to smell the leaking gas. Loss of smell in the elderly causes all food to taste the same, depriving the old person of one of life's most important remaining gratifications.

Touch In those patients confined to bed or chair for long periods, and also in those with hemisensory syndrome after a stroke, the sense of touch may be impaired. Infrequent baths or showers and changes of clothing also reduce the amount of sensory input through the skin.

Speech Barriers Many old persons are European immigrants, and some may know little English. Thus they may be socially isolated because of a language barrier. Patients having cerebrovascular disease may be aphasic and suffer an even greater social isolation.

Restriction on Mobility

Patients with fractured hips, hemiplegias, chronic arthritis, lower-limb ulcerations, and amputations make up a high percentage of nursing home residents. Many are temporarily or permanently wheelchair-bound. They often need help in transferring from bed to wheelchair and back again. Not uncommonly, wheelchairs do not operate efficiently, posing a further barrier to the patient's freedom of movement. Where patients endanger themselves through poor judgment, confusion, and agitation, restraints such as Posey jackets, sheets, or mittens may be applied. Again the result is reduction of the patients' ability to choose their own stimuli. Thus, they cannot turn on the radio or television, are unable to reach for a book, newspaper, or telephone, and cannot move to join the conversation of their fellows.

All these limitations further reduce the sensory input to the patient, not just temporarily as in the classical sensory deprivation experiments on young, healthy volunteers, but over long periods. The geriatric patient, apart from not recognizing the subtle sensory deprivation, is unable to take any steps to counter it.

Environmental Effects

The physical environment of many nursing homes is sterile, to say the least. Such an environment cannot offer the same range of visual and auditory stimuli present in the average home. In most homes, family photographs, flowers, and cherished treasures are displayed, memorabilia are kept, cooking smells arise, the noise of children is heard, and family members stop by to see how the grandparents are getting along. Outside, the sounds of cars, lawnmowers, and children at play can be heard.

By contrast, institutions are notorious for their corridors with blank walls, long vistas of floor without pattern or eye-catching features, and other bleak spaces. Rooms tend to lack homeliness, clocks, and calendars. To assure security, personal possessions are often discouraged. The organization of one day is much like that of another. Patients must be roused at an early hour whatever their preference. They must be washed, bathed, and dressed at specific times, meals are served at set times from set menus with individual preferences severely restricted, and then the patients must retire at times arranged to dovetail with the nursing shifts. A paragraph from *Old Age: The Last Segregation* (*6*) provides a graphic picture: "In many homes we observed patients gathered in the lounge waiting for dinner an hour or more before the meal time. They would sit in the auditorium waiting for a movie more than an hour before the film was scheduled to begin. The home did not even have to post the name of the film; they simply announced that a film would be shown, knowing that patients would be all too glad for any amusement to break the monotony of their day."

The point is that no matter how humane and enlightened its policy may be, an institution is forced to operate by rigid schedules because no institution can operate efficiently while respecting individual differences.

Goffman (*7*) has emphasized that institutions resist change, are impersonal, and lack the most ordinary pleasantries of life. For example, patients cannot keep a pet in an institution as they can at home, cannot have any of their own personal furniture—a rocking chair, for example—and of course cannot engage in any sexual activity. The result is to cut down further on the infinite variety of stimuli that play on the elderly living at home.

Staff Attitudes

Götestam (*8*) pointed out the importance of staff attitudes in working with geropsychiatric patients: "Good care must include tenderness and love, and these attributes are the unspecified treatment variables which every hospitalized or institutionalized individual should have the privilege to receive, equally as well as all other individuals." However, the problem of staff burnout—staff exhaustion resulting from excessive demands on energy, strength, or resources—has recently caused concern. Freudenberger (*9*) first described the somatic, psychological, and interpersonal symptoms of burnout. The interpersonal symptoms in particular may be regarded as promoting sensory deprivation in the patients through distancing maneuvers. These include treating patients strictly "by the book," avoiding them, shortening interviews, decreasing eye contact, imposing derogatory labels, and drawing sharp distinctions between personal and professional life. The net result of burnout is the transformation of a staff member from a caring, feeling, compassionate person to an unfeeling, indifferent automaton. Such a burned-out, affectively frozen staff member will reduce substantially the number of helpful stimuli offered to patients, primarily because of the defensive operations of the staff member's own ego.

Psychotropic Medication

In many nursing homes, recourse to psychotropic medications to control disturbed behavior is much too free and physician effort to diagnose the underlying cause too infrequent. In 1970, Nelson Cruikshank, President of the National Council of Senior Citizens, called on Congress to investigate the "dangerous use of tranquilizer drugs on elderly nursing home patients simply to pacify them. . . . Excessive use of tranquilizers can quickly reduce an ambulatory patient to a zombie, confining the patient to a chair or bed, causing the patient's muscles to atrophy from inaction and causing general health to deteriorate quickly" (*10*).

Senator Frank Moss, of the Special U.S. Senate Committee on Aging, wrote in the book *Too Old, Too Sick, Too Bad,* (*11*) ". . .the tranquilizer may have replaced tender loving care in many of today's long-term care facilities." By their effects on the cerebral cortex and subcortical structures, such as the reticular formation, the major tranquilizers block arousal mechanisms, thereby creating a kind of internal sensory deprivation. The observable clinical result is a patient who is apathetic, dull, lacking, in motivation, silent, asocial, and extremely dependent on the nursing staff. The danger is that a tranquilizer once prescribed for an emergency may be continued indefinitely in the absence of any critical review. It is no exaggeration to say that this continued use will over time lead to a state of chronic sensory deprivation.

CLINICAL PATTERNS OF SENSORY DEPRIVATION

Are there some recognizable patterns or syndromes possibly resulting from sensory deprivation in the geriatric inpatient population? I believe there are, and that they may be classified as follows.

The Sundowner Syndrome

At night, when sensory stimulation is reduced both visually and aurally, the old person may develop visual illusions and even hallucinations. Anxiety is often increased, leading to agitation, confusion, noisiness, and even aggressive, destructive behavior. The presence of a night nurse or family member, together with increased lighting may be enough to relieve the symptoms. In the past, similar behavior not uncommonly followed eye surgery, where the eyes of the patient were bandaged for from 24 to 48 hours.

Deafness Associated with Paranoid Symptoms

Cooper et al. (*12*) demonstrated conclusively that deafness in the elderly predisposes patients to paranoid rather than affective psychoses. The psychological mechanisms operating are probably social isolation, misinterpretations of what is said by others, and reduced sensory input—from which ideas and feelings emerge that the patient is weak, helpless, and the target of hostile forces from the human environment outside. Blindness in the elderly does not seem to be associated with paranoia to the same extent.

Institutional Neurosis (The Social Breakdown Syndrome)

In this condition, first described by Barton (*13*) and later by Gruenberg and associates (*14*), patients become apathetic and indifferent to anything not immediately personal or present and lose interest in the future. Personal habits and standards may deteriorate. Patients become resigned to the situation and resist discharge. At the Jewish Institute for Geriatric Care, we have observed that after about six months it becomes increasingly difficult to discharge a patient to a lower level of care. Originally

Barton attributed the institutional neurosis to loss of contact with the outside world, enforced idleness, authoritarian attitudes of the staff, loss of personal possessions, interruption of activities that emphasize individuality, sedation, the atmosphere on the inpatient wards, and the dwindling of future prospects. One may be tempted to include all these factors under the general heading of chronic sensory deprivation. At the same time, it must be recognized that some personalities, e.g., those with traits of severe dependency, seem much more vulnerable than others to the effects of sensory deprivation.

Regressive Behaviors

Demented patients often manifest primitive or regressed behavior. For example, they may use their fingers to eat with instead of a knife and fork, spit or soil themselves, smear food or feces, rhythmically rock their bodies, or pick at themselves incessantly. They may actually believe themselves to be much younger and call for, or even go in search of, long-dead parents. It is possible that authoritarian staff attitudes foster such regression and dependency. The expectation of dependency and regression could act as a self-fulfilling prophecy. Brink (*15*), for example, writes, "Much of what goes on in nursing homes is a systematic process of suggestion: the staff consistently tells the patient that he is too feeble to do anything on his own." The implication here is that the staff's whole range of possible attitudes and the stimuli derived from them narrow down to the single theme that the geriatric patient depends totally on the staff.

SENSORY DEPRIVATION IN THE DEVELOPMENT OF DEMENTIA

As previously mentioned, Cooper et al. (*12*) defined a substantial subgroup of paranoid patients with deafness beginning before age 45 whose personalities seemed to be less deviating and in whom the deafness possibly played a relatively specific role in causing the psychosis. Cooper pointed out that deafness starting early in life imposes handicaps on a person's social life and prospects of employment and also cause underachievement. He does not think that deafness, even that of long duration, produces any consistent change in personality that might increase the liability to psychosis. This observation suggests that deafness is an especially damaging form of stimulus deprivation, resulting not in dementia but most commonly in paranoid psychosis.

Eisdorfer (*16*) demonstrated that impaired hearing in aged subjects related to a decline in the developmental level indicated by Rorschach test responses. He concluded, "Aged individuals with impaired audition, when compared with their normally hearing peers, show a less mature perceptual approach to their environment and developmentally lower level of communication. It may thus be inferred that these subjects are exhibiting a more poorly integrated personality."

By contrast, persons with visual impairment did not show a decline in the Functional Integration score, Content score, or Index of Primitive Thought derived from the Rorschach. Findings such as these support the clinical fact that deafness is a much more malignant form of sensory deprivation than blindness because socially we are creatures of the spoken, rather than the written, word.

SENSORY STIMULATION IN PREVENTING OR REVERSING DEMENTIA

Few controlled studies have been published regarding the effect of sensory stimulation on mental disorders of the aged. Cosin and associates (*17*) in 1958 studied two groups of patients. One group comprised nine confused elderly persons, and the other consisted of three confused and six mentally well-preserved elderly. They took part in a 12-month program of domestic activities, individual crafts, social activities, full occupational therapy, and collective activities. The investigators showed that the confused patients cooperated in a variety of social and occupational programs. Although the rise in activity scores indicated that purposive and appropriate behavior increased, no long-term therapeutic benefit resulted. Maximum improvement occurred during the first months of treatment. During the last six months, scores generally fell, perhaps indicating continuing deterioration after initial improvement. The investigators finally concluded that the initial rise in scores was mainly due to increased activity, social contact, and emotional state, whereas intellectual status and skill remained constant. Even if the intellectual status did not change, the study is still of considerable importance in demonstrating that a well-planned program of social and occupational stimulation can lead, even in confused elderly patients, to observable improvement in behavior.

Bower (*18*) took 25 women suffering from senile dementia with a mean age of 76.2 years and exposed them to 4.5 hours of structured stimulation five days a week for six months. A control group of 25 demented women having a mean age of 81.9 years and confined to a geropsychiatric hospital were selected after meeting criteria for diagnosis, physical state, and initial score. Psychiatric, nursing, and occupational ratings were performed on all the patients.

Nearly half of the experimental group exposed to structured stimulation showed improvement on all the rating scales, whereas the conditions of two thirds of control group subjects deteriorated during the same timespan. Bower thought that these results proved the disease process of senile dementia was slowed because of the therapeutic measures. He emphasized that, to be effective, the stimulation program must be applied continuously, finding that a weekend rest period led to a falling-off of performance gained earlier in the week. He concluded, "Stimulation of patients who are old and becoming demented, to be therapeutically effective, must be consistent and of long duration."

Folsom (*19*) introduced reality orientation as a formal program of social interaction for demented patients. In that program, nursing aides interact with a small group, repeatedly going over personal and current information with each patient, with correct patient responses rewarded with expression of approval. Daily classes last for 30 minutes, and, as the patient improves, more complex material is added. Brook et al. (*20*) found that an experimental group receiving reality orientation improved on ward behavior rating scales, compared with ratings for a control group exposed to the same milieu but without reality orientation. Improvement in the experimental group persisted throughout the 16-week study period.

On balance, then, persistent sensory stimulation and the creation of an enriched environment are acceptable therapeutic tools in the treatment of senile dementia.

PRACTICAL ASPECTS OF SENSORY STIMULATION FOR SENILE DEMENTIA

In considering the practical aspects of sensory stimulation as a therapy for the dementias of old age—using dementia in the sense of a decline of intellectual abilities of sufficient severity to interfere with social or occupational functioning, regardless of the specific diagnosis—some essentials in sensory stimulation are as follows:

1. *The sensory stimulation must be perceived by the patient.* Aging tends to reduce the efficiency of our receptor organs, partly through reduced channel capacity and partly through the effects of disease. Therefore, clear, unambiguous stimuli are necessary at all times.
2. *The sensory stimulation must be repeated.* Long-continued stimulus repetition is the basic principle behind reality orientation, imprinting, and retaining. Essentially, a planned, conscious effort is made to maximize use of surviving functional pathways in the central nervous system. The principle is analogous to that in the rehabilitation of poliomyelitis and stroke victims, where maximum use is made of surviving muscle groups.
3. *The sensory stimulation must have significance for the patient.* Only stimuli that are within the patient's experience will have an impact. Although new learning is certainly possible at any age, considerations of time dictate that sensory stimulation programs appeal to the familiar and well known. Such appeal is the basis of reminiscing and life-review programs.
4. *The sensory stimulation must be generally acceptable to the group of patients.* To provide sensory stimulation on a one-to-one basis would be uneconomical. Hence, any program of sensory stimulation must be applicable to groups.

PROGRAMS OF SENSORY STIMULATION

Sensitivity Training for Staff

First priority should be given to developing a constructive attitude among the staff. The reason is simple: Most of the stimuli directed at the patients come from nurses, aides, orderlies, activities therapists, and food-service attendants. Some essentials to foster among the staff include:

1. Calling patients by their title and surname, recalling Dale Carnegie's observation that "the sweetest music in any man's ear is the sound of his own name."
2. Making repetition the rule by greeting a patient every time you see him. I have never met a patient who reproached me for saying "Good morning, Mr. Jones" ten times—but how woeful the effect if you forget just once!
3. Smiling often because it is a highly positive stimulus and may be reassuring when the patient has lost the ability to respond to words. One should be ever mindful that, in earliest infancy, the mother's smile elicits a response before her words do.
4. Reminding all who work with demented patients never to do anything that the patient might regard as a threat.
5. Remembering always to speak slowly, clearly, and loudly enough for patients and to allow them sufficient time to respond. Your face should be in a good light so that the patient can lip-read if necessary.

Social Groups

Visiting hours should be liberal in order to support the patients' basic feeling that they remain a member of that basic group, their family. Where visitors do not interfere with medical or nursing procedures, they should be encouraged to visit their elderly relatives and, if indicated, take them out on the grounds or to the cafeteria.

To promote social interaction, many institutions permit the partaking of alcoholic or nonalcoholic beverages in a predinner cocktail hour. Coffee breaks have the same function. Each unit in an institution should list and celebrate patients' birthdays and also celebrate public holidays. Whenever possible, patients should be allowed to attend important family celebrations.

Verbal Groups

Patients can interact verbally in several ways. Reading aloud from the daily newspaper, a magazine, or classics in prose or poetry are possibilities, followed by open discussion. Patient government is another forum to promote good relations, improve patient welfare, and allow for the airing of grievances. Reminiscing, a favorite activity of the old, can be organized, with each member of the group taking turns to recount events of his or her life.

Visual Groups

Apart from providing large clocks and calendars in patients' rooms and in public places, the large areas of corridors and unadorned walls offer an opportunity to display artifacts made by the patients themselves. Paintings, weavings, needlepoint, and other decorations can enhance the surroundings, just as in a private home.

Television sets usually abound in institutions. In these days of videocassettes, however, surprisingly little effort is made to use television in a planned way to reach old people, particularly those who have cognitive impairments. For example, videocassette programs on calisthenics, grooming, craft work, and other therapeutic activities could easily be presented on existing sets.

Film showings are another offering that patients enjoy, especially if they are wheelchair-bound. Topics must be carefully selected to appeal to the older, impaired patient.

Activities Groups

One of the most valuable therapeutic activities is calisthenics, often to music. Both ambulatory and wheelchair patients can take part. If scheduled regularly, calisthenics often achieves greater participation than verbal groups, yielding dividends in better circulation, less risk of thrombophlebitis, less constipation, improved appetite, less insomnia and need for hypnotics, and less risk of contractures from inactivity. For those able to participate, dancing is another gratifying activity and will improve grooming and dress among both men and women.

Elderly patients love to play bingo, despite the handicaps of amnesia and disorientation. Although some people regard bingo as a boring and meaningless activity, it in fact demands attention, continued observation of the card, the accurate placement of covers over the numbers called, and the ability to discern when the line or card is full and to call out the triumphant "Bingo!" The reward of a small sum of money offers an incentive to the patients, and when refreshments are included, the program is eagerly looked forward to, even among the impaired.

Musical Groups

Music is probably the best form of sensory stimulation in institutions. It provides a spectrum of benefits: rhythm, a primitive life force; nostalgia, really musical reminiscing; and, most important, an incentive to identify oneself with the group, as in singing or beating time, no matter how demented the patient may be.

Sing-alongs of familiar tunes can be organized, with the patients being given large-print copies of the words or a screen being used to carry the words and suitable visual images to reinforce the theme of each song. Patients may be supplied with maracas, cymbals, or bells with which they can beat time. On other occasions, patients may be offered music appreciation programs, using a record player or tape recorder. School orchestras and choirs are often pleased to visit an institution and give a concert for the patients. Where patients have retained some musical skill, recitals or talent shows can be organized.

Occupational Therapy Groups

For the demented patient who needs to work and can benefit from it, providing a proper "work setting" is essential. Many elderly patients in institutions suffer from a loss of role and complain that time hangs heavy. A sheltered workshop can offer creative occupation, even where the tasks are simple and repetitive. At the Jewish Institute for Geriatric Care, the patients count out small items like paperclips, rubber bands, and screws and package them. They prepare sets of flatware and napkins for use in our cafeteria. Some are able to staple papers together or stuff envelopes. They are paid at piece-work rates for their work. Many appreciate this opportunity to supplement their meager incomes, and they enjoy the social aspects of the workshop and the feeling of dignity and accomplishment that the work offers them.

CONCLUSION

Given our present state of knowledge, we cannot yet affirm that programs of sensory stimulation do anything to prevent or reverse the impairments associated with dementias of old age. However, one thing is certain: programs of sensory stimulation, unlike some other recommended treatments, do no harm to the patients. Even if careful research showed that the benefits to the patients could not be proved, the benefits to the staff caring for demented patients seem incontrovertible. Staff mood and morale are lifted when they are charged with the creative care of these patients. As indicated above, some studies have shown that the patients' behavior improves while they are participating in the programs.

Finally, health care is like justice—it must not only be done, it must also be seen to be done. Hence, when families visit and see that efforts are being made on behalf of their mentally impaired elderly relatives, their feelings of guilt and frustration are relieved. They are less prone to blame and project their hostile feelings on to the staff. Perhaps then the many relatives of these patients will eventually become part of a broad constituency supporting services for the mentally disabled elderly.

In closing, let me say that sensory stimulation is not new. Many centuries ago, its principles were anticipated in this ancient piece of Talmudic wisdom: "Respect an old man who has lost his learning; remember that the fragments of the tablets broken by Moses were preserved alongside the new."

REFERENCES

1. *Diagnostic and Statistical Manual of Mental Disorders,* 3rd edn. American Psychiatric Association, Washington, D.C., 1980.
2. E. W. Busse and D. G. Blazer, *Handbook of Geriatric Psychiatry.* Van Nostrand Reinhold, New York, 1980.
3. P. Solomon, *Sensory Deprivation.* Harvard University Press, Cambridge, Mass., 1961.
4. P. Solomon, and S. T. Kleeman, Editor's notebook: Sensory deprivation, *Am. J. Psychiat.* **127:**1546 (1971).
5. L. S. Libow, and F. T. Sherman, *The Core of Geriatric Medicine.* Mosby, St. Louis, 1981.
6. C. Townsend, *Old Age: The Last Segregation.* Bantam Books, New York, 1971.
7. E. Goffman, *Asylums.* Anchor Books, Garden City, N.Y. 1961.
8. K. G. Götestam, Behavioral and dynamic psychotherapy with the elderly, in: J. E. Birren, and R. B. Sloane, *Handbook of Mental Health and Aging.* Prentice-Hall, Englewood Cliffs, N.J., 1980.
9. H. J. Freudenberger, Staff burnout, *J. Social Issues.* **30:**159 (1974).
10. N. Cruikshank, cited in Moss and Halamandris (*11*).
11. F. Moss, and V. A. Halamandris, *Too Old, Too Sick, Too Bad.* Aspen Systems, Rockville, Md. 1977.
12. A. F. Cooper, R. F. Garside, and D.W.K. Kay, A comparison of deaf and non-deaf patients with paranoid and affective psychoses, *Br. J. Psychiat.* **129:**532 (1976).
13. R. Barton, *Institutional Neurosis,* 2nd edn. Wright, Bristol, England, 1966.
14. E. M. Gruenberg, H. B. Snow and C. L. Bennett, Preventing the social breakdown syndrome, in *Social Psychiatry* (F. C. Redlich, ed.). Williams and Wilkins, Baltimore, 1969.
15. T. L. Brink, *Geriatric Psychotherapy.* Human Sciences Press, New York, 1979.
16. C. Eisdorfer, Developmental level and sensory impairment in the aged. *J. Proj. Techniques Personality Assessment* **24:**129 (1960).
17. L. Z. Cosin, M. Mort, F. Post, C. Westropp and M. Williams, Persistent senile confusion: A study of 50 consecutive cases, *Int. J. Soc. Psychiat.* **4:**24 (1958).
18. H. M. Bower, Sensory stimulation and the treatment of senile dementia, *Med. J. Australia* **1:**1113 (1967).
19. J. C. Folsom, Reality orientation for the elderly mental patient, *J. Geriat. Psychiat.* **1:**291 (1968).
20. P. Brook, G. Degun and M. Mather, Reality orientation, a therapy for psychogeriatric patients: A controlled study, *Br. J. Psychiat.* **127:**42 (1975).

8 Sociological Risk Factors

Erdman B. Palmore

Everybody has some idea of what senility means. Dictionaries define it simply as the physical or mental infirmities of old age. Yet when we attempt to determine scientifically what its risk factors are, we run into many problems of conceptualization and measurement. Does senility refer to *any* infirmity that an old person has? Probably not, because many infirmities may be present from birth. Senility implies a *decrement* from a previously healthy condition. Does senility include acute conditions, like a fracture that will soon heal? Probably not, because senility implies an *irreversible,* or at least a chronic, decrement. Does it then refer to *all* chronic decrements that occur to any older person? Probably not, because although some chronic decrements (like allergies) may develop in old age, they are less common in old age than in the younger years. Senility implies that old age somehow *caused* the decrement or at least made the older person more susceptible to it.

Therefore, if strict criteria are set up so that senility refers only to chronic and irreversible decrements resulting from old age itself, the task of proving that the infirmities associated with old age meet all those criteria would be extremely difficult. To get around this problem, we simply examine in this chapter the sociological risk factors associated with the increased mortality, morbidity, and mental illness that occur in old age, even though they may not meet the criteria of a strict definition of senility.

MORTALITY

That many social characteristics are associated with higher mortality among the aged is now fairly certain, although the explanation for some of these associations is less than certain.

Gender

Mortality is lower among older women than among older men. In fact, this mortality differential obtains at all ages (Figure 8-1). The question is, How much of this gender difference is due to genetic differences and how much is due to lifestyle or social differences between the genders? Several facts indicate a genetic superiority of women over men in longevity:

Women have lower mortality in all developed countries and in most underdeveloped countries (*1*).

In the uterus, females survive better than do males. About one third more males than females are stillborn (*2*). This difference cannot be caused by sex role or environmental differences.

Females have greater longevity than males in every species of animals studied so far (*3*).

A study of men and women in similar Catholic teaching orders with similar health conditions and hazards found that the women still had substantially greater life expectancy (*4*).

Does this genetic superiority of females explain all of the difference in mortality between men and women? I think not. At least four pieces of

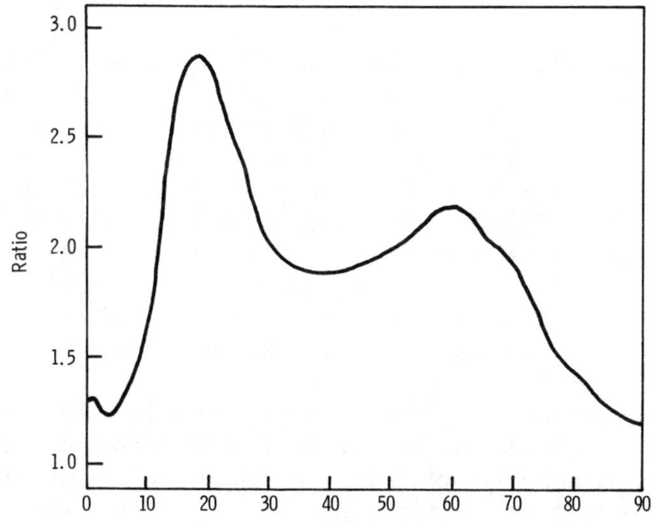

Figure 8-1. Ratio of male to female mortality by age, for the United States, 1970 (data from the Division of Vital Statistics, National Center for Health Statistics).

evidence support the theory that some, if not all, of the gender differences in mortality are caused by differences in the sex roles and social environments of men and women:

1. A later investigation of Catholic teaching orders showed that the priests tended to smoke more than the population average, to be more overweight than the average, and to experience great stress from their vows of chastity and obedience and from the other demands of their order (*5*). Each of these factors would tend to increase the mortality of the priests in comparison with that of the nuns in similar orders.
2. Males had lower mortality than females in Western countries before industrialization and continue to have lower mortality in several undeveloped countries, such as India, Pakistan, Liberia, and Nigeria. This lower mortality for males is presumably related to higher maternal mortality and the poorer living conditions of women in these countries, but it demonstrates that poor environments can counterbalance the genetic superiority of women.
3. Smoking of tobacco is a well-known cause of higher mortality from various kinds of cancer and cardiovascular disease. Until recently, substantially more men than women smoked. Indeed, one study concluded that most of the variations in mortality among men and women in the United States could be accounted for by differences in smoking habits (*6*).
4. Male mortality is one third higher than female mortality through the first five years of life, when sex roles apparently make little or no difference. However, starting at age 5, the "excess" male mortality begins to increase until it reaches a peak at ages 15 to 24, when it is almost three times that of females (Figure 8-1). Then it tends to drop, so that at ages over 75 the excess male mortality is similar to the rate of the preschool years. This drop to early-years mortality seems to indicate that sex role differences again become unimportant in mortality in late old age. The increase in excess male mortality during ages 15 to 75 may be explained by the greater risks among adult males from such things as heavier smoking and involvement with more accidents, more hazardous occupations, and more violence (including wars).

In summary, this evidence indicates that females have a genetic superiority over men in longevity but that the mortality for women during their adult years is further reduced below that of males by the facts that women smoke less, have fewer accidents, have fewer hazardous occupations, and engage in less violence.

Socioeconomic Status

I use the broader term "socioeconomic status" rather than "social class" because the latter term is often restricted to those aspects of social stratification inherited from one's family. Socioeconomic status refers to all aspects of stratification, whether inherited or acquired, such as education, occupation, and income. The differences in mortality associated with various indicators of socioeconomic status are reviewed first and followed by a discussion of the possible causes of these differences.

Occupation has been a classic indicator of socioeconomic status because it relates directly to occupational risks and to lifestyles. All studies, whether in the United States or Great Britain or elsewhere, agree that persons in (or who were in) the higher socioeconomic occupations have substantially lower mortality than do those in the lower occupations. This correlation holds for older persons as well. For example, in the United States white men aged 25 to 64 who were professional or technical workers had mortality rates 20 per cent below the population average, whereas those who were laborers or service workers had mortality rates 37 per cent above that average (*7*). An exception to this general white-collar/blue-collar difference is the fact that agricultural workers had the lowest mortality of all occupations: 24 per cent below the population average.

Of special interest is the fact that certain occupations entail unusual hazards that are greater than those attributable to their socioeconomic level. This occupational hazard relationship is shown by the substantially higher mortality among men in these occupations compared with the mortality for their wives. For example, the mortality for sandblasters was 73 per cent above the average, but that for their wives was at the average; the mortality for machine tenders was 60 per cent above the average, but that for their wives was 23 above the average.

At the other extreme, the mortality for top business executives was substantially lower than the average for managers or officials. Although the mortality for managers averaged 9 per cent below the average for all white males, the mortality for business executives listed in *Who's Who in America* was 29 per cent below the average, and the mortality for top male corporate executives in *Fortune's* list of 500 top industrial corporations was 37 per cent below the average (*8*). These data show that, within the broad occupational categories, socioeconomic status and longevity vary substantially.

Income is another accepted measure of a person's socioeconomic status and a direct measure of access to many of the things that contribute to longevity, such as good medical care, nutrition, and housing. For example, the mortality for white male family members (aged 25 to 64) with incomes below $2000 in 1960 was 51 per cent above the population average, whereas the rate for those with incomes of $10 000 or more was 16 per cent below the average. Among women, the differences are somewhat less but in the same direction.

Education is an even better indicator of socioeconomic status because it is more stable and accurate than occupation and income. One difficulty with occupation and income is that they often decline with approaching death, and therefore part of their association with mortality is explained by approaching death causing lower socioeconomic status, rather than the other way around. Education level, however, generally does not change substantially after age 25. Here again, the association between education and longevity is strongly positive. White men with one or more years of college, for example, have about three more years of life expectancy at age 25 than those with fewer than eight years of education. Women with some college have about ten more years of life expectancy than those with fewer than five years of education.

An important question is whether something about education itself contributes to greater longevity (through better understanding of the world and ability to solve crucial problems, for example) or whether more education simply leads to higher income, which in turn gives access to things that contribute to longevity. A recent analysis that controlled for income so that the independent effects of education (and vice versa) could be studied found that education and income influence mortality independently. For example, the educational differential in longevity was reduced by half when income was controlled, and the income differential was reduced by one third when education was controlled. Therefore, both are important.

Also indicating the influence of socioeconomic status on longevity are the differences between racial categories. Japanese-Americans have the highest life expectancy, whites are next, American Indians are substantially lower, and blacks have the lowest life expectancy of all. This ranking of the races by longevity correspond to their ranking by average family income. Therefore, most, if not all, of these racial differences in longevity are probably caused by socioeconomic differences.

As a final example of socioeconomic influences on mortality, consider the large differences in longevity between countries. While developing countries such as India and China have average life expectancies at birth of 46 and 53 years, respectively, Japan (in the same region and with the same racial composition as China) has an average life expectancy of over 73 years. The best record for longevity is currently held by Sweden, with an average life expectancy of almost 75 years. These differences in longevity correlate closely with differences in economic development, which indicates the strong influence of socioeconomic factors on longevity.

The Nature-Nurture Controversy

Just as there are alternate explanations of the gender differences in mortality, there are two main explanations of the socioeconomic differences in mortality. The "nature," or heredity, explanation attributes mortality differences to genetic differences. This theory argues that one's genetic constitution largely determines mortality, and that the reason that higher socioeconomic categories have lower mortality is that genetically superior persons tend to move up to, or remain in, the upper socioeconomic categories, whereas genetically inferior persons tend to move down to, or remain in, the lower categories.

This theory has substantial evidence to support it. First, in most societies, even those with fairly rigid class or caste systems, there is considerable mobility up and down socioeconomic levels. That genetically influenced abilities and health would have some influence in this process of social mobility seems plausible. Second, we know that inherited disease and disability increase mortality. We do not know how many persons are thus affected nor how much impact they have on life expectancy averages. Third, we know that some association exists between the longevity of parents and that of offspring. Several of the early studies probably exaggerated the size of this association because of various methodological defects, but nearly all agree that there is some association (*9*). The better studies indicate that the difference in life expectancy at about age 25 between persons with greater parental longevity and those with lesser parental longevity is from two to four years.

On the other hand, this estimate of the possible influence of heredity is much smaller than the ten-year gain in life expectancy at age 25 that has been achieved in the United States during this century. Because the change in genetic characteristics has been negligible during this period, this 10-year gain must have been caused mainly by changes in the environment. When one looks at changes in life expectancy at birth, the gains are even more impressive: about 20 years for white men and about 25 years for white women.

Furthermore, it is often forgotten that the association between the longevity of parents and offspring cannot be attributed entirely to genetic factors. As Dublin and associates (*2*) state:

> The survival of parents to old age means, in most cases, a more favorable life for the children. These advantages, which are spiritual, mental, and physical, undoubtedly favor longevity. A child with both parents present to look after its welfare gains by better environment, by better attention to its daily needs, and quite frequently by a better start in life through a more complete education, as compared with an orphaned child.

Even among intact families some of the association between longevity of parents and offspring can be accounted for by environment. Whatever environmental factors contributed to the greater longevity of the parents are also likely to be present for the offspring. Parents with better nutrition, housing, and medical care are likely to provide better nutrition, housing, and medical care for their offspring. Thus, it is theoretically possible that the entire association between longevity of parents and offspring could be accounted for by environmental differences.

A final argument in favor of the importance of social and environmental factors is the fact that wide differences in longevity between countries and within the same country over time cannot be explained by genetic differences. We have noted that Japan, with the same racial stock as

China, has a life expectancy at birth that is 38 per cent higher than that in China. Similarly, life expectancy at birth in the United States has increased by almost one half during this century, with little or no change in genetic characteristics.

Marital Status

We know that among the aged, as at all ages, married persons have lower death rates than persons in any of the nonmarried categories, but several puzzles remain. Never-married men have higher death rates than widowed men, but among women the widowed have higher rates than the never-married. What is the explanation of the higher mortality among the widowed compared with that among the married (for both men and women)? Is it the shock and loneliness of widowhood that increases mortality, or is it that whatever lifestyle and environmental risk factors were related to the death of the spouse tend to hasten the death of the widowed person? In the Duke Longitudinal Studies of Aging, we found little or no evidence of lasting trauma caused by widowhood. Indeed, many found the death of a chronically ill spouse to be a relief.

Retirement

There is no question that retired persons as a group have higher mortality than those who continue to be gainfully employed. However, this rate difference probably occurs because the more healthy aged continue to work whereas most ill persons retire. Studies of persons in compulsory retirement systems find no significant difference between expected and actual death rates in retirement. Thus, the association between retirement and mortality is probably explained by the fact that sick persons tend to retire, not that retirement causes sickness and death. There may well be some cases of persons who are forced to retire and who then withdraw from activity, become depressed, lose the "will to live," and therefore die earlier than if they had continued working, but these cases are probably balanced by those who are delighted by retirement from a stressful or unhealthy job, whose health improves on retirement, and who live longer because of their retirement.

Relocation

A common belief is that any residential change among the elderly is likely to be stressful and to increase mortality. Residential change is one of the potentially stressful "life events" listed in the widely used Schedule of Recent Events (*9*). However, studies of purely voluntary residential moves have generally failed to demonstrate any consequences that could not be interpreted as intended changes, i.e., the reasons for which the move was made in the first place (*10*).

The studies of involuntary moves are more inconsistent. Many studies have found no significant effects on mortality, few found beneficial effects, and a few found negative effects under certain conditions. In general, the evidence suggests that involuntary moves have little or no overall effect on mortality but that the following types of elderly are at increased risk of adverse effects: men, the very old, persons living alone and having few contacts with friends and kin, those in poor financial circumstances, those with less access to various social services, those having lived in the old neighborhood a long time, those low in morale and life satisfaction, those reacting with depression, hopelessness, and helplessness, and those in institutions with disintegrating social systems.

The Duke Longitudinal Studies

In a series of analyses to determine which factors are the strongest predictors, or risk factors, for mortality among the panelists of the Duke First Longitudinal Study of Aging (*11*), we found several significant social and behavioral risk factors after controlling for sex, age, and race. Smoking cigarettes was one of the strongest risk factors, especially among the men aged 60 to 70, who had the highest rates of smoking. Low intelligence, little education, and inadequate finances were also significant risk factors, although we cannot be sure whether causal relationships exist here, as stated above in the Nature-Nurtue section. Work satisfaction and feelings of usefulness were significant predictors of longevity, which we interpreted to mean that feelings of inadequacy, boredom, and uselessness may be risk factors in mortality through some complex psychosomatic processes. Finally, a significant pair of predictors of longevity were in the area of sexual activity. For men, the frequency of intercourse was a significant predictor, and for women the satisfaction with past intercourse was a significant predictor. This seems to mean that for men the quantity of sexual activity is important in longevity, whereas for women the quality of sexual activity is the important factor. For women, satisfaction with past intercourse remained a significant predictor even in a multiple regression that controlled for the effects of other significant predictors.

Through multiple-regression analysis we found that, when the effects of the three strongest predictors were combined, they could make a difference of up to 16 years in longevity for men and up to 23 years for women.

MORBIDITY

Age

Age is a complex risk factor that combines biological, psychological, and sociological variables. The social variables associated with old age include retirement, widowhood, reduced social interaction, lower income, and education. Thus, examining age as a social risk factor in morbidity is appropriate in this chapter because age may serve as a proxy indicator for the above social variables, which may be the underlying risk factors.

A widespread belief is that the older people get, the greater becomes their risk of illness and disability. Although such an age-illness relationship holds for total rates, it is *not* true for many types of illness. For example, there is much less acute illness among the aged than among younger persons: acute illnesses per 100 persons are less than half as frequent among those over age 65 as they are among those under 65 (*12*). Another example is the rate of injuries: the number of injuries per 100 persons is also about half that among persons under 65. This rate difference exists for all categories of injuries: in motor vehicles, at work, at home, and in other categories. True, older persons do have greater risk of restricted activity and bed disability resulting from injuries. Thus, even though they have fewer injuries, the consequences are more serious among the aged. Also, older persons have higher risks of developing chronic conditions and as a result have higher risks of disability days, limitations of activity, and hospitalization.

However, most people are unaware that many chronic conditions have a *lower* prevalence among the aged than among other age groups. Older persons have lower risk of five respiratory conditions: asthma, hayfever, chronic sinusitis, deflected nasal septum, and hypertrophy of tonsils and adenoids. There are also five categories of skin and musculoskeletal conditions that are less frequent among the aged: eczema, dermatitis, and urticaria; psoriasis; acne; displacement of intervertebral disc; and synovitis, bursitis, and tenosynovitis. Migraine is only about half as frequent among those over 65. Finally, gynecological problems (except breast) are less frequent among older women.

Gender

While gender is clearly based on biological differences, the lifestyle and social role differences between men and women may be even more important than the biological differences in affecting risks.

Although older men are clearly at greater risk of mortality than are older women, women are paradoxically at greater risk for most morbidity measures. Older women have greater risk than do older men of injury, acute conditions, restricted activity, and bed disability, and older women have longer stays in the hospital (Table 8-1). The only risks clearly lower for older women are days of work loss (since they work less) and per cent with activity limitations (since they normally have less strenuous activities). Women have slightly fewer hospital episodes each year, but slightly more days in the hospital for each person with one or more hospital stays.

How can we explain the paradox that older men die at a higher rate but older women seem to get sick more often? Part of the explanation is that in our culture men are expected and encouraged to minimize or deny

Table 8-1. Disability and Hospitalization Risks for Men and Women 65 and Over

Risk	Men	Women
Percentage of persons injured per year	16.0	19.8
Days of restricted activity associated with injury per person per year	4.9	6.4
Days of bed disability associated with injury per person per year	1.7	2.7
Days of restricted activity per person per year	38.0	44.5
Days of bed disability per person per year	13.0	14.3
Days of work loss per person per year	5.0	4.2
Percentage of persons with activity limitations	49.0	44.0
Percentage with limitations in major activity	44.0	35.9
Percentage of persons with short-stay hospital episode during the past year	18.9	17.8
Short-stay hospital days during year per person with one or more hospital stay	14.1	14.4

Source: National Center for Health Statistics, *Current Estimates from the Health Interview Survey,* Series 10. Department of HEW, Washington, D.C., 1979.

illness more than women, but it also appears that women do suffer from more of the nonfatal illnesses than men do.

Socioeconomic Status

Just as mortality is higher for the lower socioeconomic groups, so is morbidity. For example, among persons 65 and over, the incidence of acute conditions is lowest for white-collar workers; number of restricted activity days is lower for professional and technical workers, managers, and other white-collar workers; and limitations of activity due to chronic conditions are lower for professional and technical and other white-collar workers. In general, the lower educational and income groups also have higher morbidity rates.

As in the explanations for the association of mortality with lower socioeconomic status, the effect from genetic and environmental factors on this difference is uncertain. Nonetheless, it seems safe to conclude that part of the difference results from the better nutrition, housing, sanitation, and medical care of the higher socioeconomic groups.

Rural-Urban

Most of the standard indicators of health show that the rural elderly have more sickness and disability than the urban elderly (Table 8-2). Exceeding the national averages are farm elderly, who have over one fourth more acute conditions; rural nonfarm and farm elderly, who have more

Table 8-2. Morbidity Among The Rural Elderly

Category	All Residences	Rural Nonfarm	Farm
Acute conditions	1.1	1.1	1.4
Percentage with chronic activity limitation	45.9	49.1	47.2
Days of restricted activity	38.4	40.8	32.0
Work-loss days due to injury	0.9	1.2[a]	
Bed days due to injury	1.7	1.8[a]	
Total bed days	12.9	12.2	6.6

Source: National Center for Health Statistics. Unless otherwise indicated, statistics are per person per year.

[a]Combined rural nonfarm and farm. Separate statistics are not available.

chronic activity limitation; rural nonfarm elderly, who have more days of restricted activity; and rural elderly, who have more work-loss days and bed days due to injury. The only exception to this pattern is that rural elderly say they stay in bed less than the average, despite their greater incidence of acute and chronic illness. This exception may result from a stronger belief among rural elderly that one should get out of bed and carry out normal activities if at all possible.

The greater risk of morbidity among rural elderly is probably due to a combination of poorer health care (hospitalization, surgery, and physician visits are lower among the rural elderly) and the more strenuous and dangerous occupation of farming.

MENTAL ILLNESS

The study of risk factors in mental illness among the elderly is complicated by greater problems of case identification, diagnosis, and sampling than obtain for studies of mortality and morbidity. There are no nationally representative studies of mental illness among community residents in the United States. Therefore, our estimates of risk factors must be based on a series of local community studies and institutionalized populations. The findings from some of these studies disagree, and so our present conclusions are based on only the usual findings and must be considered tentative.

Age

Does total mental illness increase in old age? Most studies agree that the total prevalence rate is higher among the older ages, although two studies found this to be true of men but not of women (*13*). However, the *incidence* of new cases of mental illness did not increase with old age in two of three studies based on community case registers. This finding suggests that the risk of new mental illness does not increase with age, and so the increase in prevalence with age must be due to lower recovery rates in old age.

When the risks of specific kinds of mental illness are considered, the patterns become even more complex. Most studies agree that both the incidence and prevalence of neurosis and schizophrenia are lower in old age than at younger ages, but these declines are more than made up for by the increases in psychosomatic complaints and organic brain syndrome. Furthermore, anxiety neurosis apparently tends to be replaced by depressive neuroses and other unspecified depressions. Apparently, too, the general increase in the prevalence of total mental illness is due primarily to organically related declines, such as chronic brain syndrome and psychosomatic ailments, and secondarily to the losses and stresses of old age, which increase depression.

Gender

Most studies have found the rate of overall psychiatric impairment higher among older women than among older men (*14*). However, when specific types of mental illness are separated, there is no agreement among the studies as to whether older men or women have higher rates of organic psychoses, functional psychoses, schizophrenia, or affective illness (*15*). On the other hand, three of four studies agree that older men have higher rates of personality disorder, and five of six studies agree that older women have much higher rates of neuroses. Therefore, the higher risk of overall mental illness among older women is probably due to their higher risk of neuroses. The latter risk may be due largely to cultural expectations, whereby women are allowed to express neurotic symptoms more than men are.

Socioeconomic Status

The studies of socioeconomic status and mental illness among the elderly are inconclusive (*13*). Those studies that have found some association between mental illness and some indicators of lower socioeconomic status have usually concluded that the lower socioeconomic status is more the consequence than the cause of mental illness.

Marital Status

Many studies have found higher rates of hospital admission for the single and widowed elders for the married (*13*). However, a community study in Syracuse, New York, found that this relationship no longer existed once age, physical health, and socioeconomic status were held constant. Also, two studies found no evidence that bereavement increases mental illness. Therefore, it seems probable that the higher rates of hospital admission for the nonmarried results primarily from the fact that the nonmarried tend to be older, sicker, poorer, and less likely to have someone to care for them outside the hospital.

Isolation and Loneliness

The relations between social isolation, loneliness, and mental illness are complex (*13*). Persons who say they are lonely usually have higher rates of neuroses, but these reports of loneliness seem to be more a symptom of neuroses than a result of social isolation. Lifelong social isolation does not seem to relate to increased mental illness. When some association has been found between social isolation and mental illness, the isolation appears to be more the result than the cause of mental illness.

Psychosocial Stress

Holmes and Rahe (*9*), as well as others, have shown that increases in the number of "life change events" are often followed by increases in mental illness among the general adult population. However, this relationship has not been studied among the elderly. The Duke Second Longitudinal Study of Aging found surprisingly little effect of five major life events on various measures of adjustment, when each was considered separately (*16*). However, when several events occurred together, they tended to have significant negative effects. The existence of psychological and social resources also had significant meliorative effects that seemed to allow better adjustment to multiple life events.

CONCLUSION

Mortality risks are higher among older women than older men, partly because of genetic factors and partly because of gender roles. Older persons in the lower socioeconomic groups have higher risks of mortality, and this increase in risk is also probably due to a combination of genetic and environmental factors. Mortality risk among older married persons is lower than that for nonmarried persons, but the causal link is unclear. Retired persons have higher risks of mortality, but the increase occurs because ill persons are more likely to retire. Studies of relocation and mortality are inconsistent, and there is probably no pure relocation effect on mortality. The Duke Longitudinal Studies found higher risks of mortality among smokers and persons with low intelligence, little education, inadequate finances, low work satisfaction, feelings of uselessness, and low sexual activity (men) or dissatisfaction with past sexual experience (women).

Higher total morbidity risks are associated with older age, but older persons are at lower risk for acute illnesses and many types of chronic illnesses. Older women are at greater risk than older men for injury, acute conditions, restricted activity, and bed disability and have longer stays in hospitals; however, older women are at lower risk for days of work loss and activity limitations. Older persons from lower socioeconomic groups have greater risks of morbidity, but this increased risk is also probably due to a combination of genetic and environmental factors. Rural elderly are at higher risk of morbidity than are urban elderly, probably because of a combination of poorer health care and the greater hazards of farming.

Older persons are at greater risk for total prevalence of mental illness, but the incidence of new cases of mental illness apparently does not increase with age. Risks of neuroses and schizophrenia tend to decline with age, whereas risks of organic brain syndrome and psychosomatic complaints increase with age. Older women have higher risks of overall psychiatric impairment, primarily because of their much higher rates of neuroses. Older nonmarried persons are at higher risk of mental illness, primarily because they tend to be older, sicker, poorer, and less likely to have someone to care for them than are married persons. Multiple life events may increase the risk of mental illness among the elderly, but psychological and social resources tend to reduce the negative effects of these events.

REFERENCES

1. *Demographic Yearbook, 1980.* United Nations, New York, 1981.
2. L. Dublin, A. Lotka and M. Spiegelman, *Length of Life.* Ronald Press, New York, 1949.
3. C. Rose, Critique of longevity studies, in *Prediction of Life Span* (E. Palmore and F. Jeffers, eds.). D. C. Heath, Lexington, Mass., 1971.
4. F. Madigan, Are sex mortality differentials biologically caused? *Milbank Memorial Fund Quarterly* **35:**202 (1957).
5. F. Madigan, Role satisfaction and length of life in a closed population, *Am. J. Sociol.* **67**:640 (1962).
6. G. Grannis, Demographic perturbations secondary to cigarette smoking, *J. Gerontol.* **25:**55 (1970).
7. E. Kitagawa and P. Hauser, *Differential Mortality in the U.S.* Harvard University Press, Cambridge, Mass., 1973.
8. Metropolitan Life Insurance, Longevity of corporate executives, *Stat. Bull.* **55:**3 (1974).
9. T. Holmes and R. Rahe, The social readjustment scale, *J.Psychosomatic Res.* **11**:213 (1967).
10. S. Kasl, A. Ostfeld and G. Brody, Effects of involuntary relocation on the health and behavior of the elderly, in *Epidemiology of Aging* (S. Haynes nd M. Feinleib, eds.). GPO, Washington, D.C., 1980.
11. E. Palmore, Predictors of the longevity difference, *The Gerontologist* (in press).
12. National Center for Health Statistics, *Data from the National Health Survey,* Series 10. GPO, Washington, D.C. 1979.
13. D. Kay and K. Bergmann, Epidemiology of mental disorder among the aged in the community, *Handbook of Mental Health and Aging* (J. Birren and R. Sloane, eds.). Prentice Hall, Englewood Cliffs, N.J., 1980.

14. D. Blazer, The epidemiology of mental illness in late life, in *Handbook of Geriatric Psychiatry* (E. Busse and D. Balzer, eds.). Van Nostrand Reinhold, New York, 1980.
15. B. Dohrenwend, B. S. Dohrenwend, M. Gould, B. Link and R. Neugebauer, *Mental Illness in the United States*. Praeger, New York, 1980.
16. E. Palmore, W. Cleveland, J. Nowlin, D. Ramm, and I. Siegler, Stress and adaptation in later life, *Gerontology* **34:**541 (1979).

9 Health Risks and Lifestyle

Haitung King and Frances B. Locke

The term "style of life" was originally used by Weber to mean a primary determinent of "status of honor" or "status groups" (*1*), whereas "class status" and "social class" are, according to Weber, primarily determined by market or "economic relevant situations" (*1,2*). Amplifying Weber's concept, we use the term "lifestyle" here to mean "particular ways of living commonly shared by most constituent members of an aggregate population," such as an ethnic group or social class. We emphasize the impact of divergent living habits in various socioeconomic groups on their members' "life-chances." As an example of chance of survival, the fate of the three classes of female passengers on board the *Titanic* may be cited. As the story goes, only four of the 143 women in first class (including three who volunteered to stay on the ship) drowned. In contrast, 15 of 93 women in second class sank with the ship, as did 81 of the 179 women in third class; the heavy toll of the latter passengers was said to be attributable to their being ordered to remain below deck (*3*).

DATA AND MEASURES

The mortality data presented here derive mainly from official mortality statistics on occupations (from which social classes are primarily determined), particularly those of England and Wales; published U.S. occupational mortality figures are meager. The data refer to males with work experience, aged 15 or 20 to 64, because official data for persons aged 65 and over, even if available, are generally crude and less reliable.

Morbidity statistics for the United States derive mainly from the findings of various health surveys of noninstitutionalized civilian populations conducted by the National Center for Health Statistics (NCHS). The General Household Survey of England and Wales provides basic information on those areas of Great Britain.

Health risk measurement is expressed mainly in terms of standardized mortality ratio (SMR); other indices include incidence rate, prevalence rate, and relative risk. Whenever possible, some of the crude measures used in data sources for subgroups have been standardized by us to the total survey population to minimize the possible effect of differential age distribution between social strata.

Levels of health risk among different socioeconomic groups are expressed in terms of positive and negative (or inverse) class gradients. A positive gradient indicates that health risk increases from the lowest to the highest class. The reverse is true for a negative relationship. Thus, with a positive gradient, the higher the class, the higher the risk; with a negative gradient, the higher the class, the lower the risk.

Some limitations of the analysis should be noted. Data and space restrictions preclude a detailed cross-factor health profile (e.g., age-sex-race-social class) as well as a fuller coverage of topics under discussion, particularly some of the findings from the four parallel surveys of the nation's families, 1953–1970 (*4,5*).

SOCIAL CLASS DIFFERENCES IN HEALTH RISK

Studies of health risk in various population groups have benefited greatly from the introduction of the concept of social class. Social class stratification (five groups, as a rule) is usually based on occupational categories, although other criteria, such as income, education, tenure, census tract, and poverty level, may be used independently or in any combination. Regardless of the operational definition used, the resultant grouping of classes generally reflects common ways of living and life chances shared by class members. Thus, in commenting on the classification by the British Central Statistical Office of occupations into social classes, Semple (*6*) stated bluntly: "What counts to the classifier . . . is what you do for a living, and what happens to you as a result. Nearly half of all group I workers tend to live in detached houses. People in lower grades still tend to drink and smoke more and die earlier." In a similar vein, Dublin et al. (*7*) were of the opinion that "the work a man does, the condition under which his work is done, the wages he receives for doing it determine in great measure the circumstances of his life, the house he lives in, the clothes he wears, the food he eats and his recreation. A man's occupation is therefore one of the most potent factors, deciding the state of his health and fixing the length of life."

Admittedly, certain differences in lifestyle may exist among several occupations grouped into a given social class. Nevertheless, the general assumptions of an intricate relationship between work and lifestyle remain valid after appropriate adjustment. For example, Adelstein (*8*) recently examined British data using the measure of social class standardization; the calculated, perhaps oversimplified, results indicated that, overall, only 18 per cent of the variation in mortality from all causes was work-related—that is, more than 80 per cent was explained by social class. For circulatory and respiratory diseases, mortality associated with work was about 30 per cent, the remainder being associated with social class. Similarly, whereas only 12 per cent of the mortality due to cancer was related to work, 88 per cent was related to social class. With these figures as background, we examine the various dimensions of mortality and morbidity among different social classes.

Mortality

Standardized mortality ratios for selected causes by occupation for the United States, 1950, are given in Table 9-1. An increasing mortality from the highest to the lowest class was shown for practically all types of deaths—infectious, acute, chronic, or violent. A similar trend was reported for data classified by years of school completed (*10*). This finding is roughly in keeping with the social gradient of diseases prevailing among British subjects grouped into five or six socioeconomic strata, based on more extensive data from 1949 to 1971 (*11*). In the first ten years, a negative mortality gradient from Class I (professional) to Class V (laborer) was observed for most infectious diseases, acute and chronic respiratory conditions, and violent causes. Since 1960, however, the inverse class-mortality pattern of Great Britain extended to a number of chronic conditions, such as arteriosclerotic heart disease, vascular lesions, hypertension, and diabetes.

The two sets of data for the United States, 1950 and 1960, are not strictly comparable to each other or to the British data. Therefore, caution must be taken in interpreting the observed narrowing ratio differential between the two polar social strata for such causes as tuberculosis, influenza and pneumonia, and accidents. Other changes noted in the ten-year period include an increase in class-ratio disparity for diabetes and stabilized class-ratio differential for coronary heart disease.

The importance of socioeconomic determinants was shown in a recent analysis of the change in the impact of education on age-specific mortality in the United States (Table 9-2). For those under age 65 in both periods, a strong negative mortality gradient by education was noted. Among those aged 65 and over, however, there was no educational gradient in 1960, but by the 1970s the effect of schooling was about as strong as that for younger persons. Among other possible factors—advances in medicine, improved medical care, welfare programs, and social security benefits—educational betterment during the 13-year period may well have benefited the younger cohort (*12*).

Morbidity

The morbidity data presented here, derived mainly from survey findings, should be read with caution because of the inherent limitations of such

Table 9-1. Standardized Mortality Ratios for U.S. White Males with Work Experience, Aged 20–64, by Occupation, 1950

Cause of Death	Class I Professional[a]	Class II Technical, administration, management[b]	Class III Clerical, sales, skilled	Class IV Semiskilled	Class V Laborer[b]	Ratio[c] V/I
All causes	83[d]	84	96	97	120	1.4
Tuberculosis, all forms	36	40	69	103	158	4.4
Malignant neoplasms	89	91	106	104	116	1.3
Diabetes mellitus	98	99	110	88	90	0.9
Major Cardiovascular and renal diseases	98	94	103	93	103	1.1
Vascular lesions affecting CNS	87	79	89	80	94	1.1
Arteriosclerotic heart disease including coronary disease	115	109	116	100	103	0.9
Hypertensive heart disease	75	73	82	77	84	1.0
Influenza and pneumonia except pneumonia of newborn	57	51	73	95	153	2.7
All accidents	50	68	82	107	173	3.5

[a]Includes nonwhites.

[b]Except farm.

[c]Computed by the authors.

[d]Standardized mortality ratio: the ratio of the number of deaths observed to the number expected, expressed as a percentage. The standard population has the value 100%; in the different classes, the SMR has a value less than 100% if there is a lower mortality and greater than 100% if there is a higher mortality.

Source: Compiled from data in reference 9.

Table 9-2. Standardized Mortality Ratios for U.S. White Males, by Education

<table>
<tr><th rowspan="2">Years in School</th><th colspan="2">Age 25–64</th><th colspan="2">Age 65 and above</th></tr>
<tr><th>1960</th><th>1973–77</th><th>1960</th><th>1973–77</th></tr>
<tr><td>0–8</td><td>111</td><td>124</td><td>101</td><td>106</td></tr>
<tr><td>9–11</td><td>103</td><td>134</td><td rowspan="2">99</td><td>93</td></tr>
<tr><td>12</td><td>91</td><td>99</td><td>106</td></tr>
<tr><td>13–15</td><td>85</td><td>113</td><td rowspan="2">98</td><td>77</td></tr>
<tr><td>16 or more</td><td>70</td><td>84</td><td>77</td></tr>
</table>

Source: Compiled from data in Reference 12.

information. Of particular concern is the varying degree of completeness in data obtained from different socioeconomic groups, as higher-educated respondents generally reported more relevant information than did those with fewer years of schooling. As with mortality risk, the magnitude and severity of morbidity conditions generally showed an inverse relationship with class position.

Activity Limitation Due to Chronic Conditions By the NCHS definition, limitation of activity refers to such conditions as (a) inability to carry on the major activity of one's age-sex group, including working, keeping house, or going to school; (b) restriction on the amount or kind of major activity; or (c) restriction in relation to other services, e.g., recreational, church, or civic interests. Here we examine briefly these activity limitations in relation to social status as determined by annual family income or years of education completed.

According to a 1978 NCHS survey (Figure 9-1), among persons with an annual family income of less than $7000, about 22 per cent assessed their own health as only fair or poor, compared with 6 per cent among those with $25 000 or more income (age-adjusted); the corresponding proportions of persons with any limitation of activity due to chronic disease or impairment in the lowest and uppermost income groups were 21 per cent and 10 per cent, respectively. All other limitations also displayed an inverse relationship with income.

By specific disorder, a 1974 NCHS survey reported that the leading chronic conditions reported for the lowest income group were arthritis and rheumatism (22 per cent), followed by heart conditions (17.5 per cent) (*14*). However, the rank order of these two causes was reversed in all other five income groups. Hypertension without heart involvement was reported as the third leading condition for any income group.

The 1974 NCHS survey also showed that the proportion of persons with limitation of activity in each age group declined as educational level rose. As was true for persons classified by family income, heart conditions and arthritis and rheumatism were the two leading disorders among those with little education.

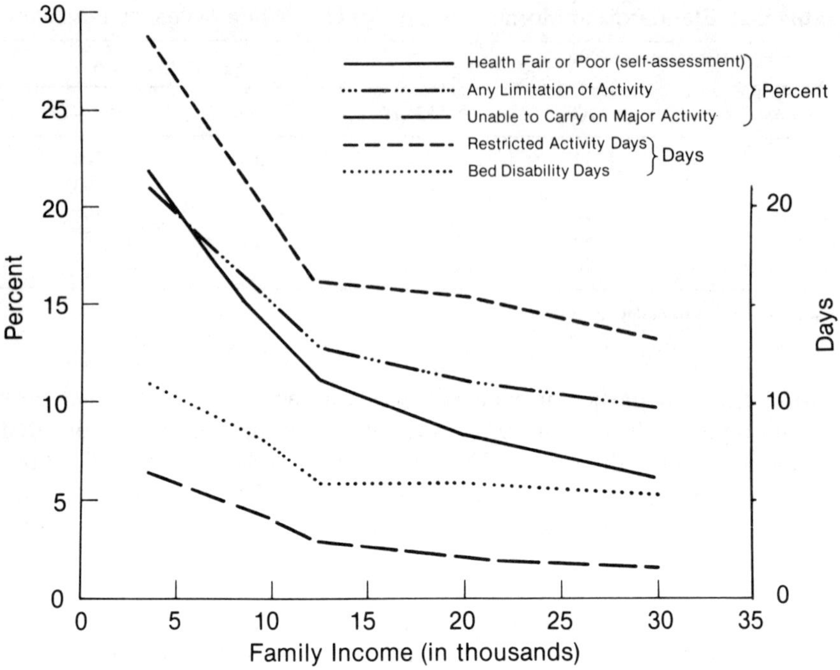

Figure 9-1 Age-adjusted percentage of persons reporting fair or poor health and with selected chronic limitation of activity, by family income, United States, 1978 (*13*).

Prevalence of Chronic Conditions by Selected System

Circulatory conditions Roberts and Rowland (*15*) showed that, as family income and education of the head of the family rose, the age-adjusted prevalence rates for cerebrovascular conditions, and particularly hypertensive disease with heart involvement, declined. For coronary heart disease, however, the prevalence rates showed little class differential by income or education, in keeping with the increasing mortality from this condition among lower classes in England and Wales.

Respiratory conditions Age-adjusted prevalence rates of selected chronic respiratory conditions are described in a 1970 NCHS survey (*16*). An inverse relationship by family income was shown for emphysema, active tuberculosis, and, to a lesser degree, bronchitis. For hay fever without asthma, however, the rates rose with elevation in family income. A negative education gradient was also noted for emphysema and active tuberculosis, in addition to hay fever without asthma. Notably, the impact of hay fever without asthma on upper or lower-class members was relatively slight, whereas that of emphysema and tuberculosis on lower-class members was considerable in terms of limitation of activity and disability days each year.

Digestive conditions Differences in prevalence of selected chronic digestive conditions by income and education are reported in a 1975 NCHS survey (*17*). Ulcers of the stomach and duodenum were the most commonly reported disorders, followed by frequent constipation, hernia of the abdominal cavity, and upper gastrointestinal disorders. All these conditions, along with nearly all other disorders reported in the survey, displayed a higher risk among lower than among upper social classes. An extremely low risk for liver disorder was noted for both upper and lower socioeconomic groups, but its impact on disability was striking. Overall, nearly 27 per cent of liver disorders caused limitation of activity and over one third necessitated bed confinement.

Other selected chronic conditions Scott (*18*) reported on the prevalence of chronic disorders of the genitourinary, nervous, endocrine, metabolic, and blood and blood-forming systems, in addition to a broad group of gynecological conditions other than those involving the breast. With one or two exceptions, a consistent negative relationship was shown for the occurrence of specific disorder and family income or educational status of the head of the family.

Cancer Cancer risk by socioeconomic status deserves special attention, mainly because of the traditional thinking of the importance of various work-related carcinogens in causing malignant neoplasms. Although our emphasis has only recently been toward lifestyle as a strong intervening variable, in England and Wales consistent differences in general mortality risks (including cancer) between social classes have been well documented for more than half a century (Figure 9-2).

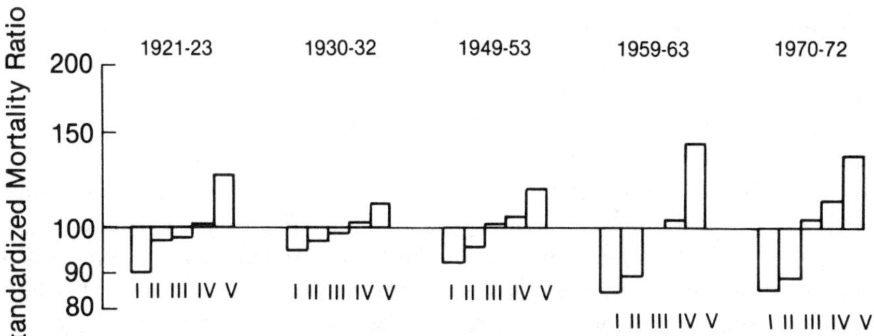

Figure 9-2 Standardized mortality ratios for males, age 15 to 64, by social class, England and Wales, 1921–72 (*19*).

The findings of cancer incidence among whites in the United States from a recent comprehensive study (*20*) generally supported the mortality gradient found among different classes of British subjects. For most cancer sites (e.g., lung, rectum, cervix, esophagus), a negative relationship by income was observed, with a reversed pattern found for female breast cancer. Differences in cancer incidence for several sites by education were also consistent with the income relationship. However, an elevated risk for cancers of the colon, prostate, and bladder was displayed among the better educated.

Symptoms of Psychological Stress Higher rates for 12 self-reported psychological, physical, or psychosomatic symptoms used as indices of psychological stress were observed among lower than among higher income-education groups (*21*). However, a less strong inverse relationship was shown for symptoms of psychological stress, such as insomnia, feeling of an impending nervous breakdown, and nightmares, than for physiological stress symptoms, such as dizziness, headaches, and heart palpitations. More significantly, when education was included as an additional variable with sex and age, many findings associated with other demographic variables were rendered insignificant.

INTERPRETATION OF FINDINGS

Frame of Reference

The findings presented above, based on limited available data, clearly show a persistent inverse relationship between social status and most specific causes of death or morbidity, as well as symptoms of psychological stress. The few findings with positive gradients, although difficult to account for, may be attributable to the more accurate and thorough diagnosis received by the upper classes or to the more complete and reliable information obtained from them.

The difference by social class could hardly be incidental, judging from the British experience of the past 50 years, during which a persistent social class mortality gradient was displayed (Figure 9-2). In accordance with our central theme, a conceptual scheme of lifestyle is suggested in Figure 9-3 for the interpretation of the findings. The scheme, emphasizing synergic effects of the various components in the shaping of a lifestyle, should also provide a basic framework for future research on this subject.

Aside from limitations in mortality data, the morbidity information on the association between a specific health condition and social status used in our analysis was derived from the less desirable cross-sectional, rather than longitudinal, investigations. For these reasons our comments on lifestyle and health risks are necessarily selective and at times conjectural.

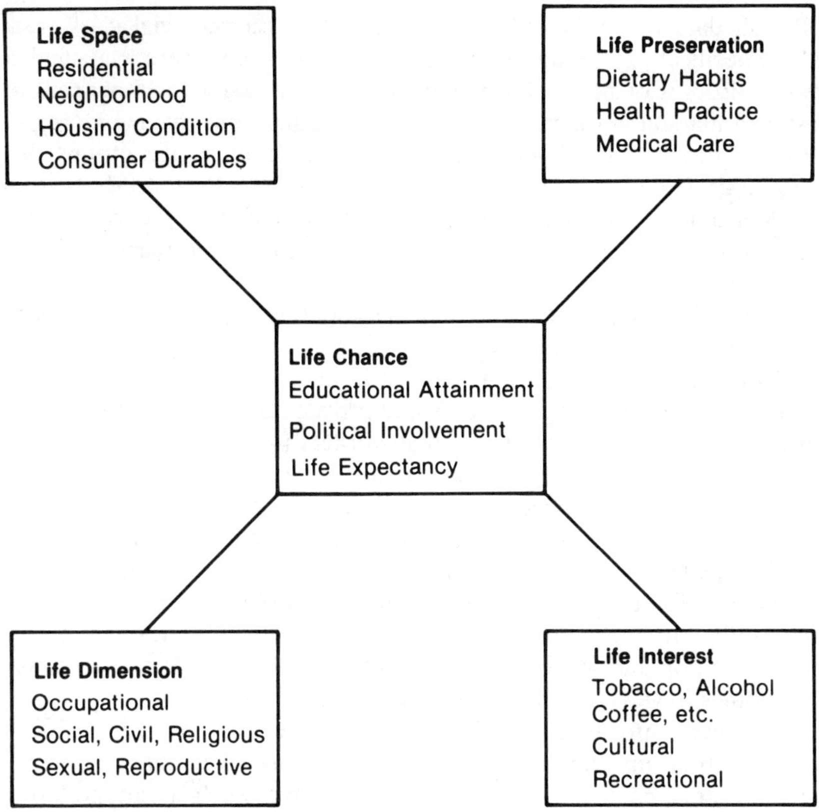

Figure 9-3 A suggested conceptual scheme for the study of health risks and lifestyle.

Implications of Findings

Life Space—Residence, Tenure, Consumer Durables The significance of amenities of life space to health risk cannot be overemphasized, judging from the large number of hours a person spends in the home and its surroundings. That the area in which lower-class persons live and the houses they live in are usually undesirable or especially conducive to health risk is well established. In addition, a sizable number of lower-class households is deprived of certain consumer durables that are essential to health maintenance. Some specific examples support our contention.

Residence A 1974 U.S. Annual Housing Survey reported that 12 per cent of households with less than $3000 income lived in units lacking some or complete plumbing facilities, compared with 0.4 per cent for households with an income of $15 000 and above (*22*). Further, according to a 1977 national outdoor recreation survey (*23*), a smaller proportion of persons in lower classes have a yard or live in areas within a 15-minute walk of a park.

British data on overcrowding also indicated drastic social class gradients. Specifically, among professionals, 37 per cent were classified as "two bedrooms or more above standard," in contrast with 15 per cent for unskilled manual workers (*19*). In addition, households having more persons per room had a higher mortality ratio for most age groups than households with one or fewer persons per room (*24*). Furthermore, excessive mortality associated with lack of bathing facilities was reflected in such causes of death as cancer, circulatory diseases, and particularly respiratory disorders, accidents, and violence.

Tenure The generally known association of tenure with health extends beyond communicable diseases. For example, cancer mortality by tenure for British men of all ages was highest in men who were public housing tenants and lowest in those who owned private homes; the difference was particularly noticeable among manual workers (*8*).

Consumer durables According to a 1973 census report, noticeably lower proportions of ownership of such appliances as freezer, refrigerator, air conditioner, and washing machine were found in households with less than $3000 income than in those with $25 000 or more (*22*). Similar social-class differences were noted in the British OPCS Longitudinal Study (*19*). Stomach cancer, which showed an elevated incidence among lower-class populations, could be attributable to the fact that fewer lower-class homes have refrigerators and freezers.

The limited information presented above, when considered along with that on other undesirable conditions prevailing over those neglected neighborhoods in which lower-class people live, such as air pollution, unsanitary atmosphere, fire traps, and high rates of violence, seems to suggest that many of the poor health risks among these populations relate to the life space they occupied.

Life Preservation—Dietary Habits, Health Practice, Medical Care

Dietary habits The link of food intake with both favorable and adverse health risks has been implicated, but adequate data are limited because of measurement problems and reporting errors. The latter are particularly true for information obtained from persons with low income and limited education.

Generally speaking, the percentage of family expenditure on food items decreased proportionately with a rise in income. Thus, the 1972–73 Consumer Expenditure Survey reported that among families with an annual income below $3400, about half of the average income before taxes was spent on food; the corresponding figure was under 10 per cent for families of $19 675 and over (*25*). Furthermore, compared with persons above the poverty level, those in the poverty class showed a consistent pattern of lower daily per capita consumption of major nutrients, especially those aged 65 and over (*26*). Some of the deficiencies reported among the poverty class are iron, calcium, vitamin A, and vitamin C, all of which could contribute, directly or indirectly, to a number of diseases observed in these populations. For example, vitamin C deficiency has been implicated in cancer risk (especially the stomach). Other essential nutrients, such as fat and animal protein, were also shown to be deficient among poverty-class persons. However, overconsumption of fat and animal protein has been incriminated in the development of heart disease and some cancers.

Recent British findings indicated that lower-income groups eat more refined carbohydrates and sugar, whereas the upper classes eat more whole-grain bread and fruit (*27*). Devesa's review of earlier U.S. data on food consumption also showed that the "use of both fresh and frozen fruits and vegetables increases with increasing income level, while canned and dried fruits and vegetables are used less frequently at the upper level" (*20*). More recent findings of the Lipid Research Clinics Study further showed that, among men aged 20 to 59, the percentage of energy from protein rose as the educational level increased (*28*).

Health practice Study findings on health practice by socioeconomic status are meager. Generally, a much lower proportion of upper-class than lower-class persons were reported to (a) get less than six hours of sleep; (b) never eat snacks; (c) be less active than others of the same age; (d) exert no control over body weight; (e) not exercise regularly; and (f) eat breakfast (*29,30*). Except for the last-mentioned, all other health practices, along with a limited consumption of alcohol and a low proportion of cigarette smokers, are consistent with the seven good health practices reported by Breslow and Enstrom (*31*).

The reported smaller proportion of lower-class than upper-class persons who engage in regular exercise in the United States was corroborated by the British experience, in which the class gradient was negative for both indoor and outdoor exercises. Such a deficiency was, according to Morris (*27*), increasingly unlikely to be made up at work among lower-class persons.

The higher degree of weight consciousness reported for upper classes was not supported by all research findings. Thus, 12 per cent of persons with less than $4000 income were reported to be on special diets, compared with 9 per cent for the top income group of $15 000 or more. However, the reported success in weight reduction was greater among the higher income group (*23*). Furthermore, among females in most age groups, a higher proportion classified as being below poverty level was reported to be obese (determined by skinfold measurement) (*23*). Obesity may contribute to the ill health status of the lower-class female population.

Medical care Family health expenses, notably dental expenses, generally increased directly with rise in family income (*32*). However, the proportion of family income spent for health decreased as income rose (*33*). As with income status, better-educated families had somewhat higher absolute expenses for health than those with less education.

As one would expect, differences in family health expenditure by socioeconomic status were reflected in disparity in the use of health services (*34*). A much higher proportion of lower-income groups never had chest x-rays, glaucoma tests, breast examinations, pap smears, or even routine physical examinations, In addition, the lower-income group had longer intervals between visits for various procedures. Moreover, the lower-income groups used dental services less frequently.

Regular use of aspirin (once a week or more) was reported to decrease with increasing educational level and family income (*35*). Also, those who used aspirin regularly had rates about twice those of the nonregular users for poor or fair health or for chronic conditions causing activity limitation. Presumably, the known high-rate use of aspirin among persons with a number of pain conditions was particularly relevant to the elevated porportion of arthritis noted previously for lower-class persons.

Regular use of sleeping pills varied by levels of income and education, with the proportion of users decreasing as income and educational status rose (*35*). Persons who used sleeping pills once a week or more reported more chronic conditions causing activity limitation than did nonregular users. In addition, a higher proportion of users rated their own health status as being only fair or poor.

Life Dimension—Occupation Besides general economic conditions and other factors, educational attainment determines the likelihood of a person having a job, the type of job, and the possibility of job advancement. For those employed, working conditions and fringe benefits also vary by occupation.

Among British workers, a person's vulnerability to unemployment (i.e., the proportion of economically active persons out of work) varied with occupational status, ranging from 1.4 per cent for Class I to 12.0 per cent for Class V (*19*). Moreover, "two-thirds of general labourers were judged to have poor prospects of obtaining long-term work, and 55 per cent of all unemployed labourers in the survey in June, 1973 were still unemployed in January, 1974." In contrast, management and professional workers had the best prospects of obtaining long-term work, with a wider range of benefits such as sick pay and off-work payment than did non-skilled and manual workers, although the latter group was more likely to be absent from work due to illnesses, accidents, strikes, and layoffs.

The employment experience in the United States has been similar. Thus, for the year 1980, the unemployment rates for persons with work experience were white-collar workers, 3.7 per cent; blue-collar workers, 10.0 per cent; service workers, 7.9 per cent; and farm workers, 4.4 per cent (*36*).

In view of these findings, the degree of stress at work would appear to be greater for blue-collar and service than for professional and management workers. Especially noteworthy are such stressors as unequal status, exclusion from decision making, domineering authority, low prospect for advancement, poor working conditions, and restrictions on behavior.

More recently, attention has been directed to ischemic heart disease among London's male civil service workers. Taking ischemic heart disease mortality in the administrative grade as 1.0, the relative risks (the ratio of a defined condition among persons exposed to a given risk factor to that among those unexposed) for the professional/executive, clerical, and other grades were 2.1, 3.2, and 4.0, respectively (*37*). These differences were partly attributed by the authors to the strong tendency for average levels of cigarette smoking and blood pressure to decrease as the employment grade increases. Comparable findings for U.S. civil service workers are not available, except that workers in the upper levels were absent from work less frequetly than those in lower levels (*38*).

Life Interest—Cigarette Smoking, Alcohol Use, Coffee Drinking

Cigarette smoking Practically all studies on smoking and health of the past 30 years have pointed to a strong risk association of varying degrees. The evidence seems to indicate that cigarette smoking is the single most important lifestyle component contributing to premature death, mainly because of the increased health risk from ischemic heart disease, respiratory cancers, and chronic obstructive pulmonary disease. Much of the elevated health risk among lower classes noted earlier could be attributable to the high proportion of cigarette smokers in those populations. For example, the findings of a recent NCHS survey reported that the proportion of smokers was much higher among male blue-collar and service workers than among white-collar workers (*35*). Also, those occupations with a high proportion of smokers showed higher averages for number of cigarettes smoked. The findings were consistent with the current British experience, which showed an inverse relationship between smoking and occupation (Table 9-3).

The NCHS survey also reported that the proportion of smokers de-

Table 9-3. Standardized Mortality Ratios for Lung Cancer and Smoking Ratio, Selected Occupational Orders, England and Wales

Occupational Order	SMR	Smoking Ratio[a]
Professional, technical workers, and artists	61	66
Administrators and managers	60	76
Clerical workers	79	87
Sales workers	85	91
Service, sport, and recreation workers	120	100
Laborers	146	133
Farmers, foresters, and fishermen	84	77

Note: Date not given in source. Presumably for the year 1977, judging from the appearance of the same data in a 1978 publication (A. J. Fox and A. M. Adelstein, Occupational mortality: Work or way of life? *J. Epidemiol. Community Health* **32:**73, 1978).

[a]Ratio of the number of smokers to the number expected on the basis of national proportion.

Source: Adapted, with changes, from Reference 8.

creased as the educational level increased. The only exception was that those having less than ninth-grade schooling were not as likely to smoke than those with some high school education. The average number of cigarettes smoked followed a similar pattern. In addition, the proportion of male smokers in the lowest family income bracket of under $5000 was 20 per cent higher than that in the top economic group of $25 000 and over (*35*).

Two recent publications on the adverse effect of smoking on health (*39,40*) showed that the proportion of persons reporting chronic and acute conditions and limitation of activity was higher among present smokers than nonsmokers. Also, an estimated 20 per cent of the total of work-loss days due to illness and injury could be attributed to the higher rates of loss among current and former smokers; the excess of days lost from work was calculated from work-loss experience of those who had never smoked cigarettes. All these data were consistent with the speculation that cigarette smoking is perhaps the single most important lifestyle component contributing to premature death among persons in the lower social classes.

Alcohol consumption Whereas the higher proportion for cigarette smoking was among lower classes, a higher proportion of alcohol imbibing was found among upper-class persons in the United States (*41*) and England and Wales (*42*). However, relatively fewer persons in the upper than in the lower socioeconomic group were classified as heavy or escape drinkers.

Coffee drinking According to an NCHS report (*35*), heavy coffee drinking (five or more cups per day) is associated with family income. Even after age adjustment, the inconsistent income and education gradients (positive by income, negative by education) shown for persons who drank five or more cups daily and the apparently better health maintained by these heavy drinkers cannot be explained. Among persons aged 20 to 44, however, those who drank fewer than five cups per day reported fewer chronic conditions causing activity limitation. The latter finding seems interesting in view of the suspected association of heavy coffee drinking with heart disease and neoplasms, including pancreatic cancer, for which a positive social class gradient was observed among persons aged 65 to 74 (*43*).

Life Chance—Educational Attainment, Political Involvement, Life Expectancy The popular belief that education has a differential influence on a person's life chances is supported by these findings: The probability of sons graduating from college relates to the educational attainment of their fathers, with a difference of over 45 per cent between college graduates whose fathers have less than eight years of education and those whose fathers have at least some college (*44*). Furthermore, a person's educational opportunity is known to be influenced by family income, as reflected in the college plans of high school seniors and in their actual enrollment in post-secondary education and type of institution attended (*23*). More recent findings further indicated that, compared with their counterparts in families having incomes of $15 000 or more, dependent members in families whose incomes were below $5000 were 2.6 times less likely to enroll in college. No less discouraging was the spurious narrowing gap observed between the two opposite groups of income during the 1967–77 decade; this narrowing was attributable to the reduced enrollment among the top income group rather than the rising attendance among the lowest level (*23*).

Educational attainment is highly related to various forms of political involvement, which in turn is one of the mechanisms for affecting political decisions. Among these decisions can be included public policy concerning matters of health and survival. Persons without a college education have been found less likely (a) to show political interest and concern; (b) to vote in elections; (c) to have ever written to a political official; (d) to give money to a political campaign; (e) to try to influence the vote of others; (f) to have been contacted by party representatives; and (g) perhaps most importantly, to believe in their effectiveness in public and political affairs (*44*). It would follow from these findings that the life chances of politically resigned persons deprived of college education would tend to rise and fall at the whim of politically active college graduates. Among the instances of differential life chances that can be cited for U.S. whites are the reported shorter years of life expectancy (for women particularly) of the noncollege group (*45*), lower survival rates of unskilled workers (*11* OPCS, 1971), and the favorable mortality observed among persons with better education, higher income, and super-grade occupation.

IMPLICATIONS FOR PREVENTION OF SENILITY

Students of health sciences and policy makers usually take what we would call a "psychographic" view on matters of health maintenance and improvement, with emphasis on individual responsibility and behavior change. The effectiveness of such measures largely depends on a person's adequate knowledge of various health subjects, high motivation, and intelligent use of health resources. Because upper-class persons generally score high on all these requirements, they naturally benefit to a greater extent than the less-health-conscious lower-class members. Furthermore, the validity of some of the "standard" practices in health recommended at a given time may be superseded by findings to the contrary. Examples of these practices include avoiding the use of marijuana and saccharin, abstinence from drinking, jogging or not jogging (particularly *not* for women), as well as the current controversies over diet and coronary heart disease and cancer risk by levels of cholesterol (*46*). Moreover, the ethical involvement of behavior intervention cannot be taken lightly. As pointed out by Kelty (*47*):

> Behavior modification procedures are generally utilized to strengthen adaptive behaviors and to lessen maladaptive behaviors. The adaptive and maladaptive behaviors often require value judgments, particularly when the etiology mechanism and motivants underlying behavior are poorly understood or are the subject of theoretical controversy.

In view of the limitations of the psychographic outlook, we therefore propose, in accordance with our examination of the health status across social classes, a forward-looking approach to matters of life prolongation and prevention of senility.

These points have been clearly presented:

1. Over time and across the nations examined, a consistent mortality and morbidity gradient pattern prevails among persons classified into various social classes by education, income, occupation, tenure, and poverty level.
2. Persons with more education generally hold better-paying jobs of higher prestige.
3. The behavorial patterns of various social classes are vividly reflected in their respective lifestyles, as distinguished by life space, life preservation, life dimension, life interest, and life chance. Evidence from examination of life chance by social class further suggests that those with a better education, when compared with the less educated, have the advantage of expressing their wishes and exerting political influences over various matters, including health maintenance.

We are therefore inclined to believe that an overall advancement of education in the general population would lead to the minimization of disparity in health risk among different population segments. Such an endeavor not only would enable more persons to choose freely in maintaining their health with minimal public intervention but also would afford them ample opportunities to share in the decision making on health matters.

The overall impact of educational betterment on the improved health status of the younger cohort in the United States, 1960–73, is noted in Table 9-2. For stomach cancer, the same cohort effect was reported to be operating in the years 1969–71, which displayed a stronger association with education than with income for the younger age groups (*20*). Incidentally, the high association between education and health observed in a recent NCHS publication (*48*) is in keeping with the general arguments and supportive data covered in this chapter. Indeed, for the country as a whole, if the entire population had similar mortality rates as those who had one year of college or more, the percentage of deaths reduced for selected causes would be astonishing. As shown in Figures 9-4 and 9-5, this kind of "excess mortality" or "unnecessary deaths" constituted 9 per cent of all deaths among white men aged 25 and older and 29 per cent among white women of that age group; the corresponding percentages for those aged 25 to 64 were 25.2 and 21.7, respectively. For certain causes of

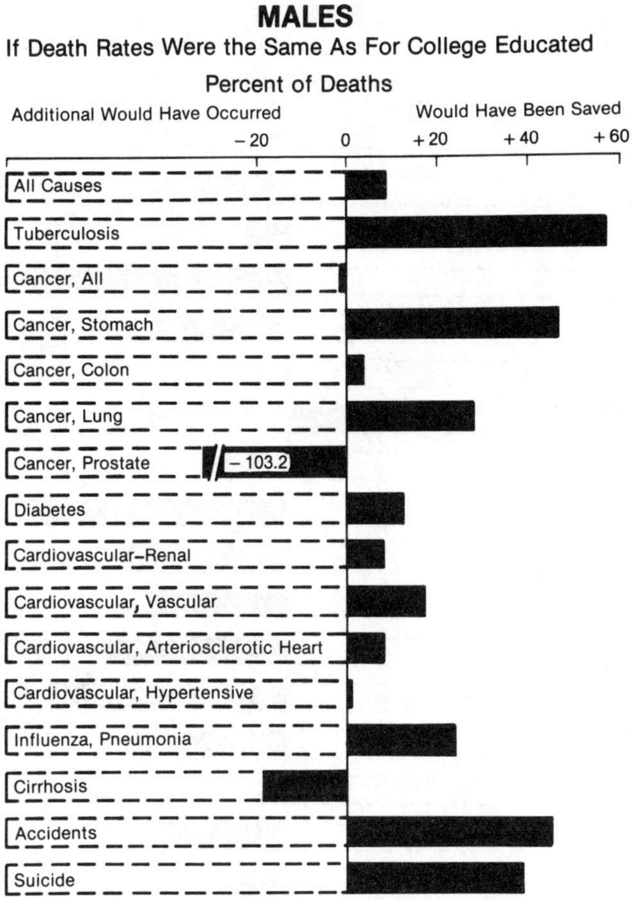

Figure 9-4 Excess deaths as percentage of total deaths, by cause, for all white males 25 years of age and over, as compared with college-educated males, United States, 1960 (*45*).

death, the excess mortality prevailing among males would have been reduced as much as from 40 to 60 per cent.

Lest a misunderstanding arise, we emphasize that we do recognize a certain usefulness in the traditional programs of health promotion, such as environment modification, mass screening, health education, and leveling of socioeconomic inequalities. However, the limitations of such measures have usually been overlooked by students of health policy. As an example, Morris (*27*) singled out socioeconomic inequalities as a major factor associated with the persistence of inequalities in health in England and Wales. This association of inequalities was evident in the fact that the introduction of the National Health Service in 1949 did not bring about a convergence in the levels of mortality across occupations (*49*). Actually it

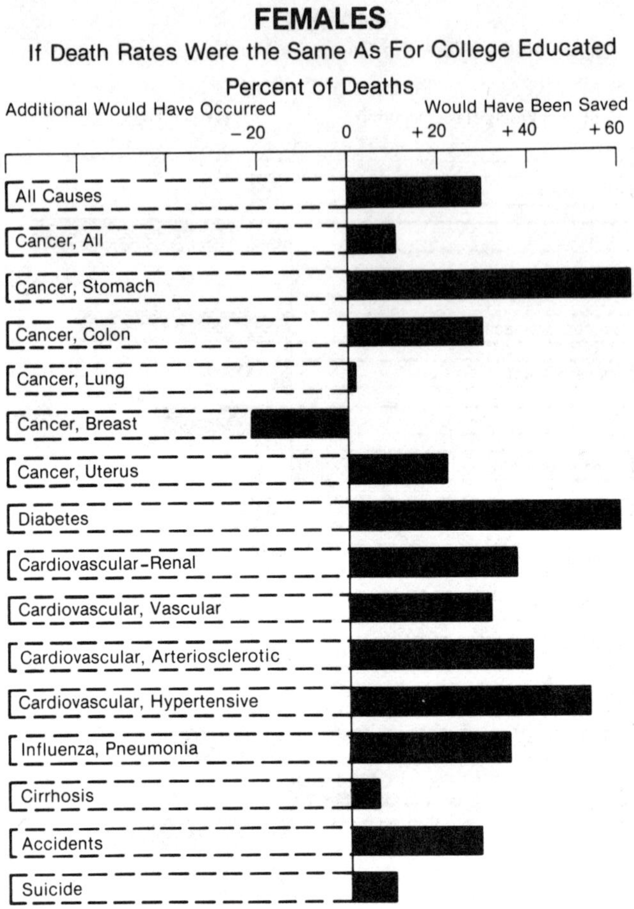

Figure 9-5 Excess deaths as percentage of total deaths, by cause, for all white females 25 years of age and over, as compared with college-educated females, United States, 1960 (*45*).

has resulted in a widening of the differences in death rates between upper and lower social classes for various broad groups of causes of death. This seemingly ironic outcome is attributed mainly to the low utilization of health care services among lower-class families (*50*). A full explanation of utility decisions was attempted by Culyer (*51*); suffice it to note that such a low demand fell far below the actual needs of lower-class persons. We are thus evermore convinced that the maximal effectiveness of most traditional programs of health promotion can be achieved only with an intelligent public interested in sharing decision making in health and other matters and competent in choosing courses of action wisely. Eberstadt (*52*) echoes this position in an editorial, that in part reads, "It is the uncounted who cannot complain and are worst at protecting themselves, who suffer most from untoward decisions from on high. Bad policy is often difficult to change, but it is impossible to change unless it is identified, analyzed, and challenged."

Finally, it is encouraging to note that in the recent past a higher educational level has been attained by each succeeding generation. In 1979, among persons 25 to 44 years of age, 82 per cent had completed high school, of whom 22 per cent were college graduates. Among persons aged 65 and over, the corresponding figures were 40 per cent and 8.5 per cent, respectively (*53*). According to the Bureau of Census, by the year 2000, the percentage of high school graduates should reach about 80 per cent for those aged 25 and above and 64 per cent for those aged 65 and over (*54*).

Acknowledgment

Jacob S. Siegel, Bureau of the Census, and Jacob A. Brody, National Institute on Aging, provided published and prepublished data on educational attainment of the U.S. population, and Marvin A. Schneiderman, the Uniformed Service University of Health Sciences, provided helpful comments for this chapter. For these courtesies we wish to express our sincere thanks.

REFERENCES

1. M. Weber, *From Max Weber: Essays in Sociology*. Oxford University Press, New York, 1946.
2. M. Weber, *The Theory of Social and Economic Organization*. Oxford University Press, New York, 1947.
3. W. Lord, *A Night to Remember*. Henry Holt, New York, 1955.
4. R. Andersen, J. Kravits, and O. W. Anderson (eds.), *Equity in Health Services: Empirical Analyses in Social Policy*. Ballinger, Cambridge, Mass., 1975.
5. R. Andersen, J. Kravits, and O. W. Anderson, *Two Decades of Health Services: Social Survey Trends in Use and Expenditure*. Ballinger, Cambridge, Mass., 1976.
6. R. B. Semple Jr., In a changing Britain, class holds the line, *New York Times,* September 13, 1975.
7. L. I. Dublin, A. J. Lotka, and M. Spiegelman, *The Length of Life,* Ronald Press, New York, 1949; cited in H. King et al., Further inquiry into Protestant mortality patterns, *J. Biosocial Science* **7**:243 (1975).
8. M. Adelstein, Life-style in occupational cancer, *J. Toxicol. Environmental Health* **6**:953 (1980).
9. L. Guralnick, *Mortality by Occupation and Industry Among Men 20 to 64 Years of Age, United States, 1950,* Vital Statistics Special Report (National Office of Vital Statistics), vol. 53, no. 5. GPO, Washington, D.C., 1963.
10. E. M. Kitagawa and P. M. Hauser, *Differential Mortality in the United States: A Study in Socioeconomic Epidemiology*. Harvard University Press, Cambridge, Mass., 1973.

11. *Occupational Mortality, England and Wales, 1951, 1961* (Office of the Registrar-General); 1971 (Office of Population Censuses and Surveys). Her Majesty's Stationery Office, London, 1957, 1971, 1977.
12. S. Rosen and P. Taubman, Changes in the impact of education and income on mortality in the U.S., in *Statistical Uses and Administrative Records with Emphasis on Mortality and Disability Research,* Selected papers given at the 1979 Annual Meeting of the American Statistical Association. Social Security Administration, Washington, D.C., 1979.
13. National Center for Health Statistics: *Health, United States, 1980.* GPO, Washington, D.C., 1980.
14. C. S. Wilder, *Limitation of Activity due to Chronic Conditions, United States, 1974,* NCHS Vital and Health Statistics, Series 10, no. 111, 1977.
15. J. Roberts and M. Rowland, *Hypertension in Adults 25–74 Years of Age, United States, 1971–1975,* NCHS Vital and Health Statistics, Series 11, no. 221, 1981.
16. C. S. Wilder, *Prevalence of Selected Chronic Respiratory Conditions, United States, 1970,* NCHS Vital and Health Statistics, Series 10, no. 84, 1973.
17. F. Drury and L. J. Howie, *Prevalence of Selected Chronic Digestive Conditions, United States, 1975,* NCHS Vital and Health Statistices, Series 10, no. 123, 1979.
18. G. Scott, *Prevalence of Chronic Conditions of the Genito-urinary, Nervous, Endocrine, Metabolic, and Blood and Blood-forming Systems and of Other Selected Chronic Conditions, United States, 1973,* NCHS Vital and Health Statistics, Series 10, no. 109, 1977.
19. Central Statistics Office, Social commentary: Social class, *Social Trends* **6:**10 (1975).
20. S. Devesa, *A Study of the Association of Cancer Incidence with Income and Education Among Whites and Blacks,* unpublished dissertation, John Hopkins University, 1979.
21. H. J. Dupuy, A. Engel, B. Devine, J. Scanlon, and L. Querec, *Selected Symptoms of Psychological Distress, United States,* NCHS Vital and Health Statistics, Series 11, no. 37, 1970.
22. Bureau of Census, *Social Indicators, 1976,* GPO, Washington, D.C., 1977.
23. Bureau of Census, *Social Indicators III.* GPO, Washington, D.C., 1980.
24. P. Goldblatt and J. Fox, Household mortality from the OPCS longitudinal study, *Population Trends* **14:** 20 (1978).
25. Bureau of Labor Statistics, Department of Labor, *Consumer Expenditure Survey: Integrated Diary and Interview Survey Data, 1972–73,* Bulletin 1992. Department of Labor, Washington D.C., 1978.
26. S. Abraham, M. Carroll, C. Dresser, and C. Johnson, *Dietary Intake Findings, United States, 1971–1974,* NCHS Vital and Health Statistics, Series 11, no. 202, 1977.
27. J. N. Morris, Social inequalities undiminished, *Lancet* **1:**87 (1979).
28. S. G. Haynes, B. Dennis, and G. Williams, Socioeconomic status and nutrient intake: Results from the Lipid Research Clinic's Study, Food and Nutrition Poster Session, Annual Meeting of the American Public Health Association, Los Angeles, November, 1981.
29. National Center for Health Statistics, *Health Practices Among Adults: United States, 1977*[a], Advance Data, No. 64. November 4, 1980.

30. L. Harris and Associates, Inc., *Health Maintenance.* Pacific Mutual Life Insurance Company, Newport Beach, California, 1978.
31. L. Breslow and J. E. Enstrom, Persistence of health habits and their relationship to mortality, *Preventive Medicine* **9:**469 (1980).
32. C. S. Wilder, *Family Health Expenses, United States—July–December 1962,* NCHS Vital and Health Statistics, Series 10, no. 41, 1967.
33. Office of Health Resources Opportunity, Health Resources Administration, *Health Status of Minorities and Low-Income Groups,* DHEW Pub. HRA 79-627. GPO, Washington D.C., 1979.
34. A. J. Moss and M. H. Wilder, *Use of Selected Medical Procedures Associated with Preventive Care, United States, 1973,* NCHS Vital and Health Statistics, Series 10, no. 110, 1977.
35. G. S. Bonham and P. E. Leaverton, *Use Habits Among Adults of Cigarettes, Coffee, Aspirin, and Sleeping Pills, United States, 1976,* NCHS Vital and Health Statistics, Series 10, no. 131, 1979.
36. Bureau of Labor Statistics, U. S. Department of Labor, *Employment and Unemployment: 1980,* Special Labor Force Report 244, 1981.
37. G. Rose and M. G. Marmot, Social class and coronary heart disease, *Br. Heart J.***45:**13 (1981).
38. M. S. Backheimer, Demographic and job characteristics as variables in absence for illness, *Public Health Reports* **83:**1929 (1968).
39. Department of Health, Education and Welfare, *Smoking and Health,* PHS 79-50066. GPO, Washington, D.C. 1979.
40. Department of Health and Human Services, *The Health Consequences of Smoking for Women,* Office on Smoking and Health, Department of Health and Human Services, Washington, D.C., 1980.
41. D. Cahalan and I. H. Cisin, American drinking practices: Summary of findings from a national probability sample. *Quarterly J. Studies Alcohol* **29:**130, (1968).
42. A. G. Cummins, A. G. Shaper, M. Walker, and C. J. Wale, Smoking and drinking by middle-aged British men: Effects of social class and town of residence, *Br. Med. J.* **283:**1497 (1981).
43. H. King and F. B. Locke, American white Protestant clergy as a low-risk population for mortality research, *J. Natl. Cancer. Inst.* **65:**1115 (1980).
44. E. K. Taylor and A. C. Wolfe, Political behavior, in *A Degree and What Else,* (S. B. Whitbey, ed.) a report prepared for the Carnegie Commission on Higher Education, McGraw-Hill, New York, 1971.
45. E. M. Kitagawa, Social and economic differences in mortality in the United States, 1960, in *International Population Conference,* London, 1969, vol 2. The International Union for the Scientific Study of Population, Liege, Belgium, 1971.
46. A. M. Lilienfeld, The human fog: Cancer and cholesterol. *Am. J. Epidemiol.* **114:**1 (1981).
47. M. F. Kelty, Ethical concerns in behavior change, in *Proceedings of the National Heart and Lung Institute Working Conference on Health Behavior,* (S. M. Weiss, ed.) May 1975, Basye, Va., 1976.
48. K. M. Danchik, et al., *Highlights from Wave I of the National Survey of Personal Health Practices and Consequences: United States, 1979,* NCHS Vital and Health Statistics, Series 15, no. 1., Washington, D.C., 1981.

49. J. R. Hollingsworth, Inequality in levels of health in England and Wales, 1891–1971, *J. Health Social Behavior* **22:**268 (1981).
50. J. LeGrand, The distribution of public expenditure: The case of health care, *Economica* **45:**125 (1978).
51. A. J. Culyer, *Need and the National Health Service,* Martin Robertson, London, 1976.
52. N. Eberstadt, The Poor? Who Are They? *New York Times,* November 16, 1981.
53. Bureau of Census, *Social and Economic Characteristics of Americans During Midlife,* Current Population Reports, Special Studies, Series P-23, no. 111, 1980.
54. J. S. Siegel, *Demographic and Socioeconomic Aspects of Aging in the United States,* Current Population Reports, Special Studies, Series P-23. Bureau of Census, in press.

10 Drug Therapy as a Risk Factor for Senility

Norman W. Pedigo Jr.

Adverse drug reactions may induce the symptoms of senility, especially when nutritional deficiencies or sensory impairments coexist. This can lead to inappropriate or premature confinement of older persons to hospitals, nursing homes, or other institutions. Thus drug interactions become a risk factor associated with iatrogenic symptoms of senility.

Administering, monitoring, and evaluating drug therapy in the elderly is substantially more complex and more critical than similar therapy for most younger adults. Geriatric patients constitute a relatively heterogeneous group in terms of physiological function and pharmacological response. Elderly persons also suffer from multiple chronic diseases and generally take more medications, including both prescription drugs and over-the-counter remedies, than any other population group. In 1970, older patients, who constituted less than 10 per cent of the U.S. population, accounted for 22 per cent of the $11.2 billion spent on drugs (*1,2*). Hence, it is not surprising that the incidence of adverse drug reactions is significantly higher in patients over 70 years of age.

DRUG INTERACTIONS IN THE AGED

A summary of the interactions discussed here is presented in Table 10-1. Drug interactions occur when one drug's effect is modified by that of a second drug administered concurrently. Although some drug interactions benefit the patient and are intentionally prescribed, others are unexpected and potentially harmful. Various studies have noted a twofold to fivefold increase in the frequency of untoward drug interactions among geriatric patients (*3*). Factors such as polypharmacy, age-related alterations of drug reponse, the presence of multiple disease states, the pathophysiological status of important organ systems, and the nutritional status of the patient may contribute to this problem. Thus, drug-induced

Table 10-1. Adverse Drug Intereactions

Drug Class	Examples	Interactions with	Possible Adverse Effects
Alcohol	Wine, beer, liquors (also some OTC preparations, including cold remedies and mouthwashes)	All other CNS depressants: narcotics, sedative-hypnotics, antidepressants, antipsychotics, and antianxiety drugs	Synergistic CNS depression
		Aspirin	Increased gastric irritation and bleeding
		Guanethidine (Ismelin)	Greater risk of orthostatic hypotension
		Disulfiram (Antabuse)	Dypsnea, tachycardia, blurred vision, flushing, hypotension, nausea
		Oral hypoglycemic drugs	Enhanced hypoglycemia, "disulfiram" reaction, especially with chlorpropamide
Analgesics, narcotic	Morphine, codeine, meperidine (Demerol), pentazocine (Talwin)	All other CNS depressants	See alcohol
		Monoamine oxidase inhibitors	Enhanced CNS depression
		Anticholinergic drugs	Additive constipation and urinary retention
Analgesics, nonnarcotic	Aspirin	See alcohol	
		Coumarin anticoagulants, methotrexate, phenylbutazone, and oral hypoglycemic drugs	Displacement from plasma proteins by aspirin
		Heparin	Additive inhibition of blood clotting
		Probenecid (Benemid) and sulfinpyrazone (Anturane)	Inhibition of uricosuric action
		Sodium bicarbonate and other urinary alkalinizers	Increased urinary excretion of aspirin
		Cholestyramine (Questran)	Inhibition of aspirin absorption

	Indomethecin (Indocin)	Coumarin anticoagulants	Enhanced blood loss and further inhibition of blood clotting
		Corticosteroids	Increased GI ulceration
		Propranalol (Inderal)	Inhibition of antihypertensive effects
	Phenylbutazone (Butazolidin), oxyphenbutazone (Tandearil)	Coumarin anticoagulants	Inhibition of warfarin (Coumadin) metabolism, increased blood loss, additive anticoagulant effects, displacement from plasma proteins
		Oral hypoglycemics	Reduced elimination of sulfonylurea drugs, displacement of tolbutamide (Orinase) from plasma proteins
		See aspirin	
Antacids	Aluminum hydroxide, magnesium hydroxide (Milk of Magnesia), calcium carbonate, sodium bicarbonate, dihydroxyaluminum sodium carbonate (Rolaids); also Maalox, Pepto Bismol, Di-gel	Tetracyclines	Formation of insoluble complex and prevention of absorption of the antibiotic
		Phenothiazines	Inhibition of absorption
		See aspirin	Urinary alkalinizers
Antianxiety agents	Diazepam (Valium), chlordiazepoxide (Librium), flurazepam (Dalmane), meprobamate (Equanil, Miltown)	All other CNS depressants	See alcohol
		Levodopa (Dopar, Larodopa)	Possible decrease in levodopa's antiparkinson effect

Drug Class	Examples	Interactions with	Possible Adverse Effects
Anticholinergics	benztropine (Cogentin), trihexyphenidyl (Artane); also antipsychotics, tricyclic antidepressants, narcotics, antihistamines with atropine-like side effects	Amantadine (Symmetrel)	Enhanced atropine-like effects with confusion and hallucinations
		Levodopa (Dopar, Larodopa)	Decreased absorption of levodopa
		Antipsychotics	tardive dyskinesia (suggested)
Anticoagulants	Warfarin (Coumadin, bishydroxycoumarin (Dicumarol)	See nonnarcotic analgesics (aspirin, indomethacin, phenylbutazone, oxyphenbutazone)	
		Anabolic steroids (Dianabol, Anadrol)	Enhanced anticoagulant effects
		Oral hypoglycemic agents	Inhibition of tolbutamide (Orinase) and chlorpropamide (Diabinese) excretion, and displacement of warfarin from plasma proteins by tolbutamide
		Barbiturates, glutethimide (Doriden)	Induction of hepatic microsomal enzymes, increase in metabolism of coumarin anticoagulants
		Clofibrate (Atromid-S)	Displacement of warfarin from plasma proteins
		Thyroid preparations	Inhibition of anticoagulant effects of warfarin
		Cholestyramine (Questran)	Decreased absorption of coumarin anticoagulants
	heparin	See nonnarcotic analgesics (aspirin)	
		Intramuscular injections	Can cause hematomas

Antidepressants	Tricyclic: amitriptyline (Elavil), imipramine (Tofranil), desipramine (Pertofrane), doxepin (Sinequan)	Other CNS depressants	See alcohol
		See anticholinergics	
		Guanethidine (Ismelin)	Inhibition of antihypertensive effects of guanethidine by blocking its uptake into neurons
		Epinephrine (Adrenalin), norepinephrine (Levophed)	Enhanced pressor response to these drugs
	Monoamine oxidase inhibitors: pargyline (Eutonyl), tranyl-cypromine (Parnate), phenelzine (Nardil)	Other CNS depressants	See alcohol
		Foods and beverages containing tyramine (some wines, beers, cheeses, chocolate)	Enhanced pressor effects of norepine-phrine released by tyramine
		Indirect sympathomimetics, i.e., ephedrine (Neo-Synephrine), metaraminol (Aramine), phenylephrine and phenylpropa-nolamine found in many OTC preparations	Same as tyramine-containing foods
		Hypoglycemic agents	Enhanced and prolonged hypoglycemic response to insulin and sulfonylurea drugs
		See narcotic analgesics	
Antihypertensive	Propranalol (Inderal)	Other antihypertensives	Additive lowering of blood pressure
		Oral hypoglycemic agents and insulin	Enhanced hypoglycemic effects and severe reflex hypertension
		Barbiturates	May increase propranalol metabolism
		Epinephrine (Adrenalin)	Vasoconstriction without cardic stimulation (resulting in hypertension and bradycardia)
		Skeletal muscle relaxants	Enhanced neuromuscular blockade

Drug Class	Examples	Interactions with	Possible Adverse Effects
	Guanethidine (Ismelin)	See alcohol	
		See tricyclic antidepressants	
		Other antihypertensives	See propranalol
		Resperpine (Serpasil)	Excessive orthostatic hypotension, bradycardia, and mental depression
		Oral hypoglycemics	Enhanced hypoglycemia
		Norepinephrine (Levophed)	Enhanced pressor response
		Chlorpromazine (Thorazine)	Inhibition of guanethidine's antihypertensive effects
	Reserpine (Serpasil)	Other antihypertensives	See propranalol
		See guanethidine	
		Levodopa (Dopar, Larodopa)	Reduced effect of levodopa
		Cardiac glycosides	Increased risk of arrhythmias
		Monoamine oxidase inhibitors	Excitation and hypertension in patients on MAOI given reserpine
	Methyldopa (Aldomet)	Other antihypertensives	See propranalol
		Levodopa (Dopar, Larodopa)	Enhanced effects of each drug
	Clonidine (Catapres)	Other antihypertensives, especially propranalol	See propranalol
		Levodopa (Dopar, Larodopa)	Inhibition of levodopa's antiparkinson effects
Antimicrobials	penicillins (PenicillinV, Bicillin, Syncillin, Orbenin, Staphcillin, Polycillin)	Tetracyclines, chloramphenicol (Chloromycetin)	Possible impairment of the antibacterial effects of penicillin
		Sulfonamides	Inhibition of the GI absorption of oxacillin (Prostaphylin)

	tetracyclines (Aureomycin, Vibramycin, Tetracyn, Achromycin)	Any orally administered medication containing calcium, magnesium, or aluminum (see antacids)	Inhibition of tetracycline absorption
		Barbiturates	Possible enhancement of metabolism of doxycycline (Vibramycin)
		Methoxyflurane (Penthrane)	Possible combined renal toxicity
	aminoglycosides: gentamicin (Garamycin), streptomycin, neomycin (Neosporin)	Ethacrynic acid (Edecrin)	Combined ototoxicity
		Skeletal muscle relaxants	Respiratory arrest due to enhanced neuromuscular blockade
		Cephalosporins, amphotericin B (Fungizone), methoxyflurane (Penthrane)	Combined renal toxicity
Antipsychotics	Chlorpromazine(Thorazine), haloperidol (Haldol), prochloperazine (Compazine), trifluoperazine (Stelazine), thioridazine (Mellaril)	All other CNS depressants	See alcohol
		See anticholinergics	
		Other antihypertensive drugs	See propranalol
		Levodopa (Dopar, Larodopa)	Inhibited action of levodopa
Cardiac glycosides	digitalis, dioxin, digitoxin	Amphotericin B. (Fungizone) and potassium depleting diuretics, i.e., hydrochlorothiazide (HydroDiuril), furosemide (Lasix), chlorthalidone (Hygroton)	Hypokalemia leading to enhanced toxicity of cardiac glycosides, especially arrhythmias

Drug Class	Examples	Interactions with	Possible Adverse Effects
		Barbiturates	Possible increase in metabolism of cardiac glycosides
		Cholestyramine (Questran) and colestipol (Colestid)	Possible binding of cardiac glycosides and prevention of their GI absorption
		See reserpine	
Diuretics	Potassium-depleting diuretics: hydrochlorothiazide (HydroDiuril), chlorthiazide (Diuril), furosemide (Lasix) ethacrynic acid (Edecin), chlorthalidone (Hygroton)	See cardiac glycosides	
		Oral hypoglycemics	Thiazides elevate blood glucose and impair hypoglycemic activity
		Cholestyramine (Questran) and colestipol (Colestia)	Possible prevention of GI absorption of thiazid
		Lithium carbonate	Decreased excretion and enhanced toxicity of lithium
	Potassium-sparing diuretics: spirone-lactone (Aldactone), triamterene (Dyrenium)	Potassium chloride preparations or high-potassium diets	Hyperkalemia
Hyperlipidemia agents	Cholestyramine (Questran), colestipol (Colestid)	See cardiac glycosides, diuretics, anticoagulants, aspirin	Inhibition of GI absorption of many acidic drugs by cholestyramine and colestipol
		Coumarin anticoagulants	Inhibition of vitamin K absorption may enhance anticoagulant effects

Laxatives	Mineral oil, bisacodyl (Dulcolax), dioctyl sodium sulfosuccinate (Colace), phenophthalein (Ex-lax)	Antacids	Possible premature disintegration of enteric coating of bisacodyl tablets
		Many drugs	Possible inhibition of absorption due to reduced GI transit time
Oral Hypoglycemics	sulfonylureas: chlorpropamide (Diabinese), tolbutamide (Orinase), tolazamide (Tolinase), acetohexamide (Dymelor)	See alcohol See phenylbutazone See propranalol See coumarin anticoagulants See diuretics	
		Monoamine oxidase inhibitors	Enhanced hypoglycemic effects
Sedative hypnotics	Barbiturates:	All other CNS depressants	See alcohol
	phenobarbital, secobarbital (Seconal), pentobarbital (Nembutal)	See coumarin anticoagulants, cardiac glycosides, tetracyclines; also sulfonamide and corticosteroids	Barbiturates induce hepatic microsomal enzymes and enhance the metabolism of these and other drugs
	Chloral hydrate (Noctec),	All other CNS depressants	See alcohol
	glutethimide (Doriden), flurazepam (Dalmane)	Coumarin anticoagulants	Displaced from plasma proteins by chloral hydrate and increased elimination after glutethimide

mental confusion, irritability, nervousness, or insomnia should not be regarded as unavoidable symptoms of senility.

The frequency of drug interactions increases considerably with the number of drugs a patient is taking. It has been estimated that elderly patients institutionalized in nursing homes receive an average of six or seven different drugs daily (*3*). In addition, those over age 65 use a disproportionate amount of over-the-counter drugs, especially laxatives, antacids, analgesics, sleep aids, cold remedies, and vitamins. Thus, the two principal factors that contribute to polypharmacy in older persons are (1) the frequent presence of multiple, chronic diseases that necessitate use of a variety of therapeutic regimens and (2) age-related declines in physiological function for which the patient tries to compensate by using different drugs.

Therapeutic Perspectives

Before the various mechanisms of drug interactions are described, this subject must be put in proper perspective with regard to the needs of the geriatric patient. Multiple-drug therapy may be required to treat multiple, chronic diseases that afflict the elderly. In situations where adverse drug interactions are predicted, certain precautions can minimize the severity of such complications. In many cases, different drugs have similar therapeutic actions but do not interact dangerously. Adjusting the dosage for either or both interactive drugs and careful monitoring of the patient can also reduce the severity of adverse drug interactions. However, to achieve beneficial effects from combination drug therapy and to anticipate possible adverse drug interactions, the mechanism of action and pharmacokinetic profile of the drugs being administered must be understood.

Pharmacokinetic Interactions

Although drugs interact through many diverse mechanisms, such interactions may be generally classified as either pharmacokinetic or pharmacodynamic. Most pharmacokinetic interactions ultimately result in a change in the free (unbound) plasma concentration of a drug induced by the concurrent administration of another drug. Increasing the drug's free plasma concentration increases its availability at its site of action, tissue storage sites, and biotransformation and excretion sites. Hence, the drug's therapeutic and toxic effects are enhanced; however, the duration of action of most drugs is reduced. The opposite is true for drug interactions that decrease the free plasma concentration of a drug.

Pharmacokinetic interactions may result from induced alterations by one drug in the absorption, distribution, biotransformation, or excretion of another drug. Drug interactions that can modify the absorption of a drug include direct physical and chemical interactions and alteration of gastrointestinal contents or motility. An example of direct, physicochemical drug interaction is the precipitation of various acidic drugs (diazepam, secobarbital) by cholestyramine or colestipol. Drugs that increase or decrease gastrointestinal motility also affect transit time of other drugs in the gastrointestinal tract. People over 65 years of age use many drugs having anticholinergic properties, which may decrease gastrointestinal motility, as well as laxatives and cathartics, which decidedly increase gastrointestinal motility and significantly reduce transit time in the gastrointestinal tract.

Drug competition for binding sites on plasma proteins is a potential means of drug interaction in all patients, but it can be especially important in the elderly, whose concentration of plasma albumin may be decreased. In the elderly, different drugs compete for fewer sites and smaller doses of a competing drug are needed to displace another drug from plasma proteins.

Elderly patients also metabolize drugs more slowly than do younger adults, primarily because of a reduction in blood flow to the liver. Drugs that inhibit hepatic microsomal enzymes (such as coumarin anticoagulants, cimetidine, isoniazid, methylphenidate, oral antidiabetics, and some sulfonamides) may further reduce the rate of metabolism of a wide variety of psychoactive drugs. In contrast, chronic administration of some drugs (barbiturates, alcohol, meprobamate, glutethimide, or chlopromazine) induces microsomal enzymes, thus increasing their concentration in liver cells and thereby stimulating the metabolism of many drugs. Some current evidence suggests, however, that the degree of microsomal enzyme induction can be reduced in those over 70 years of age (*4*).

Severe drug interactions are also likely when one drug alters the renal excretion of another, especially in older persons whose renal function may be impaired and who may consequently eliminate drugs more slowly than do younger adults. Drugs that alter the pH of the urine can certainly affect the rate of elimination of weakly acidic or weakly basic drugs. The rate of urinary excretion of weak acids, such as diazepam and phenobarbital, will be considerably increased in basic urine and reduced in acidic urine. The opposite is true for weakly basic drugs, such as amphetamine, meperidine, or imipramine. Furthermore, any drugs that cause nephrotoxicity or decreases blood flow to the kidneys—already reduced in geriatric patients—would be expected to reduce the rate of elimination of many drugs.

Pharmacodynamic Interactions

Two drugs administered concurrently may have additive, potentiative, or antagonistic actions as a result of their interaction at the receptor level, that is, when their plasma concentrations are essentially unchanged. Possible mechanisms for such pharmacodynamic interactions include modification of a drug's access to its receptor, alterations in the number of receptors available, and changes in the concentration of intracellular mediators of drug-receptor coupling. A common mechanism of pharmacodynamic interaction occurs when pharmacological antagonists block specific receptors and inhibit the action of agonist drugs and endogenous substances. For example, the muscarinic antagonist atropine inhibits endogenously released acetylcholine, thereby reducing parasympathetic activity, and also blocks the pharmacological action of cholinergic agonists, such as bethanechol, pilocarpine, and neostigmine. Many drugs (neuroleptics, tricyclic antidepressants, antiparkinsonism drugs) with divergent therapeutic actions may have potentially additive anticholinergic or atropine-like side effects. This additive effect may be of particular importance in geriatric patients, where atropine-like side effects (such as dryness of the mouth, urinary retention, constipation, blurred vision, and increased intraocular pressure) may exacerbate similar problems associated with advanced age.

Another pharmacodynamic interaction that may be especially relevant in elderly patients occurs between the antihypertensive drug guanethidine and the tricyclic antidepressants (TCA), such as desipramine and amitriptyline. In a patient taking guanethidine and a TCA, the antihypertensive effects of guanethidine will be greatly diminished; the TCA prevents neuronal uptake of guanethidine and thus blocks that drug's access to its site of action at synaptic vesicles in the nerve terminal. In some elderly patients the efficacy of methyldopa may be similarly decreased if TCA drugs are administered concurrently.

Drugs that alter the concentration of endogenous hormones or intracellular mediators may also alter the pharmacological response of another concomitantly administered drug. One well-known drug interaction is that between monoamine oxidase inhibitors (MAOI), which inhibit the enzymatic degradation of biogenic amines, and indirect-acting sympathomimetics. Such an interaction could result in a hypertensive crisis. The prevalence of sympathomimetic drugs in over-the-counter medications and foods almost certainly precludes the use of MAOI drugs in elderly patients, except under the most rigidly controlled hospital settings.

A final example of a pharmacodynamic interaction is the synergistic CNS depression seen with many centrally active drugs. The adverse interactions between alcohol, narcotics, sedative-hypnotics, antipsychotics, antihistamines, and antianxiety drugs may produce excessive sedation, lethargy, mental confusion, orthostatic hypotension, dizziness, and headache. These symptoms may be exaggerated in geriatric patients, who are generally more sensitive to CNS depressants than are younger adults.

IATROGENIC RISK FACTORS FOR SENILITY

Drug-induced symptoms of memory impairment, insomnia, irritability, delirium, or depression are easily recognized in young adults but may be misinterpreted as irreversible signs of dementia or psychosis in geriatric patients. Factors contributing to the elderly's iatrogenic symptoms of senility include their high level of drug use, their increased sensitivity to psychoactive substances, and age-related alterations in the distribution, metabolism, and excretion of various drugs. Many medications commonly used in geriatrics have the potential to disrupt cognitive functions or to alter behavior and personality in older persons.

Sedative-Hypnotics

Persons over 70 years of age are often extremely sensitive to the sedative action of all CNS depressants, especially when two or more such drugs are used concurrently. This sensitivity could be due, in part, to reduced numbers of functioning neurons or to diminished cerebral blood flow (*5*). Distribution and elimination of sedative-hypnotic drugs, especially barbiturates, may also be altered in the elderly. Chronic use of these drugs can lead to apathy, confusion, insomnia, and diminished mental acuity, any of which might be inappropriately identified as a sign of senility in geriatric patients. In contrast, some elderly patients may show paradoxical excitement, anxiety, restlessness, hostility, and confusion in response to sedative-hypnotic drug therapy; such reactions could be misconstrued as psychotic behavior.

Barbiturates or glutethimide are often given to elderly patients who experience insomnia. These drugs may be useful as occasional hypnotics, but their long-term use is contraindicated because they may actually disturb natural sleep. Although insomnia is a frequent complaint among the elderly, the best remedies include alleviation of underlying causes (e.g., depression or pain) and nondrug therapy, such as enhancing comfort and encouraging flexible sleep patterns. The high risk of tolerance and addiction characteristic of barbiturates and glutethimide further limits their chronic use.

Antianxiety Drugs

Benzodiazapines, notably chlordiazepoxide (Librium), diazepam (Valium), and flurazepam (Dalmane), are used extensively by persons of all ages to relieve symptoms of anxiety, agitation, and insomnia. In one study of elderly patients treated for adverse drug reactions, diazepam was cited as the most commonly misused drug (*6*). Even relatively small doses of diazepam can cause stuporous sleep, sluggishness, drowsiness, impaired gait, and decreased memory and intellectual function in patients over 75 years old (*7*). Additionally, after taking flurazepam, geriatric patients frequently experience ataxia, confusion, and, possibly, hallucinations; symptoms may not appear for up to three weeks because of the drug's unusually long half-life in the elderly.

Many of the toxic CNS side effects associated with benzodiazapine therapy could be mistaken for symptoms of dementia or psychosis. Nevertheless, diazepam is more useful than barbiturates for treating acute anxiety or agitation in the elderly because its incidence or habituation and fatal overdose is lower (*8*). One should note, however, that few well-controlled clinical studies have been done to compare the effects, therapeutic and toxic, of benzodiazapines and barbiturate drugs in geriatric patients. The widespread use of neuroleptics for their tranquilizing effects in the elderly is, in many cases, inappropriate because these drugs have a high incidence of extrapyramidal side effects and may induce tardive dyskinesia.

Antidepressants

The two major classes of antidepressant drugs are monoamine oxidase inhibitors (MAOI) and tricyclic antidepressants (TCA). MAOI drugs are of limited value and should be used by geriatric patients only in a carefully controlled, institutional setting. These drugs have a high incidence of adverse interaction with many over-the-counter sympathomimetics and even some foods, and any interaction may result in a severe, perhaps fatal, hypertensive crisis (*9*). TCA drugs, either sedating (doxepin and amytriptyline) or nonsedating (desipramine and imipramine), are beneficial for treating endogenous depression, but their anticholinergic side effects and the induction of arrhythmias preclude their use in some older patients (*10,11*). These drugs are also contraindicted in patients taking guanethidine because TCAs block guanethidine's antihypertensive effects.

It has been suggested that, in the elderly, neuroleptic drugs (thiothixene) have a therapeutic efficacy equal to that of the TCAs, with a similar incidence of side effects (*12*). However, neuroleptics and TCAs should not be used concurrently because of their additive anticholinergic properties, which may include confusion and memory loss.

Neuroleptics

Antipsychotic drugs are potent CNS depressants that should be used only in those elderly patients who have chronic schizophrenic psychoses or recurring hallucinations. Use of these drugs for treatment of organic brain syndrome is questionable, and other, less toxic agents may be equally useful in acute cases of agitation, aggression, or violent reactions (*5*).

The incidence and severity of neuroleptic-induced side effects increase greatly for patients over 60 years old. Reportedly half of the elderly patients taking neuroleptic drugs experience extrapyramidal side effects (*13*). In addition, up to 40 per cent of geriatric patients taking phenothiazines may develop tardive dyskinesia (*9,14*). Older persons are also more sensitive to the sedative actions of these drugs, especially when other CNS depressants are coadministered. Other toxic effects of some antipsychotic drugs include orthostatic hypotension, irregular heart beat, and hyperthermia or hypothermia. Finally, many neuroleptics have atropine-like side effects or are given with anticholinergic drugs.

Other Drugs

Alcohol and narcotic drugs, such as morphine and meperidine, are CNS depressants that can produce sedation, ataxia, and confusion in the elderly. Alcohol use is a major source of adverse drug interactions in older patients and may produce a synergistic CNS depression with neuroleptics, antianxiety drugs, anesthetics, antidepressants, or narcotics. Chronic alcoholism is not uncommon in the elderly and may be a significant factor in the pathogenesis of organic brain diseases and dementia. Finally, alcoholic delerium may occur in some geriatric patients and could present symptoms similar to paranoid psychosis.

Electrolyte imbalances, especially hypokalemia, may accompany treatment with diuretics and can lead to anorexia, muscle weakness, and confusion. Metabolic abnormalities resulting from oral antidiabetics or insulin, thyroid preparations, and digitalis may also mimic symptoms of dementia or psychosis. Antihypertensive drugs, alone or through various drug interactions, may produce cerebral anoxia leading to confusion, disorientation, and fainting. Guanethidine and reserpine can also induce severe suicidal depression.

Because many elderly persons eat infrequent or poorly balanced meals, malnutrition is a common cause of psychotic or confused behavior. The excessive use of laxatives and cathartics may further impair the nutritional status by reducing the absorption of foods and by causing serious dehydration. Conversely, many drugs with anticholinergic side effects produce constipation and water retention, which may lead to loss of appetite. Use of appetite-suppressant drugs can also result in nutritional deficiencies.

Many over-the-counter drugs contain sympathomimetic agents that can induce cardiac arrhythmias, hypertension, CNS excitation, and, possibly, psychotic behavior. Nonprescription sleeping aids, antihistamines, and allergy pills all have atropine-like side effects that can be especially serious in geriatric patients. Misuse of social drugs, such as alcohol, caffeine, and nicotine, may also have serious consequences. Overuse of caffeine, for example, can lead to disruption of natural sleep, irritability, agitation, confusion, and aggressive behavior.

PHARMACOKINETIC RISK FACTORS

Pharmacokinetics refers to the absorption, distribution, biotransformation, and excretion of drugs. Many physiological changes associated with advanced age can alter the pharmacokinetics of various drugs. Such alterations of the pharmacokinetic profile of psychoactive substances undoubtedly contribute to the increased incidence of adverse drug reactions among geriatric patients.

Drug Absorption

Absorption of drugs, after oral administration, can be modified by age-related alterations in the physiology of the gastrointestinal tract. For example, secretion of gastric acids is often reduced in elderly patients and so the stomach becomes less acidic. This decreased acidity theoretically could reduce the rate of absorption of weakly acidic drugs, such as barbiturates and glutethimide, and increase the rate of absorption of weakly basic drugs, such as tricyclic antidepressants, narcotics, and phenothiazines. The decreased acidity of the stomach could also facilitate gastric emptying and thereby deliver drugs more rapidly to the small intestine. However, in many geriatric patients gastric emptying is somewhat delayed. Although the rate of drug absorption may vary in older persons, the absorption is nonetheless usually complete, perhaps due to a relative decrease in intestinal motility and the consequent increased drug transit time through the gastrointestinal tract.

The patient's age probably affects absorption of drugs administered intramuscularly or subcutaneously less than it does absorption of drugs given orally. However, blood flow in skin and skeletal muscles may be reduced in the elderly, and the rate of drug absorption from these sites may be somewhat slowed. The ultimate clinical significance of these pharmacokinetic variables remains unclear. However, one may generally assume complete absorption of most drugs in geriatric patients (*15*).

Drug Distribution

Several age-related factors can affect the degree of protein binding or tissue availability and hence the distribution of drugs. As the amount of plasma albumin decreases with age, the proportion of drug bound to plasma proteins is reduced. Different drugs competing for fewer plasma protein binding sites may result in more frequent instances of adverse drug interactions.

Older persons are generally smaller and lighter than young adults, and drug dosage must therefore be adjusted accordingly. With advanced age, also, the amount of body fat increases and muscle mass is generally reduced. Hence, highly lipophilic drugs, such as the barbiturates, may be concentrated in fatty tissues, possibly requiring higher initial doses of these drugs (*16*). Plasma volume, extracellular fluid volume, and total body water are also decreased with advanced age, but the clinical significance of such changes is unknown. In summary, initial and maintenance doses of many drugs should be reduced in the elderly to compensate for age-related decreases in body weight, plasma protein binding, plasma volume, and drug elimination.

Drug Metabolism

The two most important factors influencing drug metabolism by geriatric patients are the rate of blood flow to the liver and the concentration of hepatic drug-metabolizing enzymes, especially the microsomal (cytochrome P450) enzymes. Blood flow to the liver may be reduced by as much as 40 per cent in elderly persons, consequently slowing the rate of elimination of drugs metabolized by hepatic enzymes (*16*). Although definitive clinical evidence is lacking, the concentration of hepatic microsomal enzymes may decrease in later life, and the induction of these enzymes after chronic treatment with a drug like phenobarbital may be reduced. Because many drugs are metabolized by these microsomal enzymes, the possibilities of reduced rates of drug biotransformation in elderly patients, and therefore increased duration of action and drug accumulation, are important. Again, if the patient is over 65 years of age, a wise course would be to reduce the dose or frequency of administration of drugs that are extensively metabolized in the liver, especially if other signs of diminished hepatic function are present.

Drug Excretion

The kidneys are the most important route of elimination for most drugs and drug metabolites. In the elderly, alterations of renal function are critical in determining an individual patient's response to a particular therapeutic regimen. Age-related reductions in renal blood flow and in the number of viable renal cells often compromise the ability of the kidneys to excrete drugs. Impairment of renal excretion in the elderly can lead to higher-than-expected plasma levels of drugs. A lower rate of elimination of a drug increases its plasma half-life and therefore the time necessary to reach plateau drug levels during maintenance therapy. The half-life of a drug also defines the time necessary to reach new plateau levels after a change in dosage regimen or clearance rate of the drug and the time required to remove the drug from the body after discontinuation of therapy. These factors could partially account for the enhanced sensitivity of elderly patients to many psychoactive drugs and for their increased risk of adverse drug effects.

PHARMACODYNAMIC RISK FACTORS

The interaction between a drug and its receptor and the resultant physiological response is termed pharmacodynamics. Elderly patients may show increased or decreased sensitivity to drugs at the receptor, tissue, organ, or systems levels. A great number of patients over 70 years of age respond to low doses of drug (hyperreactivity) or require high doses to produce therapeutic effects (hyporeactivity). In addition, elderly patients may show atypical responses to certain drugs, such as the paradoxical excitement and insomnia after administration of sedative-hypnotics. Quantitative differences in drug action are common in older patients and may reflect more diverse drug sensitivities of the geriatric population as compared with younger adults. This observation should not be surprising, since the aging process is highly individual.

Many elderly patients are highly sensitive to certain medications. This sensitivity is especially true for CNS depressants, which can cause excessive sedation, drowsiness, behavioral disturbances, memory impairment, respiratory depression, and orthostatic hypotension.

Receptor Alterations

Although the effects of aging on pharmacokinetic parameters are only poorly understood, still less is known about pharmacodynamic functions in the elderly. At least part of the different response to certain drugs could be due to age-related changes in drug-receptor interactions. Receptors are generally membrane-bound proteins or intracellular enzymes, which are often the site of action of endogenous substances as well as therapeutic drugs. Receptor alterations with aging could therefore underlie a wide variety of physiological changes and could also substantially modify a person's response to a drug. Basic research in laboratory animals shows that many hormone receptors decline in number during senescence, whereas others decrease early in adulthood and a few actually increase with advanced age (*17*).

Receptors exist not as static entities but in a state of dynamic equilibrium. The number of hormone receptors fluctuates in response to different concentrations of endogenous substances, to chronic drug therapy, or to pathological states. The phenomenon of denervation supersensitivity (i.e., a compensatory increase in the number of receptors after the loss of specific neurons) is well documented. Similarly, chronic treatment with receptor-blocking drugs may also result in up-regulation (due to an increased number) of receptors. Such a mechanism may be the cause of tardive dyskinesia, an iatrogenic disease characterized by persistent involuntary choreiform movements. Tardive dyskinesia is most often observed in older psychiatric patients who have received long-term, continuous neuroleptic therapy. Neuroleptic (antipsychotic) drugs are known to block central dopaminergic receptors, and tardive dyskinesia may be related to a kind of "pharmacological" denervation supersensitivity that induces an increase in the number of dopaminergic receptors.

The opposite process can also occur, i.e., receptor desensitization or down-regulation. Recent speculation from experimental studies with animals relates desensitization of central beta-adrenergic receptors to the mechanism of antidepressant drug action (*18*). Chronic treatment (two to three weeks) with tricyclic antidepressants or monoamine oxidase inhibitors may significantly decrease the density of beta-receptors in rat brain (*19*). The time course of this drug action corresponds closely to the length of treatment required in humans for therapeutic (antidepressant) effects. One crucial question that remains is whether or not the elderly retain the same ability to regulate receptors as to do younger adults.

Drug Tolerance

An important aspect of pharmacological tolerance may be the dynamic adjustment of hormone receptors during chronic drug therapy. Pharmacological tolerance occurs when previous exposure to a particular drug, or to a closely related drug, diminishes the original pharmacological response, despite the equivalency of drug concentrations at the site of action. This phenomenon may result from a drug-induced decrease in receptor sites or from changes in intracellular messengers, such as cyclic-3′,5′-adenosine monophoshate (cyclic AMP), which may moderate receptor-mediated events. Pharmacological tolerance is common after the chronic administration of CNS depressants and often occurs simultaneously with the development of physical dependence on narcotics, barbiturates, and ethanol. Because drug abuse, especially alcoholism, is not uncommon in the elderly, these issues are certainly relevant to geriatric therapy. To speculate that the increased sensitivity of older patients to CNS depressants could relate to an impaired ability to develop pharmacological tolerance to these drugs is also interesting.

In summary, possible pharmacodynamic changes that could account for the different effects of certain drugs in the elderly include fewer hormonal receptors or age-related alterations in receptor regulation. Such variables could affect the response of a geriatric patient both acutely and after chronic drug therapy. Current evidence further suggests that many pathological and iatrogenic diseases of aging, including tardive dyskinesia, depression, and schizophrenia, may involve hormonal receptor dysfunctions.

CONCLUSIONS

Elderly patients are at risk for developing iatrogenic symptoms of dementia, depression, delirium, and psychoses. Numerous risk factors account for their enhanced vulnerability to drug-induced manifestations of senescence. The elderly take a disproportionately high number of prescription and over-the-counter medications and many also misuse social drugs such as alcohol, caffeine, and nicotine. Many of these drugs are psychoactive substances or induce significant CNS side effects. Furthermore, the incidence of idiosyncratic drug reactions may be higher for geriatric patients, possibly reflecting the increased heterogeneity of this population.

Drugs used by the elderly may differ in their onset or duration of action and intensity of effect compared with their actions in younger adults. Age-related changes in the absorption, distribution, metabolism, and excretion of drugs, pharmacodynamic alterations in older persons, and an increased frequency of drug interactions are additional risk factors common to geriatric patients.

Clinicians have the imperative, therefore, to evaluate carefully each patient over 60 years of age for iatrogenic symptoms of senescence. Also crucial is that drug side effects not be treated by prescribing other, more potent psychoactive medications. The health professional's enhanced awareness of such risk factors will ultimately improve the quality of life for persons in their later years.

REFERENCES

1. D. L. Rabin, Use of medicine: A review of prescribed and nonprescribed medicine use. Department of Health, Education and Welfare, USPHS Pub. 73-3012, Washington, D.C., 1972.
2. I. Burnside, *Nursing and the Aged.* McGraw-Hill, New York, 1981.
3. A. M. Kratz, B. Schwaninger, R. A. Henry, and D. A. Hussar, *Geriatric Drug Interactions,* Sandoz, Morris Plains, N.J., 1979.
4. M.R.P. Hall, Use of drugs in elderly patients, *NY State J. Med.* **75:**67 (1975).
5. W. D. Poe and D. A. Holloway, *Drugs and the Aged.* McGraw-Hill, New York, 1980.
6. D. M. Peterson and C. W. Thomas, Acute drug reactions among the elderly, *J. Gerontol.* **30:**552 (1975).
7. C. Salzman, R. I. Shader, J. Harmatz and L. Robertson, Psychopharmacologic investigations in elderly volunteers: Effect of diazepam in males, *J. Am. Geriat. Soc.* **23:**451 (1975).
8. M. Raskin and C. E. Eisdorfer, Psychopharmacology of the aged, in *Drug Treatment of Mental Disorders* (L. L. Simpson, ed.). Raven Press, New York, 1976.
9. L. J. Epstein, Anxiolytics, antidepressants, and neuroleptics in the treatment of geriatric patients, in *Psychopharmacology: A Generation of Progress* (M. A. Lipton, A. DiMascio, and K. F. Killam, eds.). Raven Press, New York, 1978.
10. R. D. Friedel, Effects of age on the pharmacology of tricyclic antidepressants, in *Age and the Pharmacology of Psychoactive Drugs* (A. Raskin, D. S. Robinson, and J. Levine, eds.). Elsevier/North Holland, New York, 1981.
11. J. J. Schildkraut, Tricyclic antidepressants and the aging process: Discussion of selected pharmacodynamic and pharmacokinetic issues, in *Age and the Pharmacology of Psychoactive Drugs* (A. Raskin, D. S. Robinson and J. Levine, eds.). Elsevier/North Holland, New York, 1981.
12. A. Kiev, Double-blind comparison of thiothixene and protriptyline in psychotic depression, *Dis. Nerv. Syst.* **33:**811 (1972).
13. F. J. Ayd, A survey of drug-induced extrapyramidal reactions, *J. Am. Med. Assoc.* **175:**1054 (1961).
14. G. E. Crane, Tardive dyskinesia in patients treated with major neuoleptics: A review of the literature, *Am. J. Psychiat.* **124:**40 (1968).
15. B. L. Beattie and E. M. Sellers, Psychoactive drug use in the elderly: The pharmacokinetics, *Psychosomatics* **20:**474 (1979).
16. Sandoz, Inc., *Physiologic and Pharmacokinetic Factors as Determinants of Drug Response in the Elderly,* Sandoz, Morris Plaines, N.J., 1980.
17. G. S. Roth, Hormone receptor changes during adulthood and senescence: Significance for aging research, *Fed. Proc.* **38:**1910 (1979).
18. P. L. Mobley and F. Sulser, Down-regulation of central noradrenegic receptor systems by antidepressant therapies: Biochemical and clinical aspects, in

Antidepressants: Neurochemical, Behavioral and Clinical Perspectives (S. J. Enna, J. B. Malick and E. Richardson eds.). Raven Press, New York, 1981.

19. A. Maggi, D. C. U'Prichard and S. J. Enna, Differential effects of antidepressant treatment on brain monoaminergic receptors, *Eur. J. Pharmacol.* **61:**91, 1980.

11 Cardiovascular Changes as Risk Factors For Senility

Seymour Eisenberg

Age-associated changes in the cardiovascular system may play a major role in diminishing vigor and limiting life-span. However, knowledge is insufficient to assess accurately the relative contribution of various organ systems to this general decremental process. As the biology of aging is currently understood, no single system determines one's ultimate frailty or vigor. On the other hand, the cardiovascular system—clearly not designated for infinite survival—deserves some consideration for this critical limiting role. Alterations in collagen, elastin, and muscle in this system lead to physical changes that ultimately compromise its basic oxygen delivering function. These changes in physical characteristics and performance conceivably could be crucial to the entire aging process, that is, to the multisystem decrements that culminate in death.

In this chapter I consider these age-associated changes in the cardiovascular system as possible risk factors in the senility complex. Wherever possible, true aging changes must be distinguished from disease-caused changes and deconditioning changes. Furthermore, disease-caused changes that are directly responsible for symptoms and signs similar to those of senility, as well as diseases that are almost certain to result in premature death, must be excluded from consideration as risk factors. Both in a sense constitute negative risk factors for future senility changes by precluding vigor and/or survival.

As noted in Chapter 1, true aging changes, by definition, are universal, irreversible, and not preventable. Disease changes are common in the elderly but are not universal; they are preventable, treatable, and to some extent reversible. Aging changes probably in some way enable most of these diseases to develop. The ultimate deconditioning changes are those resulting from a completely sedentary existence; theoretically, every decrement could be prevented by a full conditioning program. Any conclusions regarding reversibility drawn from the results of an activity program in someone over 70 are of dubious credibility because of the possibility that some of the deconditioning changes might not be reversible after several years of sedentariness.

The changes in performance that occur in the elderly, but still competing, marathon runner would be pure aging changes—in the absence of undetected disease. Thus, her or his times would slowly increase and oxygen uptake and maximum attainable heart rate slowly decrease with time. Deconditioning changes could be measured if by chance this marathon runner had an identical twin who had ceased running 20 years earlier. The sedentary twin would have undergone both aging changes and deconditioning changes that could be compared with the pure aging changes of the active twin. No such data exist, but longitudinal comparisons may permit a reasonable assessment of these two types of change.

AGING CHANGES

Anatomical

Aging causes notable anatomical changes in the cardiovascular system. These changes, adequately detailed in gerontological texts and monographs (*1,2*), are only summarized here.

Studies of heart size and of heart muscle, collagen, and elastic tissue in autopsy material from persons who died in old age have yielded conflicting data (*3*). In humans only the results of cross-sectional studies are available, and the prevailing opinion is that the heart gradually enlarges decade by decade until age 90, with perhaps some atrophy thereafter. Whether this gradual hypertrophy is a true aging change, and thus universal and not preventable, remains unknown. If some of the ongoing noninvasive studies show that a substantial number of persons have no evidence of hypertrophy in the absence of illness or atrophy, cardiomegaly will not qualify as an aging correlate. On the other hand, it may be a true aging change that permits ventricular emptying. Ultimately this survival mechanism could become a survival-limiting factor by virtue of decreasing compliance—a "musclebound" syndrome of the ventricular myocardium. Longitudinal noninvasive studies of moderately active elderly persons who are normotensive and disease-free may answer the important question of whether cardiomegaly is an aging correlate and a factor in survival.

Minor changes in the amount of cardiac collagen and elastic tissue have been reported (*4*), but no specific qualitative changes have been identified consistently. Further histological and histochemical studies are needed in as much as the increasing stiffness of the heart could be due to molecular changes in collagen, changes that occur throughout the body, particularly affecting the supportive system but including the heart and vascular tree as well. The collagen/elastin ratio is increased in the aorta of elderly humans, with fragmentation and loss of resiliency of the elastin. The number of cross-linkages of collagen increases, altering compliance and, perhaps, the diffusion of nutrients (*1*). The aorta stiffens and dilates—or dilates and stiffens. Dilatation in the disease-free aorta is apparently complete by age 60. The increase in capacitance of the thoracic aorta mitigates changes in wall tension with the volume increments of left ventricular systole. The aorta becomes increasingly less extendible, so that further volume increments induce large pressure changes. With these changes, aortic impedance, originally lessened by the changes in capacitance, gradually increases, ultimately assuming increasing importance after maximal dilatation has occurred. The flow characteristics of blood gradually change, from almost continuous flow through an elastic system to a more pulsatile, intermittent flow through a semirigid one. In summary, the great vessels gradually change in size, relative content of elastic tissue, and distensibility. These are unambiguous aging changes, although whether they are progressive after age 60 (when, in the absence of disease, dilatation apparently is maximal) remains unclear.

Performance

Distinct changes in performance characterize the aging cardiovascular system. Most of these are true aging changes, perhaps as pure as any identified in the intact organism. However, the possibility of independent disease change cannot be excluded, particularly in humans. The changes in performance of the heart and great vessels are essentially what might be predicted from the anatomical changes outlined above, i.e., the stiffened, probably hypertrophied left ventricle pumping against the increasing resistance of the inelastic aorta and vascular tree.

Changes in the vascular tree could represent the primary event. Exposure of the aorta and its major tributaries to what is deemed to be "normal" intravascular pressure ultimately results in fragmentation of the elastic tissue. The elastic fiber microfibrils change in appearance, become disarrayed, and lose their resilience, so that ultimately they contribute only rigid structural support. Beyond the point of maximal aortic dilatation, volume increments result in an abrupt increase in wall tension because further dilatation of the collagen-dominated vessel wall requires a significant increase in pressure. This dilatation/pressure relationship perhaps explains the gradual increase in systolic/pressure and the slight decline in diastolic pressure usually observed in aging persons. Vascular resistance also increases beyond the major tributaries, the precise cause of which is not clear. The net effect, however, is apparent in the decreased perfusion of most organs and tissues. There are putative changes in smaller vessels and perhaps in oxygen diffusion across aging capillaries, but the evidence for these changes is not completely convincing.

Changes in the heart are also predictable from the anatomical changes noted. There is little question that the aging heart, although adequate at rest almost until the end of life, is incapable of responding adequately to the basic characteristic of the aging process—having to cope with stress.

That the left ventricle likely becomes hypertrophied and measurably stiffened has been noted. Although enzymatic changes may occur that could exert a negative influence on contractility, these are inconsistent and likely of only marginal importance. Moreover, it is possible that the increasing oxygen requirements of the stiffening, often hypertrophied cardiac muscle exceed the capabilities of its own oxygen delivery system, the coronary circulation.

Weisfeldt (*2*) summarized the important factors contributing to the aging changes in left ventricular function:

1. Prolonged ventricular contraction, particularly of the relaxation phase
2. Decreased sympathetic responsiveness in terms of chronotropic, inotropic, and vasodilating capacity
3. Decreased left ventricular diastolic compliance
4. Increased impedance to left ventricular ejection

The following are among the more important measurable changes in cardiovascular performance with age (the more important changes are those elicited by exertion; few changes in function are actually perceivable at rest).

Peripheral vascular resistance gradually increases (Figure 11-1) (*5*).

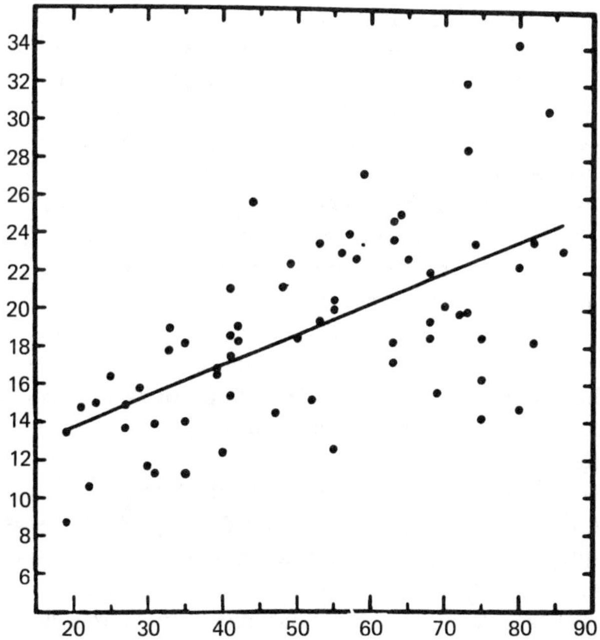

Figure 11-1. Estimated total peripheral resistance of the great circulation in relation to surface area versus age.

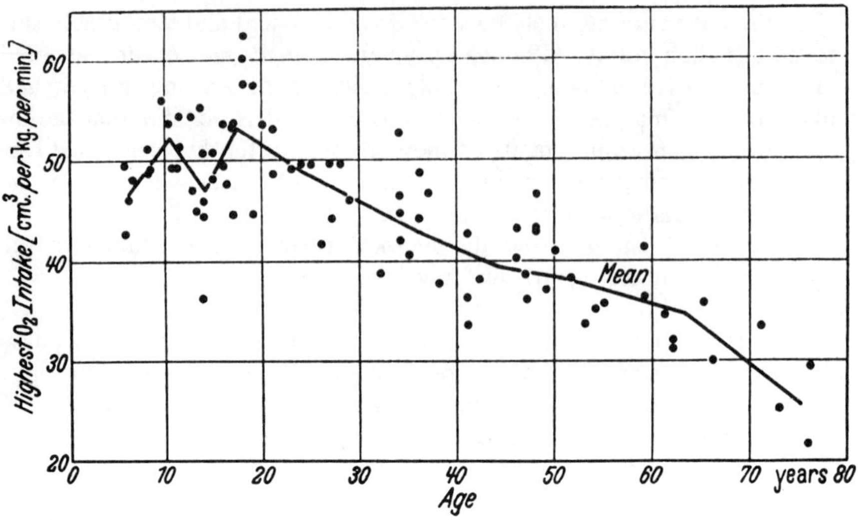

Figure 11-2. The highest oxygen intake attained during maximal work.

The decline in maximum oxygen uptake (Figure 11-2) (*6*), mostly a reflection of the limited increase in cardiac output with stress, is unrelenting. At rest, when factors such as change in body mass and composition are considered, cardiac output in the elderly is probably unchanged from that of normal younger adults; with exercise, output—both heart rate and stroke volume—increases only slightly. Resting heart rate may decrease slightly with age. Of greater importance, however, is the well-documented decrease in maximum heart rate (Figure 11-3) (*6*). The cause of this decrease is not clear; anatomical changes in the SA node have been suggested, but Weisfeldt (*2*) and others (*7*) seem to favor the view that the decrease is a failure of chronotropic response to the adrenergic surge that is itself one of the more important components of the response to maximal exercise. Some investigators have suggested that the decrease might represent a decline in either number or responsiveness of beta-adrenergic receptors; however, Abrass and colleagues (*8*) were unable to demonstrate a decrease in number or affinity of these receptors and suggested that the decreased responsiveness is at a level other than the receptor site.

Systole is prolonged, primarily as a result of delayed relaxation (Figure 11-4 shows the typical alteration in contraction) (*2*). Relaxation is likely an active process related to the rate of uptake of calcium ion by the sarcoplasmic reticulum. Animal studies have suggested that physical conditioning may accelerate the rate of relaxation; if this is true, it might account for some of the improvement in cardiac performance after a vigorous exercise program. This delay in relaxation likely plays a key role in limiting maximum cardiac output and the intolerance of elderly sub-

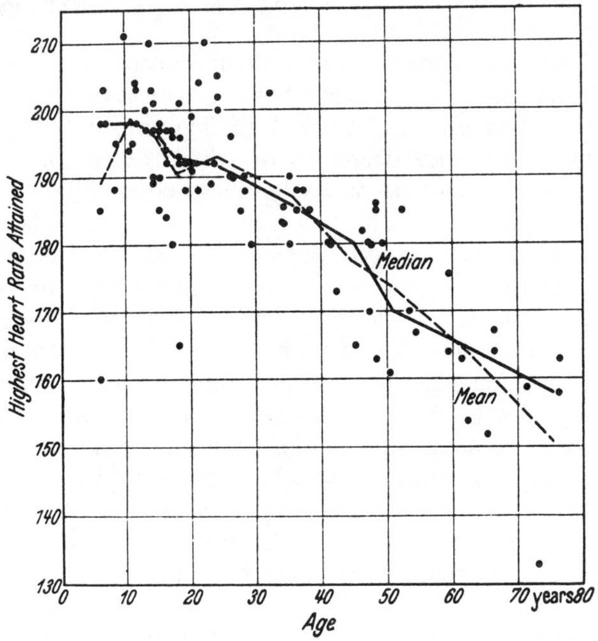

Figure 11-3. Highest heart rate attained during maximal work.

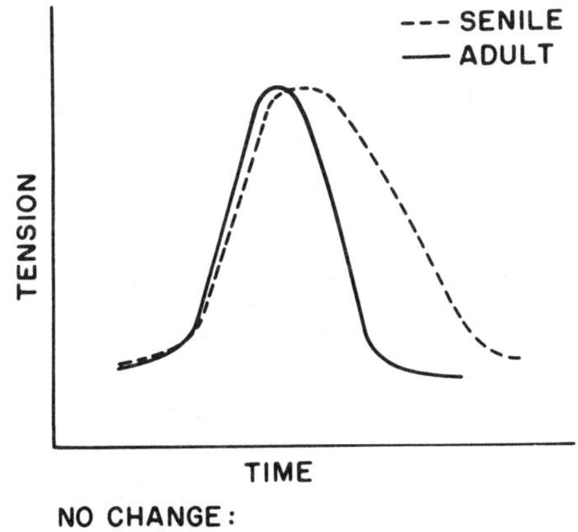

Figure 11-4. Representative isometric contraction at the length at which contractile tension is maximal in muscle from adult and senile rats. The major age changes are in the time course of the twitch rather than in the rate of tension development or the maximal tension developed.

jects to ectopic tachycardias. Under circumstances of a considerable increase in heart rate, systole might begin before relaxation is complete, resulting in an increse in left ventricular filling pressure.

Myocardial compliance decreases or stiffness increases. This altered physical property cannot be precisely measured in the intact human. A stiffness index has been established from actual versus calculated alterations in pressure/volume relationships. The exact cause of the change in compliance is not clear. As noted, only minor quantitative changes are seen in left ventricular collagen, and the amounts of elastic tissue in the ventricle are insufficient for such changes to be a contributory factor. Qualitative aging changes in collagen probably occur throughout the body, perhaps due to alterations in molecular composition or configuration. One other possible explanation is the previously mentioned hypertrophy of ventricular muscle. Models of hypertrophy, such as that induced by aortic binding, display many of the qualities of the aging ventricle; this fact at least raises the possibility that the problem is ultimately the thickened muscle, which is in turn a result of outflow impedance.

Left ventricular ejection fraction declines with exercise. According to Port and associates (*9*), the ejection fraction, a common measure of left ventricular function that is determined by noninvasive radionuclide study, is normal at rest in elderly subjects but diminishes consistently after exercise (Figure 11-5). This decrease in ejection fraction with exer-

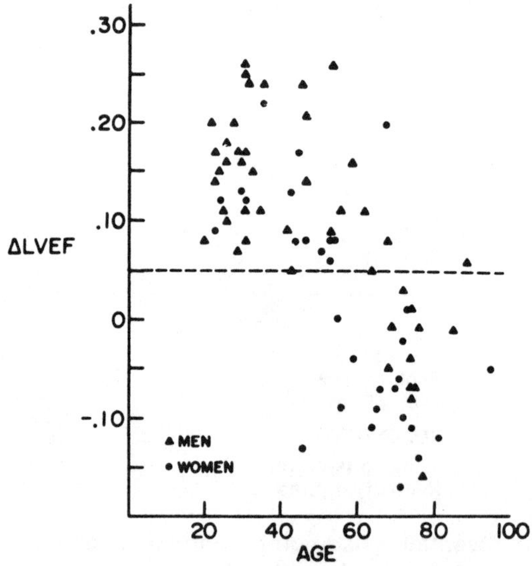

Figure 11-5. Change in left ventricular ejection plotted against age for 46 men and 31 women. Dashed line indicates an ejection fraction change of 0.05, the normal minimum increase.

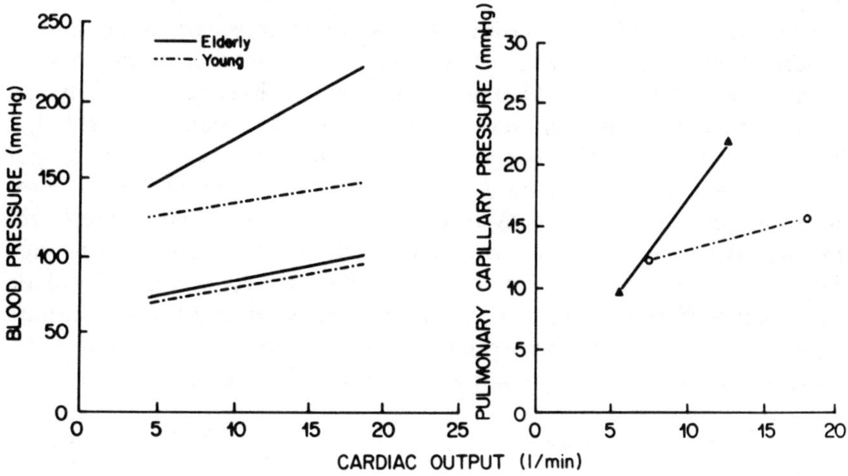

Figure 11-6. Age-related changes in blood pressure and pulmonary capillary pressure with exercise.

cise is also characteristic of the response of the ischemic heart, and Weisfeldt has suggested that Port's sharp separation of young and old was likely due to the presence of undetected coronary artery disease in the "normal" elderly. This unresolved issue is important inasmuch as ejection fraction decline with exercise could provide an aging marker with predictive capability.

In an important study, Granath et al. (*10*) performed cardiac catheterizations in apparently healthy human subjects and clearly showed that, during exercise in elderly subjects, the pulmonary capillary wedge pressure rises sharply to heights usually associated with diminished lung compliance and dyspnea (Figure 11-6). In young adults, exercise induces only a slight rise in pressure. The implications of this reaction to stress are far-reaching—from a pivotal role in the aging process to at least a marker of impending physical limitation and enfeeblement. What remains unknown is whether or not this pressure rise is a progressive, relentless change that, carried to the ultimate, is incompatible with life. If this hypothesis is true, myocardial stiffness could be among the important factors establishing an individual's maximum life-span.

With advancing age, the systolic blood pressure tends to increase gradually and diastolic pressure either remains the same or declines. Therefore, any increase would have to be considered a disease change rather than an aging change.

Deconditioning

The inadequacy of long-term, longitudinal comparisons of sedentary versus active persons, the fact that general performance and cardiovascular function improve with exercise programs, and a considerable amount of anecdotal material available all confuse the question of deconditioning changes. The data are conflicting, but inactivity is likely associated with a decline in cardiac function. Such deconditioning has been documented in two studies (*11,12*). Whether actual cardiac performance in elderly subjects can be enhanced by an exercise program is disputed. Several programs are currently addressing this issue, and perhaps answers are forthcoming. Aggressive exercise programs begun early and continued may delay some aging changes. Nonetheless, the gradual decline in athletic performance indicates that basic aging changes, such as stiffness, continue inexorably; perhaps the performers are basically preventing ony true deconditioning changes and merely delaying disease changes.

Disease

Heart disease is the leading cause of death in elderly patients; coronary artery disease, congestive heart failure, and hypertension and its consequences are widespread. The impact of underlying disease of the cardiovascular system on the process of senility is difficult to assess without including everything inimical to cardiac performance and organ perfusion. Statistics for hypertension are available, and this disorder has clearly been associated with an increased incidence of stroke (*13*), dementia, renal failure, congestive heart failure, and death (*14*). Coronary artery disease impairs contractility and general cardiac function, limits activity, and promotes deconditioning by virtue of activity-limiting pain. It also induces serious arrhythmias and conduction disorders. Many of these problems may be indolent and do not sharply curtail life-span. In this way symptomatic but nonlethal coronary artery disease could limit life-style, activity, and the general pursuit of maximum conditioning. One might conclude that a 70-year-old person with angina pectoris, although seemingly in symbiosis with a nonprogressive disorder, will be much more likely to develop senility changes at 85 than a person without these problems who is active, vigorous, and involved in the pursuit of a full life.

Risk Factors for Cardiovascular Disease

The risk factors that in themselves substantially increase the chances of having or later developing serious cardiovascular disease are pertinent to these considerations. Data adduced by the Framingham study (*15*) clearly indicated that high-risk men 65 years of age have about an 82 per cent chance of developing cardiovascular disease in eight years, contrasted with 9 per cent chance in low-risk men in the same age group. It would seem appropriate, therefore, to examine these putative cardiovascular risk factors that, by their very presence, could have important implications regarding the future well-being and vigor of those just entering the elderly group. We also assess the significance of perceived but asymptomatic cardiovascular abnormalities to establish some idea of their potential for affecting future vigor—might they, in fact, predispose to senility without inducing the overt clinical disorders usually associated with their presence? The risk factors to be considered are family history, hypertension, diabetes mellitus, abnormal serum lipids, smoking, and obesity. The cardiac abnormalities to be considered are ectopic rhythms, conduction disorders, and seemingly insignificant heart murmurs.

Family History The conventional wisdom is that a positive family history ceases to be an important risk factor for cardiovascular disease in persons over 65 years of age. The decrease in importance of genetic influences may be more apparent than real inasmuch as the frequency of cardiovascular events in the elderly tend to overwhelm the detectable importance of any isolated factor. A more important question would be whether a negative family history for cardiovascular disease exerts a permissive effect on longevity and vigor, or, stated differently, whether the descendants of vigorous elderly persons without cardiovascular disease tend to remain vigorous and relatively free of cardiovascular disease. The influence of environmental, dietary and other factors complicate the development of such a concept.

Diabetes Mellitus In this extremely common disorder in the elderly, unambiguous cardiovascular complications are almost the rule. The most common associated problem is obliterative peripheral vascular disease with its potential for severe disability; in addition, the incidence of associated cardiovascular and cerebrovascular events is remarkably increased in all persons with intermittent claudication (*15*), whether or not they have diabetes. The frequency of these serious associated disorders does not auger well for sustained vigor once carbohydrate intolerance supervenes.

Alterations in Serum Lipids Persons with serious lipid disorders do not tend to survive to become candidates for senility. Those with moderate disorders, such as heterozygote familial hypercholesterolemics, may, with good management and good fortune, survive to a fairly advanced age. Their potential for cardiovascular disease and ultimate debility and senility is extremely high.

Obesity The usual victim of the senility complex is frail and poorly nourished, so that obesity might be perceived as a negative risk factor. On the other hand, it could be argued that obese persons do not survive; moreover, there is a tendency toward weight loss with advancing age. Up to a point, this weight loss could be beneficial were it to consist mostly of adipose tissue; ultimately, however, there is a loss of muscle mass, which likely plays an important role in the genesis of the asthenia of senility.

Smoking By the age of 65 or 70, proving that cigarette smoking plays an important role in atherogenesis would be difficult. Smoking would be more important as an acute, precipitating factor in cerebral and cardiovascular events and could further compromise blood flow and increase the likelihood of gangrene in extremeties where blood supply is precarious.

Previous Cardiovascular Events Previous cardiovascular or cerebrovascular events, even though there has been apparently complete functional recovery, increase the likelihood of subsequent events. Thus, myocardial infarction, arrhythmias, stroke, and transient ischemic attacks constitute unambiguous risk factors for future disabling problems and senility. The person with repeated small strokes is particularly likely to develop a syndrome not unlike senility, although it should not be subsumed under this rubric. Even in the absence of subsequent events, impairment from the original injury may assume increasing importance as compensatory mechanisms become less efficient with advancing age.

Hypertension There is little question that sustained, poorly controlled hypertension constitutes the most important cardiovascular risk factor—if strokes are included with cardiovascular disease—and, by the same token, protracted low levels of blood pressure impute relative freedom from these illnesses. Some clinicians support the view that mild hypertension is essential for adequate organ perfusion, particularly that of the brain, but clear evidence of this concept has not been shown. Perhaps abrupt lowering of blood pressure does not permit prompt activation of counter-regulatory mechanisms, however inefficient, but this ineffectiveness does not imply benefit from higher levels of blood pressure. There is controversy regarding this issue.

Conduction Disturbances and Arrhythmias The widespread use of cardiac pacemakers and the introduction of better-tolerated and more effective antiarrhythmic agents have decidely affected survival; however, the net effect on protracting vigor is uncertain. The proper use of these treatments does tend to reverse the debilitating manifestations of the immediate problem, many of which might simulte the senility syndrome. In a certain sense, though, what they may be doing is permitting the survival of persons whose lives three decades earlier would likely have been shortened, so that survival of the moderately impaired person is now possible. If the bradycardia or heart block is due to isolated disease of the conduction system and if the arrhythmia is not a reflection of underlying diffuse heart disease, proper management can represent an antisenility intervention. On the other hand, if the conduction and rhythm disorders reflect more widespread myocardial disease, chances for future senility are enhanced. Use of these treatments in the elderly is not questioned; all patients should be considered candidates for the benefits of modern therapeutic interventions. It is evident though that, as a rule, conduction abnormalities, severe bradycardia, and recurrent arrhythmias decrease the likelihood of sustained vigor.

Valvular Heart Disease Valvular heart disease of sufficient severity to cause congestive heart failure leads to protracted disability and premature death; surgical correction may delay death and attenuate symptoms. A common problem, however, is the seemingly "innocent" systolic murmur and the presence of valvular deformity of insufficient severity to induce overt heart failure or to warrant surgery. The possibility exits that under such circumstances hemodynamic alterations may be present that are inimical to protracted vigor and that, by their long-term but nonlethal effects, are conducive to the development of the senility complex. This conduciveness is both conjectural and hypothetical; many vigorous octogenarians with calcific disease of the aortic valve have no manifestations of senility. These are perhaps the favored ones, the survivors. The more important and more difficult problem is to predict the future course of mild-to-moderate abnormalities perceived at age 65. There is always the possibility of progressively worsening valvular obstruction or insufficiency to a degree consistent with survival but not full vigor and, ultimately, overt congestive heart failure. It is difficult to distinguish between the ominous and the benign at this point.

In summary, it is perhaps best simply to accept the fact that age-associated decrements in cardiac performance and organ perfusion do occur for a variety (and likely a combination) of reasons and then try to establish these changes as harbingers of impending senility. One could argue that the decrease in organ perfusion is causal rather than simply an effect of decreased metabolic requirement and that organs actually suffer from slowly progressive ischemia. The opposing view is that diminishing intrinsic organ function mandates redistribution of blood flow by autoregulatory mechanisms so that perfusion/function ratios are maintained, i.e., the atrophic limb or organ requires less blood. To define a primary role for diminished cardiovascular performance and ischemia, decreased venous oxygen levels, or a greater arteriovenous (AV) oxygen difference would at some point prevail. Blood flow is the reciprocal of the AV difference if metabolism remains constant during the measurement interval. If flow is diminished, increased oxygen extraction occurs and venous oxygen levels decrease. Such observations would have to be done longitudinally, with samples drawn during a protracted period. Nonetheless, the critical ischemic period might be missed, and thus such a hypothesis is extremely difficult to prove.

DISCUSSION

The effects of aging on the cardiovascular system should raise for consideration the distinct possibility that herein may lie an explanation for much of the physical decline and frailty associated with aging. The question at issue, however, is whether or not age-associated changes perceived in still-vigorous persons constitute reasonable risk factors for senility at a later date. Severe disease, in that it is a cause of premature death, is a negative senility risk factor; although manifestations of disease may mimic senility and cause premature frailty, these would not constitute risk factors as the term is conventionally used, meaning to bode future impairment.

A useful purpose would be served by identifying the changes and diseases that might best be used as physiological age markers and predictors of impending senility—assuming avoidance of premature death from other causes. If a person is relatively free of cardiovascular disease and shows only minimal aging changes with stress, perhaps it can be predicted that he or she is destined for prolonged mental and physical vigor if malignant neoplasm, pneumonia, or trauma does not supervene.

The prime candidate for survival with vigor would be a "young elderly" person with low normal blood pressure; having no cardiomegaly, murmurs, or vascular bruits; and showing a normal electrocardiogram. Post-exercise ejection fraction would equal or exceed the resting value, and the person would be able to achieve a heart rate exceeding that predicted for his or her age without evidence of ischemia. Maximum oxygen uptake would be that predicted for a 55-year-old or younger person. Muscle mass would be well maintained. Such a person would have many positive health habits—a vigorous exercise program, no smoking, only modest alcohol consumption, a well-balanced diet, adequate sleep, and absence of obesity. All of these are negative risk factors and are conducive to prolonged vigor. The converse of each finding would constitute a senility risk factor.

No studies have yet compared large numbers of these two extremes of the cardiovascular risk and performance spectrum. Therefore, no incontrovertible evidence exists that duration of vigor—or onset of frailty—can be so predicted. There are dramatic differences in survival between groups according to the number of positive health habits (Figure 11-7) (*16*). Extrapolation from premature death to early disability and frailty necessitates that one assume that lethal events are likely to be preceded by a period of compromised performance.

Particular attention has been given here to distinctions between true aging changes, disease changes, and deconditioning changes. Because our quest for eternal life is obviously fruitless, the next highest goal is retention of as much vigor as possible for the maximum time—about 110 years. Conceivably, everyone has his or her own maximum life-span, probably genetically controlled. One group of siblings may be programed for 110 years, another for 92 years. Death before either time would be premature for those persons, likely the result of disease or trauma, possibly by deconditioning and negative health habits. Were these latter two factors successfully thwarted by the appropriate measures, one could then remain vigorous until aging changes develop to a point incompatible with life. Freis (*17*) has suggested the same possibilities for future generations of

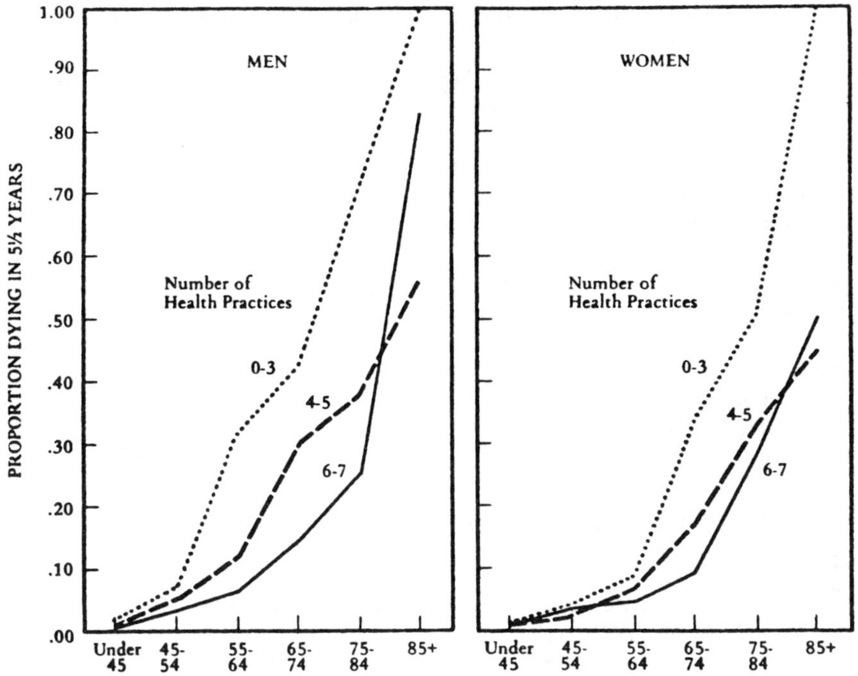

Figure 11-7. Age-specific mortality rates in a study population of men and women, in relation to number of health practices. The death rates are notably lower in both men and women with six or seven favorable health practices.

elderly, although he did not stress the role of the cardiovascular system. These considerations are highly speculative and are contingent on the hypothesis that the cardiovascular system plays a central role either in maintaining vigor or in permitting frailty. That those who are least impaired or unimpaired will function better in the future than those who are moderately impaired seems a reasonable assumption, and such persons in turn should fare better than those whose stress-elicited impairments are more overt. Measurements of degree of failure to respond to stress might provide predictive data for a senility/antisenility profile.

REFERENCES

1. I. Rossman, *Clinical Geriatrics*. Lippincott, Philadelphia, 1979.
2. M. L. Weisfeldt, *The Aging Heart*. Raven Press, New York, 1980.
3. G. M. Hutchins, Structure of the aging heart, in *The Aging Heart,* (M. L. Weisfeldt, ed.). Raven Press, New York, 1979.
4. D. E. Oken and R. J. Boucek, Quantitation of collagen in human myocardium, *Circulation Res.* **5**:357 (1957).
5. M. Landowne, M. Brandfonbrenner, and N. W. Shock, The relation of age

to certain measures of performance of the heart and the circulation, *Circulation* **12:**567 (1955).

6. S. Robinson, Experimental studies of physical fitness in relation to age, in *Zeitschrift fur die Physiologie der menschen bei Arbeit und Sport.* Verlag Von Julius Springer, Berlin, 1939.
7. F.C.P. Yin, G. S. Raizes, T. Guarnieri, H. A. Spurgeon, E. G. Lakatta, K. J. Fortuin, and M. L. Weisfeldt, Age-associated decrease in ventricular response to haemodynamic stress during beta-adrenergic blockade, *Br. Heart J.* **40:**1349 (1978).
8. I. B. Abrass, J. L. Davis, and P. J. Scarpace, Isoproterenol responsiveness and myocardial β-adrenergic receptors in young and old rats, *J. Gerontology* **37:**156 (1982).
9. S. Port, F. R. Cobb, R. E. Coleman, and R. H. Jones, Effect of age on the response of the left ventricular ejection fraction to exercise, *N. Engl. J. Med.* **303:**1133 (1980).
10. A. Granath, B. Jonsson, and T. Strandell, Circulation in healthy old men studied by right-heart catheterization at rest and during exercise in supine and sitting positions, in *Medicine and Sport: Physical Activity and Aging* (D. Brunner and E. Jokl, eds.). University Park Press, Baltimore, Md., 1970.
11. B. Saltin, G. Blomqvist, J. H. Mitchell, R. L. Johnson, K. Wildenthal, and C. B. Chapman, Response to exercise after bed rest and after training, *Circulation* **27/28** (suppl.7):1 (1968).
12. H. L. Taylor, A. Henschel, J. Brozek, and A. Keys, Effects of bed rest on cardiovascular function and work performance, *J. App. Physiol.* **2:**223 (1949).
13. R. B. Shekelle, A. M. Ostfeld, and H. L. Klawans, Hypertension and risk of stroke in an elderly population, *Stroke* **5:**71 (1974).
14. W. B. Kannel, Some lessons in cardiovascular epidemiology from Framingham, *Am. J. Cardiol,* **37:**269 (1976).
15. C. N. Peabody, W. B. Kannel, and P. M. McNamara, Intermittent claudication: Surgical significance, *Arch. Surg.* **109:**693 (1974).
16. N. B. Belloc, Relationship of health practices and mortality, *Prev. Med.* **2:**67 (1973).
17. J. F. Freis, Aging, natural death, and the compression of morbidity, *N. Engl. J. Med.* **303:**130 (1980).

12 Physical Activity and Aging

Alfredo Lopez-S

Use legs and have legs.
Proverbs 20:29

Interest in the influence of exercise on aging is as old as the history of medicine. Plato in his *Dialogue* quotes Socrates as asking the question, "And is not bodily habit spoiled by rest and illness, but preserved for a long time by motion and exercise?"

Hippocrates advanced the concept that aging is caused by a decrease in "body heat," which is generated and maintained by food and air. He further stated that food and exercise work together to produce health. This concept was further developed by Galen, who compared the production of heat from food to combustion outside the body and described aging as a change in body humors that causes dryness and coldness.

Avicenna's *Canon of Medicine* is considered the first textbook of medicine. It is also the first book containing instructions for the care of old people, including exercise, which it recommends be individualized: "The factors to consider in regard to exercise in old age are the various bodily statuses of different people, the sequels likely to arise from their ailments, and their previous habit as regards exercise."

Maimonides said that death occurs when air is prevented from entering the lungs. The body, like a burning lamp, needs not only fuel (that is, food) but also air. Thus, absense of air brings death, in the same way a lamp is extinguished.

The concept of the need for appropriate nutrient supply via the cardiovascular system to maintain life is still valid today. Physicians through the ages, and investigators in more recent times, have been impressed with the apparent decline in physical fitness with age and its improvement with exercise. Elderly persons seem to show the characteristics of younger subjects who are physically unfit. Skinner (*1*) has shown that some of the circulatory system changes that occur with training and chronic physical activity are opposite those seen with aging. Much of the work relating exercise, or lack of it, to aging is concerned with determining functional capacity of the respiratory and circulatory systems and the response of these systems to exercise (Chapter 13).

Knowing how exercise affects life-span could be useful in our understanding of the basic nature of the aging process. In this regard, two major points need clarification: whether lack of exercise shortens life-span or, alternatively, whether exercise increases life-span. No direct effect of exercise on aging would necessarily be implied by either point. For example, inactivity could result in reduced work capacity and diminished cardiorespiratory function, which would adversely affect all body functions. In such circumstances, exercise would only counteract the adverse effects of inactivity in the same way antibiotics prolong average life-span shortened by infection. No one would defend the thesis that antibiotics are involved in the basic mechanism of prolonging life.

If the effect of exercise on aging is merely to reduce the mortality risk imposed by inactivity, then exercise most likely tends to increase average life-span but has no effect on maximum life-span. If exercise can affect the basic mechanism of aging, however, then it would increase maximum life-span.

Another alternative is that exercise may exert its effect on aging-related chronic disorders (such as coronary heart disease and cancer). Although these disorders should be considered distinct from physiological aging, they seem to accelerate the last steps of aging, and apparently they can also be modulated through exercise. For these reasons, studies of the effect of exercise on these conditions could provide information on the mechanism of aging.

EXPERIMENTAL EVIDENCE

Review of the literature clarifies what is known about the effects of exercise on aging in both animals and humans.

Animal Studies

The findings from McCay's classical and impressive experiments (Chapter 13) on life-span prolongation remain unexplained at the basic level. Whether findings in captive laboratory animals apply to free-living populations of animals (or to humans) is arguable. Comfort (*2*) suggested that the ability of many animals species to reach old age is largely a function of domestication, and, in domestication, important changes occur not only in diet but also in exercise. Ross and Lustbader (*3*) studied dietary practices and growth responses as predictors of longevity in rats and concluded that body weight variables relate more closely to life-span than do dietary variables. By implication, exercise, which is an important variable affecting weight, could in this way relate to life-span.

Although Slonaker in 1912 (*4*) reported that rats allowed to exercise had shorter life-spans than control animals, more recent studies show a general trend toward increased life-span in animals that exercise regularly. Retzlaff et al. (*5*) showed that controlled early exercise increased the mean life-span of both male and female rats.

Many reports on the relationship between exercise and aging have considered the implications of such factors as serum lipid levels and obesity, but many of these reports are controversial, contradictory and, on the whole, inconclusive. However, some findings from these studies seem especially pertinent to the process of aging. For example, Edington et al. (*6*) showed that, when undergoing forced treadmill exercise, animals that began exercise at an early age had higher survival rates than those that began at a late age. They also showed that, above a certain "threshold age," beginning an exercise program at a late age may be disadvantageous not only for rat survival rate but also for rat longevity (*7*).

In a series of experiments on animals involving voluntary exercise, Goodrick showed that this type of exercise increases mean longevity in hybrid male mice (*8*) and in both male and female rats (*9*); he also found that growth duration related positively to longevity but growth rate related negatively. Observed changes in growth rates and growth duration associated with exercised rats agree with the data obtained by McCay et al. (*10,11*) on restricted animals.

The reports just cited can be important to our understanding of the effect of exercise on the mechanism of aging. For example, in his experiments with mice, Goodrick showed that exercising animals had prolonged life-span, lower peak body weight, and increased metabolic rate. Storer (*12*) reported a direct relationship between oxygen consumption (metabolism) and life-span in mice. More recently, Sacher and Duffy (*13*) reported a positive correlation between life-span and a longevity factor dependent on the partition of energy between the phasic metabolism of activity and the metabolism of continuous maintenance. A relationship between the factors that regulate basic metabolism and aging is further suggested by the experiments of Leto et al.(*14*), who showed that mice whose life-spans were increased by a low-protein diet had an increased oxygen consumption relative to that of shorter-life-span controls.

Human Studies

There is no conclusive evidence that physical activity alters the rate of aging in humans. Nonetheless, enough evidence is available to justify further investigation toward defining the role of exercise in longevity. This evidence has been derived from several major lines of investigation: populations reported to have high proportions of older citizens, the longevity characteristics of athletes, the relationship between exercise and physical fitness, and the relationship between exercise and health/longevity in the general population:

1. Only two things have been found to be common among the Villacambia, Alkasiansan, and Hunza—peoples reported to have high proportios of very old citizens—vigorous physical activity and long-lived ancestors (Chapter 1).
2. Several investigators have tried to evaluate the relationship between athletics and longevity. The available information can be summarized as follows:
   a. "Brute" exercise seems to have a deleterious effect on life-span, whereas endurance exercise, as in sports, seems to lengthen life-span (*15*), with higher survival rates for track and field participants, followed by baseball players, boxers, and football players.
   b. Continued exercise in later years seems to have an important effect on lengthening the life-span of former athletes (*15*). Saltin et al. (*16*) showed the effect of three weeks of bed rest in young, well-conditioned men: cardiac output decreased by 26 per cent and ventilatory capacity by 30 per cent. These changes are equivalent to the reported decreases in functions in normal persons during 30 years. These findings are important in light of findings that, until very recently, only 10 per cent of previously physically active married men aged 23 to 30 continued with regular activity (*17*).
   c. There is apparently a correlation between exercise and somatotype. Endomesomorphic athletes seem to have a shorter life-span than ectomorphic ones, following the trend observed in the general population (*18,19*).
   d. Exercise affects other factors known to relate to longevity, such as obesity, smoking, blood pressure, and other lifestyle risk factors.
   e. In humans as in animals, it has been observed that, for exercise to have an effect on longevity or on longevity-related health factors, the exercise must reach certain thresholds that may relate to the person's fitness (*21*).
   f. Exercise has been shown to increase the basal metabolic rate (BMR), which remains elevated 15 hours after heavy exercise ends (*22*). We have also observed an increase in BMR in young males participating for seven weeks in a program of four daily 30-minute sessions of intense physical exercise per week (Figure 12-1). These findings are of interest in view of animal experiments (*22*) showing a correlation between prolongation of life-span by diet restriction or exercise with BMR.
3. In the general population the findings of Belloc et al. showed a strong negative relationship between physical health and age (*23*) and a positive relationship (*24*) between physical activity and health. They concluded that a correlation exists between physical health and human longevity.

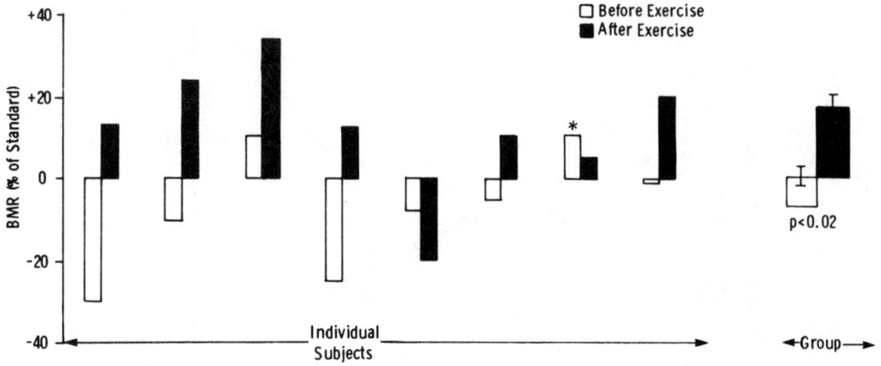

Figure 12-1. Effect of seven weeks of exercise on BMR. Participant indicated by the asterisk became sick two days before the second determination of BMR.

This protective effect of exercise on longevity may be the result of exercise's effect on the cardiorespiratory system and ultimately on the functional capacity of the whole organism at the cellular level.

RECENT OBSERVATIONS

The current popularity of exercise may be one of the reasons for the observed decrease in total and cardiovascular mortality, and increased life expectancy, observed in the United States since 1968 (Figures 12-2 and

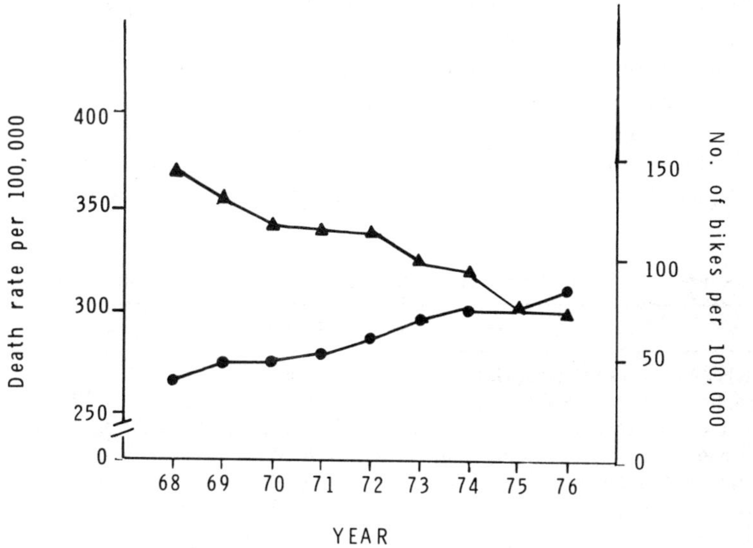

Figure 12-2. Age-adjusted cardiovascular mortality versus number of bicycles in use (United States).

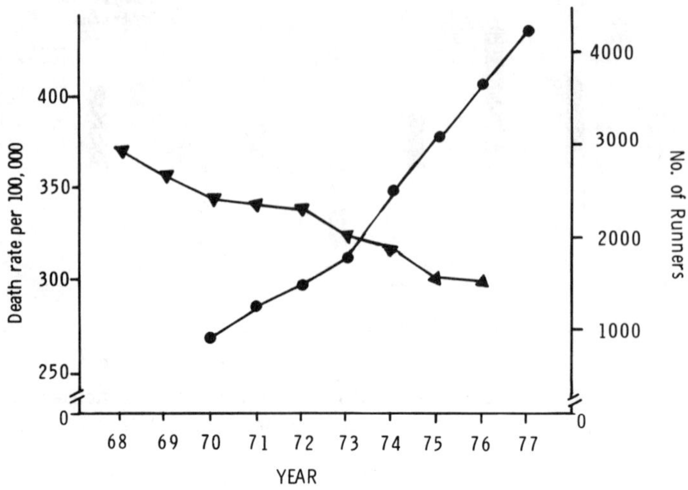

Figure 12-3. Age-adjusted cardiovascular mortality versus number of runners in 3000-m races (United States).

12-3). Other putative factors are improved treatment of high blood pressure and advances in antiarrhythmic therapy. That physical activity can be a contributory factor can be explained by its effect on known factors in coronary heart disease.

I found that exercise significantly affected some coronary risk factors (Table 12-1) in young persons participating in a program for four daily 30-minute sessions of intense (5 to 7 metabolic units) physical exercise each week. This exercise effect is of such magnitude that it can decidedly lower the risk of coronary heart disease. For example, using the table issued by the American Heart Association (*25*) to calculate coronary heart disease risk (Table 12-2), one observes that, in the hypothetical case of a 40-year-old man with a high initial risk of 7.3 per cent (according to the values of the different risk factors), the total

Table 12-1. Effect of Exercise on Some Coronary Heart Disease Risk Factors

Factor	Control	Trained
Systolic blood pressure (mm Hg)	113 ± 6	116 ±6
Diastolic blood pressure (mm Hg)	78 ± 2b	67 ±5[a]
Pulse rate (per minute)	74.9 ±9.2	68.5 ±6.1[a]
Maximum oxygen uptake (ml/kg/min)	36.8 ±5.4	43.0 ±4.0[a]
Cholesterol (mg/100 ml)	169 ±22	159 ±22
Triglycerides (mg/100 ml)	110 ±36	97 ± 36[a]
Blood Sugar		
Fasting (mg/100 ml)	75 ± 6	67 ±3[a]
2 hours postprandial (mg/100 ml)	64.7 ± 13.0	54 ± 5[a]

[a]Statistically significant.

Table 12-2. Potential Change in Risk with Exercise in High-Risk 40-Year-Old Men

Factor	Initial Level	Exercise[a] Hypothetical Effect on Each Factor			
Systolic blood pressure (mm)	165	150	150	150	150
Cholesterol (mg/dl)	260	—	235	235	235
Glucose (mg/dl)	125	—	—	115	115
Smoking	(+)	—	—	—	(−)
Risk (%)	7.3[b]	6.1	4.6	3.6	2.3

[a]Level of exertion increases from left to right.

[b]Framingham men aged 40 had an average probability of 2.3 per cent for developing coronary heart disease in six years.

risk can be reduced to normal as the effect of chronic exercise reduces each risk factor.

In general, levels of serum cholesterol and triglycerides are higher and those of high-density lipoprotein (HDL) are lower in older persons and in those with reduced activity. We (*26*) have shown that exercise increases HDL levels, and other have reported an inverse correlation between HDL levels and life-span. Recently Matter et al. (*27*) showed that older persons with higher maximum aerobic capacity tend to maintain HDL profiles comparable to those of younger persons; furthermore, older persons have been found to improve their maximum oxygen intake by proper exercise. These reports suggest that exercise, through its effect on HDL concentrations, could affect longevity. Other reports propose that HDL levels relate inversely to incidence of coronary heart disease (*28*) and directly to longevity (*29*).

Rose and Cohen (*30*) analyzed the predictive value of exercise for longevity in 500 men. They found that, as a predictor of longevity, off-the-job physical activity, was more important than on-the-job activity. They reported that "those in occupations requiring lighter physical exertion, but who indulged in heavier off-the-job physical activity, lived an average of 3.8 years longer than those who were light in both on and off-the-job activity." In addition, those who were heavy in off-the-job exercise during their 20s and 40s lived 4.6 years longer that those who engaged in light off-the-job exercise during both periods.

Even more dramatic was the fact that those who engaged in heavy exercise during both periods lived 7.1 years longer than those who changed from heavy exercise in their 20s to light exercise in their 40s. Rose and Cohen also described that, among 69 specific variables, off-the-job activity during the third and fifth decades of life ranked ninth (Table 12-3). Only one other variable (smoking) that can be affected at will ranked higher than exercise.

Table 12-3. Partial Correlation Between Selected Variables Related to Age More Strongly than to Exercise

Variable	Partial
Younger appearance ⩾40	0.47
Mean illnesses	−0.46
Smoking <40	−0.29
Smoking ⩾40	−0.28
Worried	−0.28
Younger appearance ⩽40	0.25
Urban vs. rural residence	0.24
Occupational level	0.24
Off-job activity, 40–49	0.23
Off-job activity, mean	0.18
Activity compared with that of others	0.17
On-job activity, mean	0.08

After Rose and Cohen (*30*).

CONCLUSION

Enough suggestive evidence from animal and human experiments exists to have reasonable assurance that physical activity begun early in life and continued during adulthood at a level sufficient to maintain proper body composition and cardiorespiratory fitness can significantly delay age-related diseases and/or extend average life exepectancy.

The evidence reviewed in this chapter, along with the information given in Chapter 13, suggests that exercise has the potential for decreasing death risk in high-risk persons, for prolonging life-span, and for delaying the onset of infirmity.

REFERENCES

1. J. S. Skinner, The cardiovascular system with aging and exercise, *Medicine and Sports* (D. Brunner and E. Jocker, eds.) vol. 4. Karger, New York, 1970.
2. A. Comfort, Basic research in gerontology, *Gerontologia* **16:**48 (1970).
3. M. H. Ross and E. Lustbader, Dietary practices and growth responses as predictors of longevity, *Nature* **262:**548 (1976).
4. J. R. Slonaker, The normal activity of the albino rat from birth to natural death, its rate of growth and the duration of life, *J. Animal Behavior* **2:**20 (1912).
5. E. Retzlaff, J. Fontaine, and W. Furnta, Effect of daily exercise on life-span of albino rats, *Geriatrics* **21:**171 (1966).
6. D.E.E.W. Edington, A. C. Cosman and W. B. McCafferty, Exercise and longevity: Evidence for a threshold age. **27:**341 (1972).
7. W. B. McCafferty and D. W. Edington, Skeletal muscle and organ weights of aged and trained male rats, *Gerontology* **20:**44 (1974).
8. C. L. Goodrick, The effect of exercise on longevity and behavior of hybrid mice which differ in coat color, *J. Gerontologia* **29:**129 (1974).

9. C.H.L. Goodrick, Effects of long-term voluntary wheel exercise on male and female Wistar rats: I. Longevity, body weight, as metabolic ratio, *Gerontology* **26:**22 (1980).
10. C. M. McCay, M. F. Crowell, and L. A. Maynard, The effect of retarded growth upon the length of life-span and upon the ultimate body size, *J. Nutrition* **10:**63 (1935).
11. C. M. McCay, E. Pope, and W. Lansford, Experimental prolongation of the life-span, *Bull. N.Y. Acad. Med.* **32:**91 (1956).
12. J. B. Storer, Relationship of life-span to brain weight, body weight and metabolic rates among inbred mouse strains, *Exp. Gerontol.* **2:**173 (1967).
13. G. A. Sacher, and P. H. Duffy, Genetic relation of life-span to metabolic rate of inbred mouse strains and their hybrids, *Fed. Proc.* **38**(2):184 (1979).
14. S. Leto, G. C. Kokkonen, and C. H. Barrows, Dietary protein, life-span and physiological variable in female mice, *J. Gerontol.* **31:**149 (1976).
15. M. J. Karkoken, Sports and longevity, *Advances in Cardiology* **18:**243 (1976).
16. B. Saltin, G. Blomqvist, J. H. Mitchell, R. L. Johnson, K. Wildenthal, and C. B. Chapman, *Response to Exercise After Bed Rest and After Training.* Monograph No. 23, American Heart Association, New York, 1968.
17. D.D.H. Howell, and H. L. Denis, The meaning of physical fitness: Introduction. *Proc. R. Soc. Med.* **62:**1155 (1969).
18. P. A. Polednak, Longevity and cariovascular mortality among former college athletes, *Circulation* **46:**649 (1972).
19. G. A. Sheehan, Longevity of athletes, *Am Heart J.* **86:**425 (1973).
20. A. R. Behnke, and J. H. Willmore, Alteration in body composition with physical activity, in *Evaluation and Regulation of Body Build and Composition,* (A. R. Behnke and J. H. Willmore, eds.) Prentice-Hall, Englewood cliffs, N.J., 1974.
21. J. L. Hodgson, and E. R. Burgkurk, Physical fitness and age with emphasis on cardiovascular function in the elderly, *J. Am. Geriat. Soc.* **25:**385 (1977).
22. H. T. Edwards, A. Thorndike Jr., and D. B. Dill, The energy requirements in strenuous muscular exercise, *N. Engl. J. Med.* **213:**532 (1935).
23. N. B. Belloc, L. Breslow, and J. Hochstim, Measurement of physical health in a general population survey, *Am. J. Epidemiol.* **93:**328 (1971).
24. N. B. Belloc, and L. Breslow, Relationship of physical health status and health practices, *Preventive Med.* **1:**409 (1972).
25. American Heart Association, Estimating risk of coronary heart disease in daily practice, in *Coronary Risk Handbook.* New York, 1973.
26. A. Lopez-S, R. Vial, L. Balart, and G. Arroyave, Effect of exercise and physical fitness on serum lipids and lipoproteins, *Atherosclerosis* **20:**1 (1974).
27. S. Matter, B. A. Stanford, and A. Weltman, Age, diet, maximal aerobic capacity and serum lipids, *J. Gerontol.* **35:**532 (1980).
28. W. P. Castelli, J. T. Royle, T. Gordon, C. G. Hames, M. C. Hjortland, S. B. Hulley, A. Kagan, and W. J. Zukel, HDL-cholesterol and other lipids in coronary heart disease: The cooperative lipoprotein phenotyping study, *Circulation* **55:**767 (1977).
29. C.J. Glueck, P. Gartside, R. W. Fallat, J. Sielski, and P. M. Steiner, Longevity syndrome: Familial hypobeta- and familial hyperalphalipoproteinemia, *J. Lab. Clin. Med.* **88:**941 (1976).
30. C. L. Rose, and M. E. Cohen, Relative importance of physical activity for longevity, *Ann N.Y. Acad. Sciences.* **301:**671 (1977).

13 Physical Inactivity: A Risk Factor for Senility

Herbert A. deVries

The non-disease-related biological causes of the aging process have been the central focus of investigations in our laboratory since its inception 16 years ago. Our frame of reference is the physiology of exercise, and we have been particularly interested in testing the hypothesis that a considerable part of the functional losses reported in the medical and gerontological literature as the effects of aging may be more closely related to a lifestyle that grows more sedentary with age. Indeed, from present knowledge, a reinvestigation of the effect of aging on all physiological variables likely to be altered by physical conditioning or, more important, by its inverse, "detraining," seems necessary.

Until recently, the prevailing opinions on physiology of exercise and medicine ignored physical fitness programs for the elderly because the general belief was that older citizens were untrainable. A newer body of knowledge, however, now not only supports the concept of physical conditioning for all ages but also shows the healthy elderly are just as trainable as the healthy young. Although the physiological responses to the challenge of exercise differ somewhat among the elderly (*1*), there is no longer any doubt that the health benefits to be derived by the elderly are entirely similar to those derived by young and middle-aged persons.

Yet we cannot be so naive as to believe that a program of planned activity is a "fountain of youth." As Shock and his colleagues at the National Institute on Aging have pointed out so well, all available scientific evidence shows that, as a person grows older, he or she does suffer losses in functional capacity at the cellular, tissue, organ, and system levels. The best-defined losses in function are seen when the total organism is stressed by physical work or exercise (*2*).

PHYSICAL DECLINE ACCOMPANYING AGING

In the cardiovascular system, the most important losses are those related to heart function (Chapter 11). On the average, maximum cardiac output declines about 8 per cent per decade throughout adulthood (*3*). Typically, with age, blood pressure (at least in Western cultures) increases, the coronary arteries gradually occlude with fatty deposits, and the circulation in general slows down.

In respiration, vital capacity and thoracic wall compliance decrease and lung compliance increases. Breathing therefore requires more muscular effort so that maximum ventilation is reduced with age. The middle-aged person now has to huff and puff at chores that seemed only moderate challenges to the breathing functions in youth.

Skeletal muscles decrease gradually in strength, and some capacity for muscular endurance is also lost. Indeed, humans lose 3 to 5 per cent of total muscle tissue per decade as they grow older.

All those losses combine to create a considerable loss in the ability to transport oxygen to the consumer cells and to utilize it at the cellular level. This loss in maximum oxygen consumption capability translates into what the layperson observes as a loss in vigor. Men lose about 50 per cent of this capacity by age 75, and women follow a similar course (*4,5*).

However, and this is the critical point, research has shown that similar functional losses can be brought about in *young, well-conditioned* people in as little as three weeks by the simple expedient of enforced bed rest. One of the seminal studies in this area showed that in three weeks of bed rest, the maximum values for cardiac output decreased by 26 per cent, the ventilatory capacity by 30 per cent, oxygen consumption by 30 per cent, and even the amount of active tissue by 1.5 per cent (*6*). Thus, one might say that changes roughly equivalent to three decades of aging were brought about by simply remaining motionless for three weeks.

From the available evidence, then, one may hypothesize that the functional losses reported in the scientific literature as age changes really should be considered as resulting from at least three contributing factors: (1) an increasingly sedentary lifestyle, (2) unrecognized, incipient disease processes, and (3) true aging changes. The first factor, which might be called a "risk factor for senility," is the one over which a person can exert the greatest control by virtue of physical conditioning. The reduction of this one important factor, sedentariness, can in turn significantly reduce other risk factors important to the prevention of premature age-related deterioration.

THE EFFECTS OF PHYSICAL CONDITIONING

Table 13-1 summarizes the recent research dealing with the effects of physical conditioning in slowing down the age-related losses in functional capacities in the elderly (here defined as persons over 60). With regard to

Table 13-1. Effects of Physical Conditioning on the Functional Capacities of Older Persons (Mean Age over 60)

Measurement	Sex	Number of Subjects	% Improvement	Reference
		Cardiovascular system		
Decrease in heart rate at submaximum workload	M F	5 3	19	*(8)*
	M	8	3–5	*(12)*
	F	7	3	*(12)*
Oxygen pulse	M	13	11	*(9)*
	M	48	4 (6 weeks)	*(10)*
	M	5	29 (42 weeks)	*(10)*
	F	17	7 (12 weeks)	*(7)*
	M	8	1–5 (11 weeks)	*(11)*
	F	7	0–3 (11 weeks)	*(11)*
Increased blood volume	M	13	9	*(9)*
Increased total Hb	M	13	7	*(9)*
Cardiac output at	M	34	0	*(10)*
submaximum workload	M	8	9	*(12)*
	F	7	0	*(12)*
Stroke volume at	M	34	6	*(10)*
submaximum workload	M	8	0	*(12)*
	F	7	0	*(12)*
Resting systolic pressure	M F	5 3	13	*(8)*
	M	66	2	*(7)*
	F	17	0	*(7)*
Resting diastolic pressure	M F	5 3	6	*(8)*
	M	66	4	*(10)*
	F	17	0	*(7)*
Regression of ECG abnormalities	M F	5 3	50% of abnormalities definitely improved	*(8)*

the cardiovascular system, reasonable agreement exists that bodily effort with any given submaximum workload results in a significantly lower working heart rate. That effect in turn results in an improvement in the oxygen economy of the heart (*7–11*). Agreement also exists that the oxygen pulse increases at submaximum workload, suggesting improvement in oxygen transport (*9–11*). Increases in blood volume and total hemoglobin have been reported (*9*). However, no experimental data are available for this age group as to the maximum cardiac output changes possible with training, and the available data (*10–12*) suggest there is no significant change in cardiac output at submaximum workloads. Resting blood pressure appears to be reduced in those who are hypertensive (*8*), but the change for normotensive subjects is small, though statistically significant if the group trained is large (*10*). One group of investigators

Measurement	Sex	Number of Subjects	% Improvement	Reference
		Respiratory system		
Vital capacity	M	5	0	*(8)*
	F	3		
	M	66	5 (6 weeks)	*(10)*
	M	8	20 (42 weeks)	*(10)*
	F	17	0	*(7)*
Maximum ventilation during exercise	M	47	12 (6 weeks)	*(10)*
	M	7	35 (42 weeks)	*(10)*
	M	5	50	*(8)*
	F	3		
	M	13	0	*(9)*
	F	17	0	*(7)*
		Physical work capacity, $\dot{V}O_2max$		
	M	61	9 (6 weeks)	*(10)*
	M	8	16 (42 weeks)	*(10)*
	F	17	37	*(7)*
	M	5	76	*(8)*
	F	3		
	M	14	29	*(13)*
	F	28	29	*(13)*
	M	14	11	*(15)*
	F	12	12	*(15)*
		Muscular strength		
	M	68	6 (6 weeks)	*(10)*
	M	8	12 (42 weeks)	*(10)*
	M	5	50	*(16)*
	F	15		

has also reported regression of electrocardiographic abnormalities as a result of moderate aerobic exercise (*8*).

Improvement in respiratory function is less certain. Although we have found large and significant improvement in vital capacity in older men (*10*) but not in older women (*7*), Barry et al. (*8*) found no change in either sex. We hypothesize that the difference in findings may be due to differing emphasis on improvement of flexibility in the thoracic wall, which was emphasized in our work with older men (*10*). As to the capacity for maximum ventilation, both Barry et al. (*8*) and we (*10*) found large improvement, 50 and 35 per cent respectively, although Benestad reported no change (*9*) and our own data with older women (*7*) also showed no change.

There seems little doubt that exercise can improve significantly the physical working capacity of the older person. All available data agree that such improvement does occur (*7,8,10,13–15*). There is also good agreement on the improvement of strength (*1,10,16*) for older men and women. However, recent work in our laboratory has shown that, although the percentage gains in strength are similar in old and young when the training stimulus is equated, the physiological bases differ considerably because the elderly have little potential for hypertrophy (*1*).

Important effects of physical conditioning on bone and connective tissue have also been reported. An extremely serious problem for older persons, especially older women, is the loss of bony tissue (osteoporosis). Smith and Reddan (*14*) showed that 20 women having a mean age of 82 *gained* 4.2 per cent in bone mineral composition as the result of exercise, compared with controls, who lost 2.5 per cent during the 36-month experiment.

Loss of joint mobility is another serious problem for the elderly. Here again, appropriate exercise can result in significant improvement (*17*).

THE TRANQUILIZER EFFECT OF EXERCISE

In our laboratory, interest was piqued some years ago by the prevalent notion that a good physical exercise bout would relieve nervous tension. The importance of testing this hypothesis is clear from several vantage points. First, the popular press has reported that in 1964 the yearly expenditure in the United States for tranquilizers was $327 million. By 1975, Californians were spending $104 million for Medi-Cal Valium prescriptions alone. One can reasonably believe, on these bases, that the national U.S. expenditure for tranquilizer drugs must be approaching $1 billion per year! The cost of excessive stress in Canada was estimated to be nearly $11 billion in 1979—about $6 billion in lost job productivity and another $5 billion for treatment.

Second, the recent medical literature includes many reports of clinical and laboratory studies that strongly suggest that none of the currently used tranquilizer drugs can be taken without hazard of serious side effects and/or the possibility of addiction.

Third, for the older population reaction time and movement time, which are so important to their safey as either motorists or pedestrians, are already compromised as the result of aging. Further slowing of responses brought about by tranquilizers may seriously increase the hazards in walking or driving.

In 1968 we reported on a series of three experiments using electromyographic techniques similar to those used by Jacobson, the pioneer in this area (*18*). In the first, a pilot study, reduced levels of neuromuscular activity were found in eight young subjects as the result of a 20-minute ride on a bicycle ergometer at a light workload. The changes were small, however, as might be expected in normal young students, and, because the number of subjects was also small, this reduction was not significant.

To furnish a better test for the hypothesis while still using normal persons, we had 29 subjects (PE students) make two visits to the laboratory on consecutive days. On one day they exercised at bench-stepping for five minutes and on the other day they acted as their own controls. The electrical activity in the right elbow flexor group showed a 58 per cent mean decrease on the exercise day and a 1.5 per cent decrease on the control day, a statistically significant difference (*18*).

To evaluate the chronic effect of physical exercise, 18 members of our faculty conditioning group and 7 controls who maintained a constant level of physical activity were tested and retested over a period in which the experimentals had 17 workouts of weight training and interval running. During that period, the controls increased in tension level by 24 per cent and the experimentals decreased by 25 per cent (*18*).

The latter two experiments both provided statistically significant data in favor of the tranquilizing effect of exercise. However, the experiment dealing with the immediate effect was not designed to take into consideration the fact that subjects showed an anticipatory electromyographic response on the exercise day but not on the control day. Thus the pretest levels were considerably higher on the exercise day; this finding might be considered a result of a flaw in experimental design.

For this and other reasons, another experiment was set up in which a more powerful test of the hypothesis was provided (*19*). To assure the potential for a reduction in neuromuscular tension, 10 elderly subjects were selected from 60 volunteers who considered themselves to have anxiety-tension problems. All ten subjects showed electromyographic evidence of residual neuromuscular tension. The treatment effects to be tested were

1. Exercise (walking type) at a heart rate of 100
2. The same exercise but at a heart rate of 120
3. Meprobamate 400 mg, commonly prescribed as Miltown or Equanil
4. 400 mg lactose (placebo)
5. Control

Each subject took each treatment three times. The tranquilizer drug and placebo were administered double-blind, and the anticipatory effect of the earlier experiment was eliminated by deciding on the treatment to be administered on any given day by chance and only after the pretest data had been recorded. With this design and the elimination of previous problems, the differences among treatments were highly significant. Pairwise analysis of the treatment effect showed that exercise at heart rate 100 lowered electrical activity by 20, 23, and 20 per cent at the first, second, and third post-tests, respectively (30, 60, and 90 minutes after pretest). The changes were significantly different from those of controls. Neither meprobamate nor the placebo findings were significantly different from those of controls. Interestingly, exercise at the higher heart rate approached, but did not achieve, statistical significance. Thus, we concluded that, at least in single doses, exercise of the appropriate type and intensity has a significantly greater effect on resting musculature than does meprobamate, one of the most frequently prescribed tranquilizer drugs at that time.

More recently, we undertook a re-investigation of this subject with two entirely different experimental paradigms. By using the change in spinal reflex activation level as the criterion variable, we avoided the differences of opinion with regard to the choice of muscle for electromyographic sampling.

In one study (*20*) ten subjects acted as their own controls in an experiment where each subject was tested three times before and after exercise and three times before and after quiet sitting (control). Exercise consisted of 20 minutes of cycling on an ergometer with the load adjusted to elicit a heart rate of rest rate plus 40 per cent of the value between resting and maximum. Testing consisted of electrical stimulation of the tibial nerve in the popliteal fossa to elicit Hoffmann reflexes (H waves) and directly propagated waves (M waves). The H/M ratio was calculated as in the method of Angel and Hoffmann (*21*). The reliability of this method was evaluated by ten test-retests on one subject in one day. The coefficient of variation for these data was 9.3 per cent. Biological variability was evaluated post hoc, with correlations between 21 pairs of repeated data showing $0.83<r<0.97$.

The mean of the change in H/M ratio for the three exercise days was compared with the mean change for the three control days. All ten subjects showed a fall in H/M ratio after exercise (mean = −18.2%). On the control days, six subjects showed a small rise and four showed a small drop that in no case approached the decrease seen on the exercise day (mean = +1.2%). The difference in these responses was highly significant: $t = 5.6379$ ($p<.001$).

In the second experiment, we (*22*) examined the effect of exercise on mechanically induced monosynaptic spinal reflex responses by measured tendon taps to the Achilles tendon. Six young, healthy, asymptomatic subjects were tested on two days before and after exercise and on two other occasions before and after control (equivalent period of rest). The mean depression of response after exercise was 15.3 per cent ($p<.05$). Changes on control days were consistently upward.

These findings confirm our earlier resting electromyographic results and those of other investigators who have found a tranquilizing effect. The deviant findings appear to be the result of using the frontalis muscle, which apparently should not be considered representative of the general musculature.

CONCLUSION

A close examination of the available data suggests substantial agreement with respect to the tranquilizing effect of exercise. The evidence comes from several different approaches: surveys of expert opinion (medical profession, including general practitioners and psychiatrists), use of questionnaires in controlled experiments, and, now, controlled physiological experiments using three different paradigms, viz., (1) resting electromyographic levels, (2) Hoffmann reflex activiation, and (3) spinal reflex activation levels as measured by mechanical stimulation of the Achilles tendon reflex.

Although one would like to have much more corroborative evidence than is presently available, a cautious conclusion can and probably should (in the interest of practice) be drawn that appropriate type, intensity, and duration of exercise can have a significant tranquilizing effect. We have shown this effect in young, middle-aged, and elderly subjects, and we have observed a chronic as well as an immediate effect. With regard to the dose-response characteristics, I can only say that, on the basis of our data, rhythmic exercise, such as walking, jogging, cycling, and bench-stepping, of duration from 5 to 30 minutes and intensity 30 to 60 per cent of maximum is effective in reducing tension. Contrariwise, it is possible—though not proved—that extremely high levels of work may be counterproductive.

REFERENCES

1. T. Moritani, and H. A. deVries, Potential for gross muscle hypertrophy in older men, *J. Geront.* **35:**672 (1980).
2. N. W. Shock, Current concepts of the aging process, *JAMA* **175:**654 (1961).
3. S. Julius, A. Amery, L. S. Whitlock and J. Conway, Influence of age on the hemodynamic response to exercise, *Circulation* **36:**222 (1967).
4. I. Astrand, Aerobic work capacity in men and women with special reference to age, *Acta Physiol. Scand.* **49**(suppl.):169 (1960).
5. S. Robinson, Experimental studies of physical fitness in relation to age, *Arbeitsphysiologie* **10:**251 (1938).
6. B. Saltin, G. Blomquist, J. H. Mitchell, R. L. Johnson, K. Wildenthal, and C. B. Chapman, *Response to Exercise After Bed Rest and After Training,* A.H.A. Monograph 23. American Heart Association, New York, 1968.
7. G. M. Adams and H. A. de Vries, Physiological effects of an exercise training regimen upon women aged 52–79, *J. Geront.* **28:**50 (1973).
8. A. J. Barry, J. W. Daly, E.D.R. Pruett, J. R. Steinmetz, H. F. Page, N. C. Birkhead, and K. Rodahl: The effects of physical conditioning on older individuals, *J. Geront.* **21:**182 (1966).
9. A. M. Benestad, Trainability of old men, *Acta Med. Scand.* **178:**321 (1965).
10. H. A. deVries, Physiological effects of an exercise training regimen upon men aged 52–88, *J. Geront.* **25:**325 (1970).
11. V. Niinimaa, and R. J. Shephard, Training and oxygen conductance in the elderly: I.The respiratory system, *J. Geront.* **33:**354 (1978).
12. V. Niinimaa, and R. J. Shephard, Training and oxygen conductance in the elderly: II. The cardiovascular system, *J Geront.* **33:**362 (1978).
13. K. H. Sidney, and R. J. Shephard, Frequency and intensity of exercise training for elderly subjects, *Med Sci. Sport* **10:**125 (1978).

14. E. L. Smith, and W. Reddan, Physical activity: A modality for bone accretion in the aged, *Am. J. Roentgen Radium Therapy Nuclear Med.* **126:**1297 (1977).
15. H. Suominen, E. Heikkinen, H. Liesen, D. Michel, and W. Hollmann, Effects of 8 weeks endurance training on skeletal muscle metabolism in 56–70-year-old sedentary men, *Eur. J. Appl. Physiol.* **37:**173 (1977).
16. L. C. Perkins and H. L. Kaiser, Results of short-term isotonic and isometric exercise programs in persons over 60, *Phy. Therap. Rev.* **41:**633 (1962).
17. E. A. Chapman, H. A. deVries, and R. Swezey, Joint stiffness: Effects of exercise on young and old men, *J. Geront.* **27:**218 (1972).
18. H. A. deVries, Immediate and long-term effects of exercise upon resting muscle action potential level, *J. Sports Med.* **8:**1 (1968).
19. H. A. deVries, and G. M. Adams, Electromyographic comparison of single doses of exercise and meprobamate as to effects on muscular relaxation, *Am. J. Phy. Med.* **51:**130 (1972).
20. H. A. deVries, R. A. Wiswell, R. Bulbulian, and T. Moritani, Tranquilizer effect of exercise: Acute effects of moderate aerobic exercise on spinal reflex activation level, *Am. J. Phy. Med.* **60:**57 (1981).
21. R. W. Angel and W. W. Hoffman, The H reflex in normal, spastic, and rigid subjects, *Arch. Neurol.* **8:**591 (1963).
22. H. A. deVries, C. Simard, R. A. Wiswell, E. Heckathorne, and V. Carabetta, Involvement of the muscle spindle in the tranquilizer effect of exercise, *Am. J. Phy. Med.,* **61:**111, 1982.

14 Control of Aging by Nutrition

Edward J. Masoro

Over the years four major hypotheses have evolved as to how food restriction decreases the rate of aging:

1. By prolonging immaturity
2. By decreasing the rate of and prolonging the duration of growth
3. By decreasing fat mass
4. By decreasing the rate of metabolism.

HISTORICAL PERSPECTIVE

That food restriction increases the length of life in rats was first shown unequivocally by McCay and his colleagues in 1935 (*1*). Since that time, the finding has been repeatedly confirmed and extended to include other species of laboratory rodents (*2,3*). In the study of McCay et al., the dietary restriction was enough to reduce skeletal growth severely and delay sexual maturation significantly. However, later studies have shown that levels of food restriction that have little effect on skeletal growth and sexual maturation also effectively prolong life (*4–6*).

A study in which rats were given *ad libitum* access to three different diets provides particularly striking data on the impact of food intake on longevity (*7*). It showed an inverse relationship between the amount of food the rats chose to eat and length of life (Figure 14-1).

Is the life-prolonging effect of food restriction due to the retardation of aging? Sufficient data are now available to answer this important question affirmatively. Indeed, Sacher (*8*) drew this conclusion solely from mortality data. His analysis, graphically presented in Figure 14-2, used the concept of age-specific death rates, i.e., number of deaths per unit population per unit time at specific ages. In this semilogarithmic graph, the *y* axis depicts age-specific death rate and *x* axis depicts age. The slope of

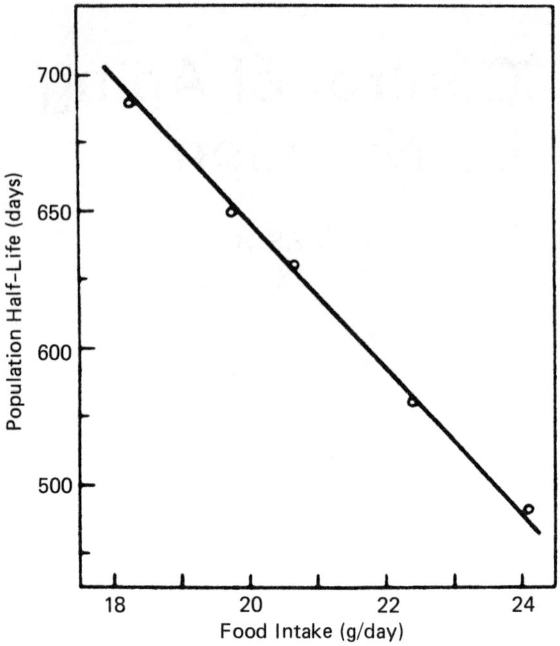

Figure 14-1. Relationship between quantity of food consumed by male rats fed *ad libitum* and length of life. (From M.H. Ross (*7*) by permission of John Wiley & Sons, Inc.)

the line from the data on *ad libitum*–fed rats is steeper than that of the rats fed restricted amounts of food. From this difference in slope, Sacher concluded that food restriction decreases the rate of aging. Further evidence for this view has emerged from studies, to be discussed below, on age-related physiological deterioration and age-related disease; both are delayed or prevented by food restriction.

It is interesting—and perhaps surprising—to compare the effect of food restriction on the longevity of rats with the effect of technology and medicine on human longevity. Although technology and medicine have increased the mean length of life in humans, they have not changed the maximum length (*9*). The maximum length of human life (Chapter 1) in ancient Rome was about 100 years (*9*), the same as in the United States today.

RESEARCH DESIGN AND DATA

Many of the data considered here were generated from our research on the effects of food restriction on aging, and thus a brief description of our research will be helpful. Weanling (28-day-old) male Fischer 344 rats, purchased from Charles River Laboratories, were fed *ad libitum* until six

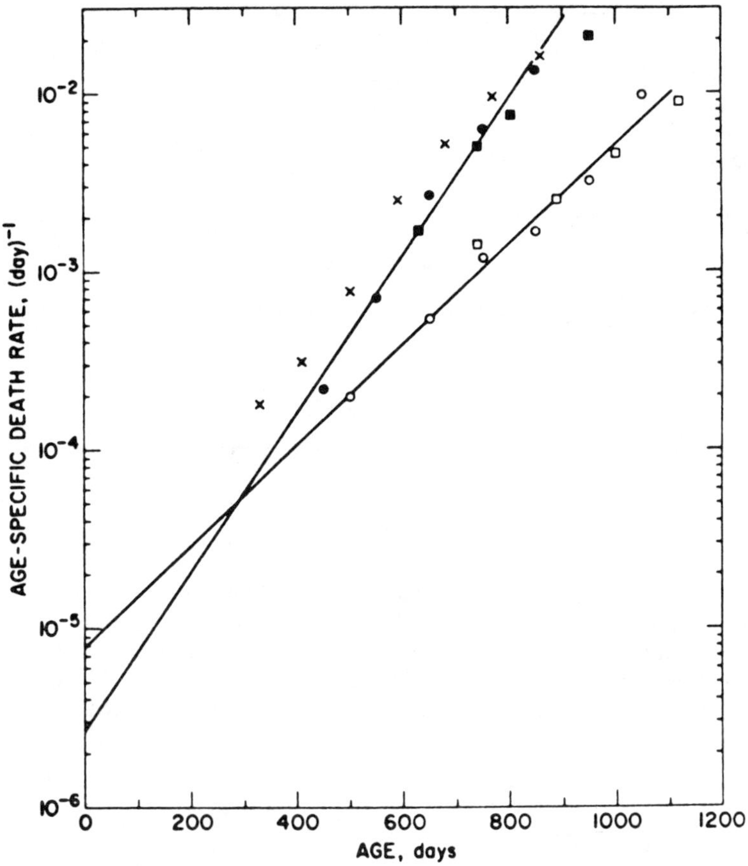

Figure 14-2. Effects of food restriction on the age-specific death rate. The *X*'s and filled circles and squares denote *ad libitum* fed rats, and the unfilled squares and circles denote food-restricted rats. (From G.A. Sacher (*8*) by permission of Van Nostrand Reinhold.)

weeks of age and then divided into two groups: group A continued to be fed *ad libitum* while group R was given 60 per cent of the *ad libitum* intake. The diet was semisynthetic, with a caloric composition of 21 per cent protein, 57 per cent carbohydrate, and 22 per cent fat (corn oil). Both groups were divided into three subgroups, one for the study of longevity, another for the longitudinal study of body composition, and a third for the cross-sectional study of physiological and biochemical variables.

Figure 14-3 shows changes in body weight during the life-span of the rats on the longevity study. Figure 14-4 summarizes the findings on longevity by means of survival curves. When the last of the 115 rats of group A died, more than 60 per cent of the group R rats were still living. The data clearly show that food restriction increased both the mean length and the maximum length of life of this strain of rat.

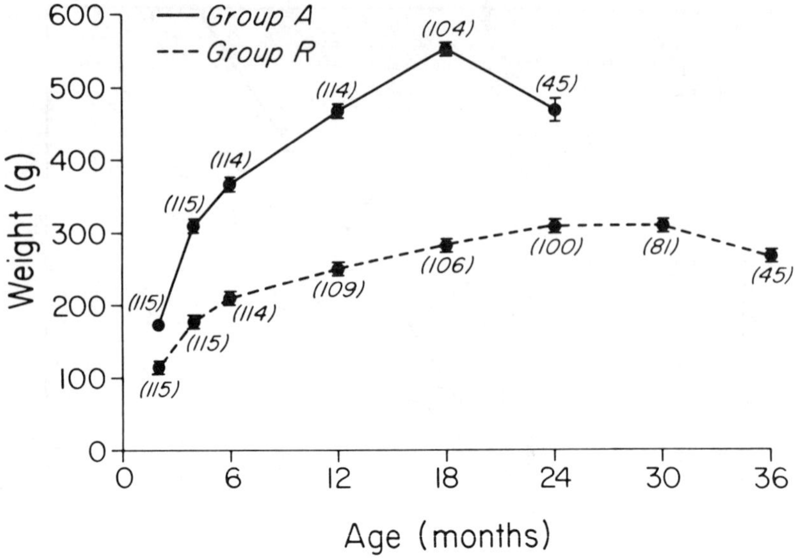

Figure 14-3. Changes in body weight during life-span of Fischer 344 rats. The data are mean values ± SE for all animals alive at a given chronological age. The numbers in parentheses show the number of animals so analyzed. (From B.P. Yu, E.J. Masoro, I Murata, H. Bertrand, and F.T. Lynd (*11*) by permission of the Gerontological Society of America, publisher of the *Journal of Gerontology.*)

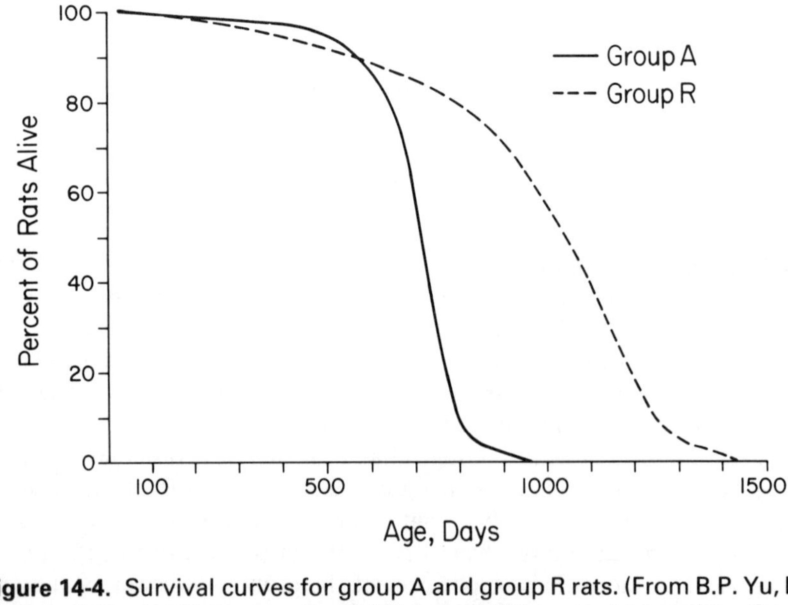

Figure 14-4. Survival curves for group A and group R rats. (From B.P. Yu, E.J. Masoro, I Murata, H. Bertrand, and F.T. Lynd (*11*) by permission of the Gerontological Society of America, publisher of the *Journal of Gerontology.*)

LEAN BODY MASS VERSUS FAT DEPOSITS

Lean body mass progressively decreases in humans from about 30 years of age onward (*10*). That loss of lean body mass is a basic aspect of aging in mammals has long been assumed, and we wondered whether food restriction could influence such loss. Therefore, we measured lean body mass in group A and group R rats throughout their life-spans; it did not decrease with age in either group (*11*). Lesser et al. (*12*) reported similar findings with Sprague-Dawley rats. Thus, a loss of lean body mass can no longer be considered a general aging characteristic in mammals.

In men and women living in developed nations, body fat increases with age, at least until late middle age (*13*). In group A and group R rats, fat mass also increased until about 70 per cent of the life-span was reached, and after that it declined with age (*14*). Group R rats had a mean fat mass smaller than that of group A rats, even in terms of per cent of body mass. Increases in fat mass can be due to adipocyte hyperplasia, to adipocyte hypertrophy, or to both.

We studied the age changes in two fat depots, epididymal and perirenal, of group A and group R rats and got somewhat unexpected results (*14*). In group A rats, both depots grew between 6 and 18 months of age, the growth in the perirenal depot occurring solely by hyperplasia and that of the epididymal depot solely by hypertrophy. In group R rats during that same age period, the growth of both of these depots involved a combination of hyperplasia and hypertrophy. At all ages studied in common, the depots of group R rats contained fewer and smaller adipocytes that did the depots of group A rats. These data disagree with the hypothesis that fat cell number is fixed in adulthood. Late in life, in both groups, the mass of these depots decreased. In the case of the epididymal depot of group A rats, this loss in mass was associated with adipocyte hyperplasia.

PHYSIOLOGICAL CHANGES

Food restriction also modulates age-related physiological changes. Probably the most striking finding is its effect on glucagon-promoted lipolysis in fat cells (*15,16*). In six-week-old group A rats, glucagon promoted lipolysis considerably, but, with increasing age, this responsiveness was rapidly lost (Figure 14-5). When these rats were six months old, their fat cells were totally unresponsive to this hormone. In contrast, fat cells from group R rats were fully responsive to glucagon through 12 months of age. Moreover, fat cells from group R rats as old as 36 months still showed a significant lipolytic response to glucagon. Because a one-month food restriction regimen started at six months of age did not have this effect, we concluded that these results were not due to the small fat cell size of group R rats or to acute food restriction.

Age-related changes in the lipolytic response of fat cells to epinephrine

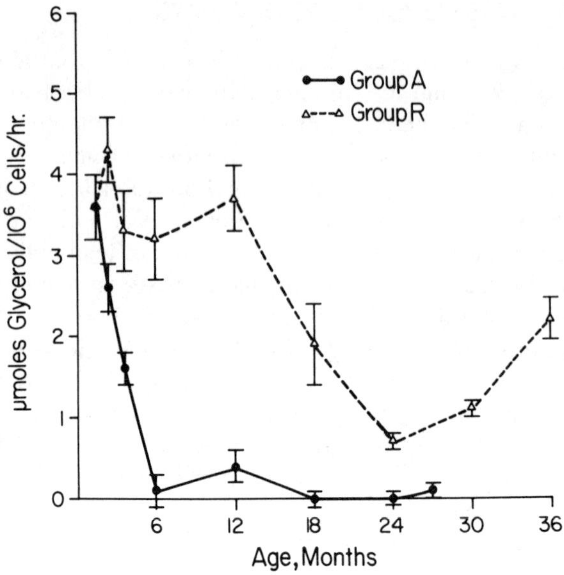

Figure 14-5. Glucagon-promoted lipolysis in adipocytes from Group A and Group R rats: the effects of age on the response of isolated adipocytes to the lipolytic action of glucagon. (From E.J. Masoro, B.P. Yu, H.A. Bertrand, and F.T. Lynd (*16*) by permission of the Federation of American Societies for Experimental Biology, publisher of *Federation Proceedings.*)

were also influenced by food restriction (*17*). In group A rats at six months of age, adipocytes had the same responsiveness to the lipolytic action of epinephrine as did group R adipocytes (Figure 14-6). However, in group A rats, a progressive loss in this responsiveness occurred from 6 to 24 months of age. In contrast, in group R rats, no loss in this responsiveness occurred until after 18 months age. Although the data in Figure 14-6 refer to 10^{-5} *M* epinephrine, similar results were found at all concentrations of ephinephrine tested.

Because fat-cell lipolysis is a basic component of fat mobilization, it seemed likely that fat mobilization would decline with age and that food restriction could modulate this age-related decline. The rate of fat mobilization is known to be activated in post-absorptive animals, and serum free fatty acid (FFA) levels serve as a good quantitative index of this action (*18*). The data on serum FFA levels in group A and group R rats, shown in Figure 14-7, are consistent with the view that fat mobilization decreases with age and that food restriction delays and partially prevents this decrease (*19*).

The age-related increase in serum cholesterol is also delayed by food restriction (*19*). As shown in Figure 14-8, serum cholesterol levels increase with age in rats as they do in humans. When the rats were six months old, the serum cholesterol levels in the two groups were similar.

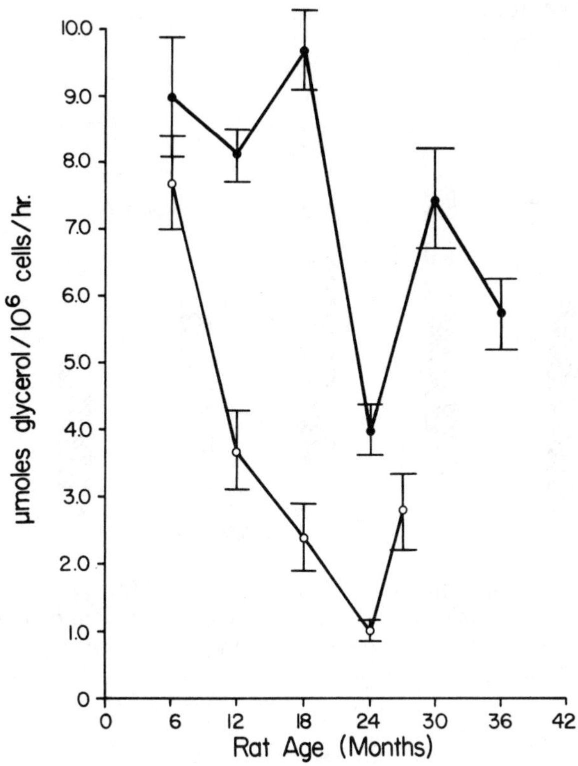

Figure 14-6. Effects of age on the lipolytic response of epididymal adipocytes to 10^{-5} *M* epinephrine. Open circles refer to cells from group A rats and closed circles to cells from group R rats. (From B.P. Yu, H.A. Bertrand, and E.J. Masoro (*17*) by permission of Grune & Stratton, Inc., publisher of *Metabolism.*)

For group A rats beyond six months of age, serum cholesterol levels increased, reaching maximum values by 18 to 24 months of age. This age-related increase in serum cholesterol was delayed considerably in group R rats. Indeed, not until age 30 months did group R have the levels of serum cholesterol reached by group A rats at 18 months of age.

The modulation of age-related change by food restriction is not limited to lipid metabolism. Loss of muscle mass occurred at later ages in group R rats than in group A rats (*11*). Moreover, loss of force development in the lateral omohyoideus muscle, which occurred by 27 months of age in group A rats, did not occur in group R rats as old as 36 months (*20*). In addition, Levin et al. (*21*), studying the effect of food restriction on dopamine receptors in brain striatal membranes of male Wistar rats, found that the number of receptors declined with age and that food restriction prevented this loss of receptors. Also, Walford and his collaborators (*22,23*) and Good and his colleagues (*24,25*) found that food re-

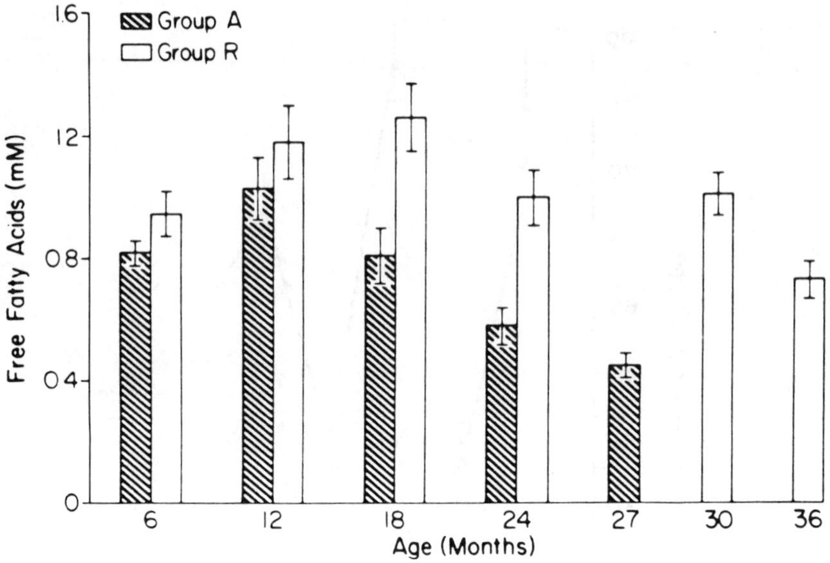

Figure 14-7. Age and the post-absorptive serum FFA levels of group A and group R rats. (From G.U. Liepa, E.J. Masoro, H.A. Bertrand, and B.P. Yu (*19*) by permission of the American Physiological Society, publisher of the *American Journal of Physiology.*)

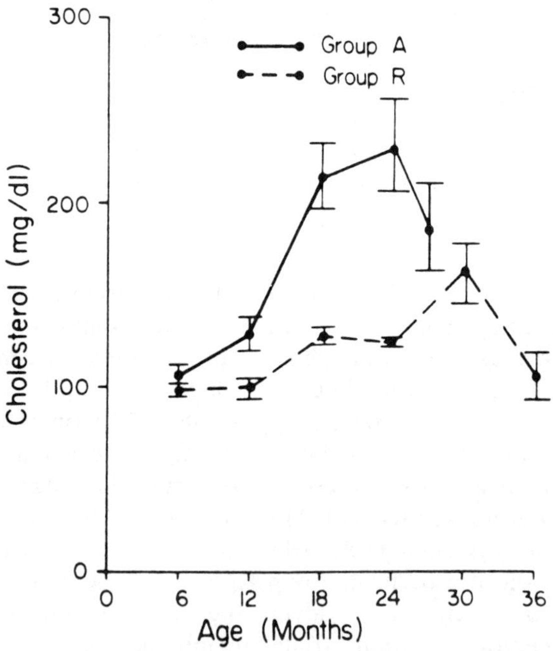

Figure 14-8. Age and post-absorptive serum total cholesterol levels of Group A and Group R rats. (From G.U. Liepa, E.J. Masoro, H.A. Bertrand, and B.P. Yu (*19*) by permission of the American Physiological Society, publisher of the *American Journal of Physiology.*)

striction in mice delayed the immune system deterioration that occurs with age. Thus, research during the last few years has shown that food restriction modulates a broad spectrum of age-related physiological changes.

EFFECT ON DISEASE

Food restriction has also been shown to delay many age-related diseases. Using Fischer 344 rats (the strain used in our research), Coleman et al. (*26*) found that chronic nephropathy increases in severity with increasing age and that death often resulted from this disease process. Our findings with the group A rats confirm their results. In addition, food restriction was found to delay the age-related increase in severity of these renal lesions. Most striking was that the death of most group A rats was associated with severe renal lesions, whereas few group R rats showed such lesions at death. Many other age-related lesions were also found to be delayed by food restriction, e.g., Leydig cell tumors, bile duct hyperplasia, myocardial fibrosis and myocardial degeneration.

FOUR HYPOTHESES: PRO AND CON

Now let us briefly review the available evidence for and against the four major hypotheses regarding modulation of aging by food restriction.

The hypothesis that led to the pioneering study of McCay et al. (*1*) was that food restriction would delay aging by delaying development and prolonging immaturity. McCay and associates found the results of their study to be consistent with this theory, but the results of recent research have shown that food restriction prolongs life in rats even when started as late as 12 months of age (*6*) and in mice when started after full growth (14 months of age) has been attained (*27*). Since in both rats and mice maturity is reached well before 12 months of age, delayed development is unlikely to be a major factor in the age-delaying action of food restriction.

The hypothesis that food restriction delays aging by reducing the rate of growth and prolonging the duration of growth is supported by studies that in mice and rats the rate of growth and length of life are inversely correlated (*28,29*). However, other studies show a direct correlation between duration of growth in rats and length of life (*29–31*). Obviously growth may be a determinant of length of life. However, it is probably not a major factor in the action of food restriction because the life-prolonging action of food restriction still occurs when initiated in adult rats and mice (*6,27*).

The hypothesis that food restriction delays aging by reducing fat mass appears to be based on the long-accepted but recently challenged view that increasing fat mass leads to premature death (*32*). There is no direct evidence to support this hypothesis, and, indeed, our work provides evidence against it. In the group A population of rats, whose fat content is greater than that of the group R rats, no significant correlation was found between fat mass and length of life, whereas in the group R rats, fat mass was found to correlate positively with length of life (*14*).

That food restriction decreases the rate of aging by decreasing the rate of metabolism was proposed by Sacher (*8*) from his analysis of a study by Ross (*33*) in which rats were offered five different diets that resulted in caloric intakes ranging from 18 to 75 Kcal per day. However, data from our recent study showed that food restriction that substantially lengthened life did not decrease the rate of energy metabolism per gram of lean body mass. Thus, our data do not support the concept that food restriction slows the rate of aging by decreasing the rate of metabolism.

CONCLUSION

Although none of the four major hypotheses can be substantiated, the conclusion to be drawn from these studies is that nutrition can greatly influence the aging process and its manifestations. Also apparent is that nutritional manipulations can provide a useful tool for exploring the basic aging process and, further, that modifying human aging by nutritional means may be possible.

REFERENCES

1. C. M. McCay, M. F. Crowell, and L. H. Maynard, The effect of retarded growth upon the length of life-span and upon the ultimate body size, *J. Nutrition* **10:**63 (1935).
2. C. H. Barrows and G. C. Kokkonen, Relationship between nutrition and aging, *Adv. Nutr. Res. 1:*253 (1977).
3. V. R. Young, Diet as a modulator of aging and longevity, *Fed. Proc.* **38:**1994 (1979).
4. B. N. Berg and H. S. Simms, Nutrition and longevity: II. Longevity and onset of disease with different levels of food intake, *J. Nutrition* **71:**255 (1960).
5. G. A. Nolen, Effect of various restricted dietary regimens on the growth, health and longevity of albino rats, *J. Nutrition* **102:**1477 (1972).
6. E. Stuchlikova, M. Juricova-Horokova, and Z. Deyl, New aspects of the dietary effects of life prolongation in rodents: What is the role of obesity in aging? *Exp. Geront.* **10:**141 (1975).
7. M. H. Ross, Nutrition and longevity in experimental animals, in *Nutrition and Aging,* (M. Winick, ed.). Wiley, New York, 1976.
8. G. A. Sacher, Life table modification and life prolongation, in *Handbook of the Biology of Aging* (C. E. Finch and L. Hayflick, eds.). Van Nostrand Reinhold, New York, 1977.
9. R. L. Walford, Immunology and aging, *Am. J. Clin. Pathol.* **74:**247 (1980).
10. G. B. Forbes, The adult decline in lean body mass, *Human Biology* **48:**161 (1976).
11. B. P. Yu, E. J. Masoro, I. Murata, H. Bertrand, and F. T. Lynd, Life-span study of SPF Fischer 344 male rats fed *ad libitum* or restricted diets: Longevity, growth, lean body mass and disease, *J. Geront.* **37:**130 (1982).

12. G. T. Lesser, S. Deutsch, and J. Markofsky, Aging in the rat: Longitudinal and cross-sectional studies of body composition, *Am. J. Physiol.* **225:**1472 (1973).
13. R. M. Malina, Quantification of fat, muscle and bone in man, *Clin Orthopaedics Related Res.* **65:**9 (1969).
14. H. A. Bertrand, F. T. Lynd, E. J. Masoro, and B. P. Yu, Changes in adipose mass and cellularity through the adult life of rats fed *ad libitum* or a life-prolonging restricted diet, *J. Geront.* **35:**827 (1980).
15. H. A. Bertrand, E. J. Masoro, and B. P. Yu, Maintenance of glucagon-promoted lipolysis in adipocytes by food restriction, *Endocrinology* **107:**591 (1980).
16. E. J. Masoro, B. P. Yu, H. A. Bertrand, and F. T. Lynd, Nutritional probe of the aging process, *Fed. Proc.* **39:**3178 (1980).
17. B. P. Yu, H. A. Bertrand, and E. J. Masoro, Nutrition-aging influence of catecholamine-promoted lipolysis, *Metabolism* **29:**438 (1980).
18. E. J. Masoro, Lipids and lipid metabolism, *Ann. Rev. Physiol.* **39:**301 (1977).
19. G. U. Liepa, E. J. Masoro, H. A. Bertrand, and B. P. Yu, Food restriction as a modulator of age-related changes in serum lipids, *Am. J. Physiol.* **238:**E253 (1980).
20. R. McCarter, B. P. Yu, and E. J. Masoro, Dynamic properties of mammalian skeletal muscle: Variation with age, *Physiologist* **22:**85 (1979).
21. P. Levin, J. K. Janda, J. A. Joseph, D. K. Ingram, and G. S. Roth, Dietary restriction retards age associated loss of rat striatal dopaminergic receptors, *Science,* **214:**561 (1981).
22. R. L. Walford, R. K. Liu, M. Delima-Berbasse, M. Mathis, and G. S. Smith, Long-term dietary restriction and immune function in mice: Response to sheep red blood cells and to mitogenic agents, *Mech. Aging Dev.* **2:**447 (1974).
23. R. H. Weindruch, J. A. Kristie, K. E. Cheney, and R. L. Walford, Influence of controlled dietary restriction on immunologic function and aging, *Fed. Proc.* **38:**2007 (1979).
24. G. Fernandes, P. Friend, E. J. Yunis, and R. A. Good, Influence of dietary restriction on immunologic function and renal disease in (NZB × NZW)F_1 mice, *Proc. Natl. Acad. Sci.* **75:**1500 (1978).
25. G. Fernandes, E. J. Yunis, and R. A. Good, Influence of diet on survival of mice, *Proc. Natl. Acad. Sci.* **73:**1279 (1976).
26. G. L. Coleman, S. W. Barthold, G. W. Osbaldiston, S. J. Foster, and A. M. Jonas, Pathological changes during aging in barrier-reared Fischer 344 male rats. *J. Geront.* **32:**258 (1977).
27. R. H. Weindruch, J. A. Kristie, and R. L. Walford, Dietary restriction imposed in middle-age mice: Life-span, disease and immunologic effects, *Gerontologist* **25:**5, Part II, 223 (1980).
28. C. L. Goodrick, Body weight change over the life-span and longevity of C57BL/6J mice and mutations which differ in maximal body weight, *Gerontology* **23:**405 (1977).
29. C. L. Goodrick, Effects of long-term voluntary wheel exercise on male and female Wistar rats: I. Longevity, *Gerontology* **26:**22 (1980).
30. A. V. Everitt and C. Webb, The relation between body weight changes and life duration in male rats, *J. Geront.* **12:**128 (1957).

31. M. H. Ross, E. Lustbader, and G. Bras, Dietary practices and growth responses as predictors of longevity, *Nature* **262:**548 (1976).
32. R. Andres, Influence of obesity on longevity in the aged, *Adv. Pathobiol.* **7:**238 (1978).
33. M. H. Ross, Aging, nutrition and hepatic enzyme activity patterns in the rat, *J. Nutr.* **97:**suppl. 1, part II, 563 (1969).

15 Metabolic and Endocrine Factors in Aging

Alfredo Lopez-S

Changes in adaptive responsiveness to hormones and other metabolic factors are characteristic of the aging organism. Whether these hormonal and metabolic alterations are causes of physiological aging, however, remains unclear. Finch (*1*) put forth the hypothesis that aging is a multifactorial process involving endocrine and metabolic changes. Such changes may occur early in life and subsequently affect life-span.

If aging-associated endocrine and metabolic changes are characteristic of aging and if their "timing" is determined, then the "risk of aging" can be evaluated and the experimental manipulation of the most effective timing may be possible. That such manipulation can be achieved is suggested by the studies of Bertrand et al (*2*), who studied the effect of diet on age-related loss of hormonally stimulated lipolysis, and those of Nelson et al. (*3*), who showed that the timing of the loss of the estrus cycle in rodents is not strictly age-related but may also be affected by degree of steroid exposure.

The suspected relation of hormones to aging is as old as endocrinology. In the past, researchers were impressed by the sharp decline in hormone output from most endocrine glands. Now most of the endocrine system is known to retain considerable reserve capacity with advancing age, and the decreased resting output reported previously could be due to decreased peripheral demands related to wasting peripheral tissues.

A common characteristic of all hormones is that they begin their action by binding to specific receptors. More than 100 studies report changes in hormone receptors with age. Of these studies, 70 per cent show decreases, 20 per cent no change, and 15 per cent increases. In the few studies showing increases, the results are difficult to interpret either because of the method used or because of how the results are expressed. One can conclude, however, that the evidence points in general to a decrease in receptor concentration per cell with aging. Recent studies by

Chang et al. (*4*) suggest that a reduced biosynthesis of receptors may represent a selective manifestation of the aging process.

Because the literature has little information about the risk factor value of endocrine and metabolic changes with regard to aging, this chapter focuses specifically on what is known about the interaction between aging and the endocrine system components, i.e., the neurohypophysis, thyroid, gonads, and adrenal glands.

HORMONAL FACTORS

Neurohypophysis

That the hypothalamus is the conductor of the endocrine orchestra has become evident during the past few years. By regulating pituitary function, it can be important in any relation between endocrine factors and aging. Apparently the function of the hypothalamic-pituitary axis remains virtually intact until extreme late age, although the response of thyroid-stimulating hormone (TSH) to thyrotropin-releasing hormone (TRH) seems to diminish with age. However, this continuity of function does not exclude the possibility that the hypothalamic-pituitary axis has an earlier role in aging because minimal or selective changes in neuroendocrine cell functions or neurotransmitters at that level can lead to cascading metabolic changes and age-correlated physical deteriorations.

Green (*5*) summarized the main neuroendocrine/aging findings (Table 15-1) and concluded that relatively little is known about the exact role of this system, which is so susceptible to physiological and environmental stimuli (including drugs). Interestingly, two of the classical theories of aging, nutritional (caloric restriction) and immunological (sensitivity change), may have a common denominator in the neuroendocrine system. Comfort (*6*) postulated that caloric restriction works via its effect on the hypothalamus and thus via hormone-sensitive molecules. Weindruch et al. (*7*) suggest that selective caloric restriction could also work through the immune system.

Although the thymus is not in a strict sense a component of the neurohypophysis, it is pertinent to include here a discussion of its potential role in the aging process. Makinodam (*8*) has reviewed the evidence suggesting the role of this organ as an endocrine gland, its relationship to the hypophysis, and its effects on pituitary-influenced adrenal secretory activity.

The neuroendocrine system and aging may also be linked through the role of the thymus in immunological response. Burnet (*9*) proposed this possibility because the thymus not only controls the function of T cells but also is one of the first organs to show involutional changes chronologically.

Although the role of the neuroendocrine system in aging seems to be a potentially important one, no risk value can as yet be assigned to any of its functions in humans.

Table 15-1. Aging and the Neuroendocrine System

Tissues	Aging changes
Suprahypothalamic nuclei and hypothalamus	↑ Neuronal size in supraoptic and paraventricular nuclei[a] ↓ Neurons in temperature and GDH regulating areas[b]
	↓ Activity enzymes involved in catecholamine metabolism[a] ↓ Norepinephrine, serotonin, dopamine content in hypothalamus[b]
	↓ GH[ab] ↓ GH in sleep[a] ↓ GH-releasing factor[a] ↓ GH response to exercise[a]
	↑ GDH (LH, FSH)[ab] ↑ GDH-releasing factor levels[ab] ↑ Prolactin-inhibiting factor[b]
	↓ Hypothalamic and hypothalamic-pituitary responsiveness to glucose[a] glucocorticoids[ab] gonadal steroids[b]
Hypothalamic-pituitary target organ	↓ Thyroxine secretion rate[a] ↓ Reduced tissue thyroxine utilizations[a] ↓ Plasma T_3[a] ↓ Pituitary response to TRH ↑ DECO[b]
	↓ Cortisol secretion rates[a] No abnormalities, basal or post-stress ACTH and cortisol levels
	↓ Sensitivity corticosteroid feedback mechanisms[ab] Defective corticosteroids receptors (?), excessive adrenocorticosteroids often cause increased aging by increased risk of various pathologies ↓ DHEA decreases with aging, related to atherosclerosis, cancer, osteoporosis Primary testicular failure inevitable eventually Testosterone therapy may cause increasing aging Castration may cause increased aging
Other	↓ Thymus

[a]Human
[b]Animal.
GH = growth hormone; LH = luteinizing hormone; FSH = follicle-stimulating hormone; TRH = thyrotrophin-releasing hormone; GDH = gonadotrophic hormone; DHEA = dehydroepiandrosterone; DECO = decreasing oxygen consumption hormone; ↑ = increased; ↓ = decreased.
Source: Modified from Green (*5*).

Thyroid

Various investigators have studied the relationship between the thyroid gland (and its hormones) and aging, as recently reviewed by Havard (*10*). With advancing age the thyroid gland changes morphologically, losing weight, follicle volume, and colloid content and increasing in proliferation of connective tissue. These findings suggest that the gland becomes less active.

Studies in animals have shown that circulating levels of thyroxine (T_4) and triiodothyronine (T_3) are diminished in aging rats. These findings can be accounted for by the reported decrease in thyroxine-binding capacity, decrease in T_4 deionization, disturbances in the regulation of TSH secretion by TRH, loss of circadian control of TSH, or accumulation of an apparently high-molecular-weight form of immunoreactive TSH that inhibits the normal thyroid response to TSH.

Apparently, elderly persons generally have lower serum T_3 concentrations and higher levels of reverse T_3 than do young persons. However, these changes in thyroid hormones could well be the consequence of disease rather than of age. Significant changes in thyroxine-binding prealbumin and thyroxine-binding globulin are well known to occur in chronically ill patients. The fact that thyroid function tests in relatively healthy elderly persons do not differ significantly from those of persons of other ages with similar degrees of illness suggests that ill health rather than aging is the major reason for the abnormal thyroid function values reported in the elderly.

Thyroid hormones are the major regulators of basal metabolic rate (BMR) in animals and humans, and a gradual decrease in BMR is usually observed with advancing age. Denckla (*11*) has postulated that this condition is caused by a substance produced by the aging pituitary and called decreasing oxygen consumption hormone (DECO). This hormone seems to restrict aging cells from properly utilizing the thyroxine that remains in abundance in the circulating system.

With the isolation or measurement of the proposed DECO hormone, a risk factor for aging may become definable because the hormone appears only with advancing age and animal experiments show that metabolic rate directly correlates with mean life-span.

Gonads

Historically the association of decreased sexuality with aging has been the basis for the implication that ovarian and testicular hormones are factors in aging. Decreased as well as constant levels of testosterone with increasing age have been reported in humans. In healthy participants in the Baltimore Longitudinal Study on Aging, serum testosterone did not decline with age (*12*). This could be due to changes in "target tissue sensitivity" occurring with advancing age, as suggested by the levels of LH reported in the elderly. Muta et al. (*13*) reported experiments suggesting that higher levels of testosterone are required to inhibit pituitary LH secretion in older men. Tsitouras et al. (*12*) also reported a weak association between serum testosterone and sexual vigor in men over 60 years of age. Contrary to ovarian function, testosterone production and spermatogenesis do not change suddenly unless a pathological process occurs.

In rats, in which lower serum levels of testosterone with advancing age have been reported more consistently, the adult testis apparently maintains undiminished testosterone secretory capability well into later life.

The age-related reduction in circulating testosterone reported by some investigators could represent, in some instances, dilution of a constant secretory rate of testosterone in an expanding blood plasma volume associated with increasing body weight with age. Other factors, such as alcoholism, chronic disease and stress, are known to contribute to lower levels of testosterone in the elderly.

In homothermic vertebrates, the ovaries age relatively early in life whereas other endocrine tissues continue to be active. The fact that there are significant differences between the male and female functions of the pituitary-gonadal axis further suggests that changes in gonadal function are not essential to the basic mechanism of aging. For example, with the reduction of estrogen production with advancing age in women, concomitant rises in FSH and LH levels are observed. No such elevation is observed in men. This difference has been attributed to the production of inhibin, which is secreted as long as sertoli cells remain functional. In mammals and birds senile involution of gonadal hormone concentrations and of sexual activity seems to be characteristic, but in invertebrates and insects the capacity for reproduction is maintained well into the late stages of life.

It is doubtful that indices of gonadal secretion will provide information about aging-associated risk because age-decreased gonadal hormone concentration seems to be associated not with the basic mechanism of aging but rather with diseases common to the elderly. Furthermore, many of the changes in gonadal steroids with advancing age could relate to changes in activity of the adrenal glands.

Adrenals

Changes in adrenal weight with age have been reported in animals. Nellor and Reigle (*14*) showed that, in cattle and goats, adrenal glands change morphologically and physiologically before any outward signs of aging appear. They also showed that, as animals grow older, the adrenal cortex becomes less responsive to circulating adrenocorticotropic hormone (ACTH) activity. Also reported was a reduced andrenocortical responsiveness to ACTH with age for men.

In progeria, considered a natural model of aging, the adrenal glands undergo severe hypoplasia, sclerosis, and mucoid degeneration.

These findings suggest that, with advancing age, the ability to mobilize adrenal cortical glucocorticoids in response to environmental or physiological stresses is functionally impaired. Nevertheless, evidence suggests that the adrenals of older persons have considerable reserve secretory capacity. Because of their decreased peripheral utilization, the adrenals of older persons may not need to function at the same high level as do the adrenals of younger persons to maintain the same circulatory levels of the hormone.

Little is known about the potential role of adrenal mineral corticoids in aging, although excesses of glucocorticoids have been reported to contribute to aging in animals.

Adrenal Androgens Information is available in the literature concerning changes in, and the role of, adrenal androgens with age. The urinary secretion of 17-ketosteroid has been described as decreasing with age, and this observation has been interpreted by investigators as suggesting a relationship between aging and the adrenals. Among the natural 17-ketosteroids, dehydroepiandrostexone (DHEA) (Figure 15-1) is quantitatively the most important. Although the adrenal cortex secretes DHEA and other C-19 androgens, dehydroepiandrosterone-sulfate (DHEA-S) is the principal C-19 steroid secreted by the adrenal gland (up to 100 mg/day) (*15*) and the one found in highest concentration in human plasma (Table 15-2). The concentration of DHEA-S in the blood is five to ten times greater than that of cortisol.

DHEA LEVELS IN AGING

Basal plasma levels of cortisone and aldosterone remain relatively unchanged with advance in age, whereas DHEA and DHEA-S levels decrease remarkably. After the second decade of life, the blood level of

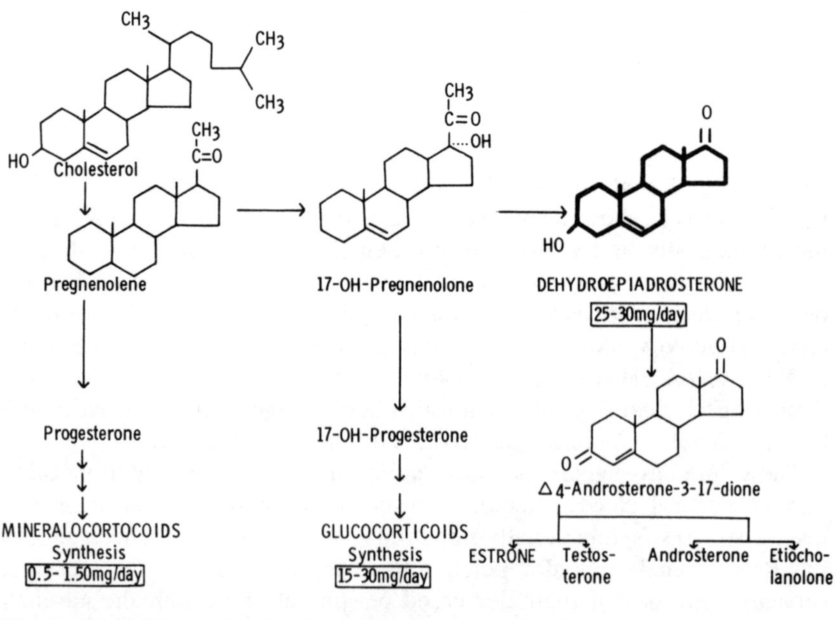

Figure 15-1. Biosynthesis of adrenal hormones.

Table 15-2. Androgens in Human Plasma

Androgen	Serum level (μg/dl)	
	Adult males	Adult females
Testosterone	559 ± 151	48 ± 14
Androstenedione	114 ± 21	180 ± 58
Dehydroepiandrosterone	553 ± 178	534 ± 157
Dihydrotestosterone	50 ± 14	22 ± 4
11-OH-androstenedione	200 ± 80	180 ± 80
Sulfates		
Dehydroepiandrosterone	126 ± 34	113 ± 28
Androsterone	43± 12	36 ± 9
Etiocholanolone	1.5 ± 0.4	1.7 ± 0.6
Testosterone	0.11 ± .05	0.02 ± 0.1
Glucuronides		
Androsterone	2.2 ± 0.6	1.5 ± 0.3
Etiocholanolone	1.8 ± 0.7	1.5 ± 0.5

Source: Adapted from Migeon (*15*).

these steroids begins to decline and, in the very old, reaches levels as low as 5 per cent of the maximum value.

Results from our laboratory (*16*) have shown that urinary excretion of DHEA correlates negatively with age. More recently, we completed a study of serum-level concentrations of DHEA in subjects aged 17 to 65 years. Again we found a negative correlation ($r = -0.28$; $P < .05$) between serum DHEA and age.

DHEA and Aging-Associated Diseases

Even if such processes as cancer, atherosclerosis, and osteoporosis differ from physiological aging, they may offer metabolic and/or endocrine clues to the normal aging process. On the other hand, these entities could represent an end of the normal aging process continuum. For example, Eggen and Solberg (*17*) reported that, among all race groups at 19 different locations, coronary atherosclerosis increased quantitatively as a function of age among persons between ages 20 and 60 years.

The effect of metabolic and environmental factors on aging-related diseases seems to be to reduce the interval (latent period) between the start of the intrinsic biological process of aging and death (*18*).

DHEA in Atherosclerosis

The potential role of the adrenals in atherosclerosis is built on these converging lines of evidence: anecdotal, experimental, and epidemiological.

From the anecdotal and historical points of view, as far back as 1908,

Goldzieher (*19*) called attention to the atrophic cortex and hypertrophic medulla he observed in patients with atherosclerosis.

Geographic (ethnic) and age differences in incidences of atherosclerosis can be explained, according to Kask (*20*), by differences in the urinary excretion of 17-ketosteroids in general and DHEA in particular.

Even more dramatic are the anecdotal reports of the small amounts of atherosclerosis in patients with Achard-Theirs syndrome. This syndrome is characterized by the presence in bearded women of diabetes and hypertension and an extremely high level of DHEA excretion.

From the experimental evidence, Kask (*20*) reported that, after the oral administration of 20 to 25 mg of DHEA daily, a patient's serum cholesterol was reduced by 37 per cent. A reduction of 21 per cent was shown by Ben-David et al. (*21*) after the oral administration of 5 mg/kg/day of DHEA to hypothyroid rats. Robinson et al. (*22*) reported that, after one year of treatment with estrogens, DHEA excretion increased 100 per cent in patients with myocardial infarct whereas no changes were observed in a control group also treated with estrogens.

From the epidemiological point of view, Kolbel et al. (*23*) reported that the serum levels of cholesterol in patients with ischemic heart disease correlated with the amount of DHEA excreted in the urine. Sonka, from the same group, later reported an inverse correlation between serum cholesterol levels and urinary DHEA in a group of 94 healthy blood donors, but this correlation was attributed to the effect of age (*24*).

Our group (*16*) concluded that the correlation between serum cholesterol and urinary DHEA could not be attributed to the effect of age because we found that the partial correlation coefficient between serum cholesterol and urinary DHEA, adjusted for age, was statistically significant. We also found negative but nonsignificant correlations between urinary DHEA level and several of the classical risk factors for coronary heart disease.

Because different factors can affect urinary steroid excretion we also studied the relationship between serum lipid levels plus other risk factors of coronary heart disease and serum concentrations of DHEA. In 92 persons aged 17 to 85 years, we found that, with advancing age, more persons tend to have higher levels of cholesterol and lower levels of DHEA. The product-moment correlation coefficient between the variables studied showed a significant negative correlation between DHEA level and triglyceride, total cholesterol, and beta-cholesterol levels (Table 15-3). When we adjusted for age, the negative correlation with total serum cholesterol persisted, but at a lower level of significance. We concluded that the association of serum levels of DHEA and several of the risk factors for coronary heart disease, mainly cholesterol level, cannot be explained totally by the effect of age, although age plays an important role.

Our group has also found (Table 15-4) that patients with myocardial infarction and controls differed significantly in the serum levels of DHEA, total cholesterol, beta- and pre-beta-cholesterol, and triglycer-

Table 15-3. Pearson Correlation Coefficients (*N*=92) Between Serum DHEA, Age, and Risk Factors for Coronary Heart Disease

	AGE	DHEA	TRI	TCHO	βCHO	HDL	SYS	DIA1	DIA2	BMI
AGE		−.28[a]	.51[a]	.48[a]	.49[a]	.16	.29[a]	.35[a]	.55[a]	.39[a]
DHEA			−.35[a]	−.31[a]	−.30[a]	−.11	.17	−.0004	−.08	−.07
TRIG				.48[a]	.51[a]	.14	.11	.09	.33	.42
TCHOL					.87[a]	.56[a]	.01	.06	.29	.23
CHOL						.11	.02	.08	.29	.32
HDL							−.06	−.02	.11	−.02
SYS								.56[a]	.45[a]	.28[a]
DIA1									.75[a]	.13
DIA2										.20
BMI										

[a]$P < .05$.

ides. All these findings suggest a possible correlation between adrenal androgens, especially DHEA, and atherosclerosis.

DHEA in Cancer

Pitot (*25*) reviewed the similarities and dissimilarities between aging and carcinogenesis and concluded that intrinsic changes of the aging process in individual cells seem to relate to later stages of carcinogenesis. If the assumption is correct, the report by Teller (*26*) becomes pertinent. In experimental animals, Teller showed a relationship between aging and spontaneous tumor incidence. From a ten-year prospective study involving more than 5000 apparently healthy women, Bulbrook et al. (*27*) concluded that women with subnormal excretory rates of androsterone and etiocholanolone had an increased rate of breast cancer. Urinary androsterone and etiocholanolone are derived primarily from adrenal DHEA and subnormal excretory rates of these two steroids reflect low plasma concentrations of DHEA.

Schwartz and Perantoni (*28*) reported that DHEA protects cultured rodent cells against dimethylbenzenanthracene (DMBA) and aflatoxin-B_1

Table 15-4 Correlation of Serum Lipids and DHEA in Myocardial Infarction Patients and Normal Controls

	MI	Controls
DHEA (mg/100ml)	51 ± 21[a]	74 ± 55
T-cholesterol (mg/100 ml)	243 ± 44[a]	182 ± 28
β-Cholesterol (mg/100 ml)	164 ± 30[a]	127 ± 30
HDL-cholesterol (mg/100 ml)	47 ± 9	49 ± 6
Triglycerides (mg/100 ml)	207 ± 119[a]	98 ± 18

[a]$P < .05$.

Table 15-5. DHEA-S in Lung Cancer Patients

	N°	DHEA-S (mg/dl)
Lung cancer patients	42[a]	87.20 ± 76
Hospital controls	42	121.67 ± 76
Nonhospital controls	42	261 ± 170

[a]$P < 0.025$.

induced cytotoxicity and transformation and inhibits the metabolism of [^{3}H]DMBA to water-soluble products. More recently, Schwartz (*29*) reported that long-term DHEA treatment of renal C3H (Avy/a) mice inhibited the formation of spontaneous breast cancer in addition to reducing weight gain.

In our laboratory we have studied the differences in metabolic variables between lung cancer patients and sex, age, and race-matched controls (hospital patients and persons from the general population). We found that patients with lung cancer have significantly lower levels of DHEA than matched controls (Table 15-5).

The fact that DHEA inhibits tumorigenesis in mice and correlates negatively with certain types of cancer in humans suggests an important role for this steroid in the basic mechanism of this age-associated process.

DHEA and Osteoporosis

In 1947, Albright (*30*) coined the terms "adrenarche" and "adrenopause." He noticed that chemicals we now know to be glucocorticoids did not change much with advancing age. However, the level of the hormone he called adrenal cortical N hormone (probably encompassing what we now know as mineral-O-corticoids and adrenal-androgens) decreased with age, and he suspected this was implicated in osteoporosis.

Marshall et al. (*31*), in reporting lower levels of estrone and androstenedione in postmenopausal osteoporotic women, postulated that this reduced sex hormone level may be an important factor in osteoporosis. They also showed that this decrease is present to a considerable degree only in younger osteoporotic patients. These patients show hormone levels comparable to those of older normal women. Whether women who become osteoporotic always had poor adrenal production of sex steroids or whether they are a population that has undergone an early decline in adrenal sex steroids production is unknown. In either case, menopause may be of importance only in uncovering the deficient adrenal activity.

These findings are important because plasma DHEA is a precursor of androstenedione (Fig. 15-1) and both DHEA and androstenedione levels decrease with age in women, even after oophorectomy, indicating a decreased production in the adrenals.

Before menopause, the predominant source of estradiol is the ovary, whereas estrone is derived in almost equal proportions from the ovary and the adrenals. Androstenedione is a precursor of estrone, and the degree of estrogen insufficiency is an important determinant of bone metabolism. Because estrogen status depends on adrenal (androstenedione) status, accelerated bone loss leading to osteoporosis in women below age 60 may be attributable to early adrenopause.

The fact that levels of plasma estrogens are generally higher in men than in post-menopausal women and decline in men at about age 60 may explain why the onset of bone loss occurs later in men than in women.

All these findings suggest an important role for the adrenal glands in general, and especially for DHEA and its metabolites, in the development of osteoporosis.

Universality of DHEA and Aging

Changes and differences in the serum level of DHEA between old and young animals have been reported for mice, rats, monkeys, and humans.

From values reported in the literature, a correlation between the lifespan of animals and their serum levels of DHEA can be seen (Figure 15-2). Interestingly, the life expectancy equivalent calculated from the linear regression equation corresponds to 3.8 μg/dl/year, close to the rate of decline in serum levels of DHEA during the adult years in men, which is about 3.2 μg/dl/year.

The facts that in different animals species serum levels of DHEA generally decrease with advancing age and that DHEA level and life expectancy seem to relate suggests that DHEA has a role in the basic mechanism of aging.

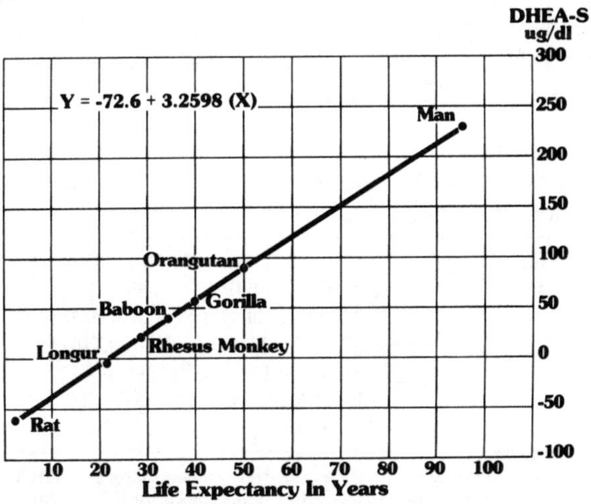

Figure 15-2. Relationship of DHEA-S to life expectancy.

DHEA as a Risk Factor of Aging

Marmorston and collaborators (*32*) reported that urinary steroid concentrations, in addition to serum lipid values, are useful in differentiating the physiological aging process and the pathological aging associated with increased risk of coronary heart disease. They studied 428 persons aged 30 to 60 years and older, including normal persons at high and low risk of coronary heart disease and patients with stabilized diagnoses of myocardial infarction.

Focusing on the relationship between age and the levels of urinary steroids and serum lipids in low-risk subjects, they used multiple linear stepwise regression analysis to select the variables most related to age. With those data they derived an equation that they then used to determine the "age index" of the subjects (Table 15-6).

DHEA was an important component of the equation. They found that the ages calculated by this index were close to the actual ages of the persons under study. The high-risk group was clearly differentiated by their age index from both the low-risk group and the MI group.

These studies show that serum DHEA level (in addition to other variables) can be used as an indicator of physiological aging and as a discriminator of pathological aging.

The first question that needs to be addressed is the mechanism involved in the decreased blood level of DHEA with advancing age. The decline of DHEA levels with age represents not an increase in metabolic clearance but a decrease in production rates. Recently, Parker et al. (*33*) showed a lack of ACTH-responsive adrenocortical reserve of DHEA-S. Their findings could be explained as (a) an age-related loss of adrenal enzymes from the cell populations producing DHEA, (b) a loss or decrease in a subpopulation of ACTH receptors specific for DHEA production, or (c) the loss of a pituitary factor necessary for DHEA-S secretion. In this regard, DHEA-S responds to injected ACTH but not in a dose-response fashion. Available evidence also suggests that a factor other than ACTH seems to be involved in DHEA-S control.

Table 15-6. Marmorston's Formula for Estimation of Aging

Estimated age	=	−0.1243 (log Andr −0.8310)/0.4758
		−0.0166 (log DHEA + 1.1461)/1.2407
		+0.0616 (log 11-OHA + 0.4481)/0.5203
		+0.0733 (log THF − 0.4886)/0.4161
		+0.0468 (log Est − 0.7848)/0.4778
		+0.1853 (log Chol − 5.3425)/0.1486
		+0.0529 (log Tg − 4.4903)/0.3348

Andr = androsterone; DHEA = dehydroepiandrosterone; 11-OHA = 11-Hydrosyandrosterone; THF = tetrahychocortisol; Est = estrogens, Chol = cholesterol; Tg = triglycerides.

Source: After Marmorston et al. (*32*).

Another factor that needs to be studied is the mechanism involved in the reported effects of DHEA and its implication on aging. In 1967 we (*34*) showed that DHEA excretion was reduced in obese persons. More recently, Schwartz (*29*) showed that long-term oral administration of DHEA effectively reduced weight gain and inhibited the formation of spontaneous mammary cancer in C3H (Avy/a) mice. Yen et al. (*35*) showed that DHEA prevented the same type of mice from becoming obese without affecting their food intake, but hepatic lipogenesis was decreased.

The question is, What is the mechanism by which DHEA affects all these processes? Investigators as early as 1960 (*36*) showed that DHEA is an important inhibitor of the enzyme glucose-6-phosphate dehydrogenease (G6PD). In a series of in vivo (*37*) and in vitro (*38*) studies, we showed that not only is DHEA a potent inhibitor of the enzyme G6PD but so are its metabolites, including androstenedione. Through its inhibitory effect, DHEA can regulate the availability of NADPH, which is required for the metabolic activation of carcinogens by mixed-function oxydases, lipid synthesis, and cholesterol synthesis. Through this mechanism, DHEA could also be involved in immunity and DNA regulation. Wang and Mays (*39*) have proposed the concept of altered regulation of G6PD as basic to the aging process. Furthermore, changes in G6PD activity have also been reported in animals and humans on calorie-restricted diets and as a result of increased physical activity.

CONCLUSION

The observations reported here are sufficient to warrant serious consideration of the role of endocrine and metabolic factors in the basic mechanisms of the aging process. The possibility exists that hormones such as DHEA and DECO, in addition to other variables, can be used to estimate risk of physiological aging (senescence) and pathological aging.

REFERENCES

1. C. E. Finch, Neuroendocrine mechanisms and aging, *Fed. Proc.* **38:**178 (1979).
2. H. A. Bertrand, E. J. Masoro, and P. B. Yu, Maintenance of glucagon-promoted lipolysis in adipocytes by food restriction, *Endocrinology* **107:**591 (1980).
3. J. F. Nelson, L. S. Felicio, and C. E. Finch, in *Aging: Its Chemistry* (A. A. Deitz, ed.), 6th ed. American Association of Clinical Chemists, Washington, D.C., 1980.
4. W. C. Chang, M. T. Hooper, and S. G. Roth, Biosynthesis rates of proteins having the characteristics of glucocorticoid receptors in adipocytes of mature and senescent rats, *J. Gerontol.* **36:**386 (1981).
5. M. Green, Aging and disease in clinics, *Endocrinol. Metab.* **10:**207 (1981).

6. A. Comfort, *The Biology of Senescence,* 3rd ed. Churchill Livingston, Edinburgh, 1979.
7. R. H. Weindruch, J. A. Kristle, K. E. Cheney, and R. L. Walford, Influence of controlled dietary restriction on immunological function and aging, *Fed. Proc.* **38:**207 (1979).
8. T. Makinodam, The thymus in aging, in *Geriatric Endocrinology* (R. B. Greenblatt, ed.). Raven Press, New York, 1978.
9. F. M. Burnet, *Immunology Surveillance.* Pergamon, New York, 1970.
10. C.W.H. Havard, The thyroid and aging, *Clin. Endocrinol. Metab.* **10:**163 (1981).
11. W. D. Denckla, Interactions between age and neuroendocrine and immune systems, *Fed. Proc.* **37:**1263 (1978).
12. P. D. Tsitouras, C. E. Martin, and S. M. Harman, Relationship of serum testosterone to sexual activity in healthy elderly men, *J. Geront.* **37:**288 (1982).
13. K. Muta, K. Kato, Y. Akamine, and H. Ibayishi, Age-related changes in the feedback regulation of gonadotropin secretion by sex steroids in men, *Acta Endocrinologica* (Copenhagen) **96:**154 (1981).
14. J. E. Nellor, and E.G.D. Reigle, Physiological and morphological changes in the adrenal gland during aging, *Fed. Proc.* **27:**449 (1968).
15. C. Migeon, Adrenal androgens in man, *Am. J. Med.* **53:**606 (1972).
16. A. Lopez-S, C. H. Wingo, and J. A. Hebert, Total serum cholesterol and urinary dehydroepiandrosterone in humans, *Atherosclerosis* **24:**471 (1976).
17. D. A. Eggen, and L. A. Solberg, Variation of Atherosclerosis with age, *Lab. Invest.* **18:**571 (1968).
18. P.R.J. Burch, Coronary heart disease: Risk factors and aging, *Gerontology* **24:**123 (1978).
19. M. A. Goldzieher, *The Adrenals.* Macmillin, New York, 1929.
20. E. Kask, 17-ketosteroids and arteriosclerosis, *Angiology* **10:**358 (1959).
21. M. Ben-David, S. Kikstein, G. Bismurth, and F. G. Sulman, Antihypocholesterolemic effect of dehydroepiandrosterone in rats, *Proc. Soc. Exp. Biol. Med.* **125:**1136 (1967).
22. R. W. Robinson, N. Higano, W. D. Cohen, R. C. Sniffen, and J. W. Sherer, Jr., Effects of estrogen therapy on hormonal functions and serum lipids in men with coronary atherosclerosis, *Circulation* **14:**365 (1956).
23. F. Kolbel, J. Gregorova, and J. Sonka, Hyperuricemia and ischemic heart disease, *Cor et vasa* **9:**11 (1967).
24. J. Sonka, M. Fassati, P. Fassati, I. Gregorova, and K. Picek, Serum lipids and dehydroepiandrosterone excretion in normal subjects, *J. Lipid Res.* **9:**768 (1968).
25. H. C. Pitot, Interactions in the natural history of aging and carcinogenesis, *Fed. Proc.* **37:**2841 (1978).
26. M. N. Teller, Interrelationships among aging, immunity and cancer, in *Tolerance, Autoimmunity and Aging* (M. M. Siegel, and R. A. Good, eds.). Charles C Thomas, Springfield, Ill., 1972.
27. R. D. Bulbrook, J. L. Hayward, and C. C. Spicer, Relation between urinary androgen and corticoid excretion and subsequent breast cancer, *Lancet* **2:**395 (1971).
28. A. G. Schwartz and A. Perantoni, Protective effect of dehydroepiandroster-

one against aflatoxin B_1 and 7,12-dimethylbenza (a) anthracene-induced cytotoxicity and transformation in cultured cells, *Cancer Res.* **35:**2482 (1975).
29. A. G. Schwartz, Inhibition of spontaneous breast cancer formation in female C3H (Avy/a) mice by long-term treatment with dehydroepiandrosterone, *Cancer Res.* **39:**1129 (1979).
30. F. Albright, Osteoporosis, *Ann. Int. Med.* **27:**861 (1947).
31. D. H. Marshall, R. G. Crilly, and B.E.C. Nordin, The relation between plasma androstenedione and oestrone levels in untreated and corticosteroid-treated post-menopausal women, *Clin. Endocrinol.* **9:**407 (1978).
32. J. Marmorston, G. C. Griffith, P. J. Geller, E. L. Fisherman, P. Welsch, and J. M. Weiner, Urinary steroids in the measurement of aging and of atherosclerosis, *J. Am. Geriatrics Soc.* **23:**481 (1975).
33. L. Parker, T. Gral, V. Perrigo, and R. Skowsky, Decreased adrenal androgen sensitivity to ACTA during aging, *Metab. Clin. Exp.* **30:**601 (1981).
34. A. Lopez-S and W. A Krehl, A possible interrelationship between glucose-6-phosphate dehydrogenase and dehydroepiandrosterone in obesity, *Lancet* **2:**485 (1967).
35. T. T. Yen, J. A. Allan, D. V. Pearson, J. M. Acton, and M. M. Greenberg, Prevention of obesity in Avy/a mice by dehydroepiandrosterone, *Lipids* **12:**409 (1977).
36. P. A. Marks and J. Banks, Inhibition of mammalian glucose-6-phosphate dehydrogenase by steroids, *Proc. Nat. Acad. Sci. USA* **46:**447 (1960).
37. A. Lopez-S and W. A. Krehl, In vivo effect of dehydroepiandrosterone in red blood cells on glucose-6-phosphate dehydrogenase, *Proc. Soc. Exp. Biol. Med.* **126:**776 (1967).
38. A. Lopez-S and A. Rene, Effect of 17-ketosteroids on glucose-6-phosphate activity (G6PD) and G6PD isoenzymes, *Proc. Soc. Exp. Biol. Med.* **142:**258 (1973).
39. R.K.J. Wang and L. L. Mays, Opposite changes in rat liver glucose-6-phosphate dehydrogenase during aging in Sprague-Dawley and Fisher 344 male rats, *Exp. Gerontol.* **12:**117 (1977).

16 Risk Factors of Senescent Sexual Adjustment

David M. Schnarch

Senescent sexuality reflects an attempt to integrate lifelong emotional needs, physiological changes, long-term attitudinal shaping, and changing life circumstances. For instance, the same performance pressure that leads some people to more sexual activity than is truly desired during midlife also leads others to less sexual contact than is truly desired in later years. Physiological, psychological, and social factors specific to later adult life encourage or discourage the nature and frequency of sexual behavior, as was true during early development. This chapter highlights those factors most relevant to senescent sexual adjustment and underscores areas worthy of further attention to maximize the dignity, richness, and fulfillment of adults in their final years.

PHYSIOLOGICAL RISK FACTORS

Hormonal Changes

Physiological changes are often assumed to be the major determinant of sexual activity patterns in advanced years of life. Ovarian estrogen and progesterone decrease markedly in women after menopause (*1*). Such changes are thought to underlie vasomotor instability (hot flashes, sweating, chills), vaginal atrophy, and emotional lability. The relationship between estrogen level and physiological functioning has been studied only recently (*2*). Post-menopausal women demonstrated decreased perivaginal blood flow, decreased quantity and modified electrolytic content of vaginal secretions, and elevated vaginal pH values. Estrogen replacement therapy significantly improved perivaginal blood flow and quantity of vaginal secretions, and it reduced vaginal pH to a more normal acidic range. The relative risks and benefits of estrogen replacement treatment are still a matter of controversy, however.

The relationship between hormonal changes in women and their overall response to cessation of menstruation is not as certain as was once assumed. From an evaluation of 152 women between the ages of 51 and 80, Weg (*3*) concluded:

> It has become increasingly evident that the psyche plays a part at least equal to, if not greater than, that of an unbalanced endocrine system in determining the sex drive of women during the postmenopausal period of their lives. If endocrine factors alone were responsible for sexual behavior in postmenopausal women (whether menopause occurs by surgical or natural means), there should be a relatively uniform response to the physiologic diminution and ultimate withdrawal of the sex hormones. However, there is no established reaction pattern to sex-steroid withdrawal.

Women whose sole function and role was mother or housewife report more distress than women who have developed additional roles for themselves through careers or outside interests (*3*). Similarly, women who believe sexuality is inseparable from reproduction may experience a more negative impact of menopause on their sexual functioning. Although incidence of dyspareunia generally increases with age-related decreases in vaginal lubrication, this phenomenon is idiosyncratic (*4*). Estimates of the intensity and frequency of complaints in the general population depend largely on the nature of inquiry. In studies specifically devoted to menopause adjustment, the frequency of complaints among women was triple that found in general health screening programs (*2*). The reason for this difference is open to speculation. In any event, there is no consistent correlation between a woman's reproductive capacity and her sexual functioning, sexual satisfaction, or capacity for orgasms.

Kolodny et al. (*5*) report that a small group of men over age 60 manifest a "male climacteric" syndrome. Such men have subnormal plasma testosterone levels and such symptoms as listlessness, weight loss, depressed libido and reduced potency, impaired concentration, weakness and instability, and these symptoms improve markedly with testosterone replacement therapy. However, these symptoms can also result from depression, severe chronic anemia, or gastrointestinal malignancy. The need for testosterone replacement therapy must be demonstrated empirically through blood analysis before it is attempted since it also presents increased risk of prostatic cancer.

The effect of testosterone reduction on sexual behavior, interest, and erectile functioning is not clear. A general reduction in plasma testosterone is noted with increased frequency in men after age 50 (*6*). However, the age of onset of reduced testosterone production varies considerably. Moreover, elderly men reporting reduced sex drive or reduced erectile ability do not always have lower testosterone levels than similarly aged men with no impairment (*7*). Testosterone replacement has also achieved ambiguous results in restoring erectile functioning in men having low testosterone levels (*8*). As with women, hormonal changes among elderly men may not be as great a risk factor to sexual adjustment as is commonly believed.

Tissue Responsiveness to Stimulation

Since the research of Masters and Johnson (*6*) on sexual response patterns of women and men over age 50 has been widely reported in the last 16 years, it will be mentioned only briefly here. Those investigators noted that, in persons over 50, nipple erection remained relatively intact, although breast engorgement decreased somewhat in women. Rectal sphincter contraction during orgasm were less common in elderly men and women than in younger subjects, and this may account for subjective reports of reduced orgasmic intensity among the aged. A relatively lower level of general muscle tension elevation in response to sexual stimulation was also noted among elderly subjects.

Post-menopausal women demonstrated reduced elevation, separation, and flattening of the labia majora, as well as reduced vasocongestive swelling of the labia minora. Preorgasmic color changes of the labia also progressively diminished with age. The walls of the vagina became thinner, less corrugated, and lighter in color as age increased. Reductions in vaginal length, width, and elasticity, as well as the amount and speed of vaginal lubrication, were noted. However, vasocongestive engorgement of the clitoral shaft and retraction of the clitoral shaft and glands during heightened sexual arousal remained unchanged with advanced age. These age-related changes in physiological response to sexual stimulation do not necessarily present a threat to sexual functioning in aging women, particularly if rapid coital coupling is not attempted. "Aging does not decrease libido or capacity to be orgasmic for women if general health is good" (*5*). For some women, sexual satisfaction and disinhibition improve in their later years.

Kolodny and associates (*5*) also report that, as in women, the physiological effects of aging in men caused a slowing down of the response pattern rather than a radical loss of functioning. As men aged, latency for penile tumescence increased two to six times over that observed during youth. More direct stimulation to the penile glands tended to be required for tumescence, and full erection was sometimes not experienced until immediately before ejaculation. When detumescence occurred before ejaculation, elderly men had more difficulty than younger men in regaining erection. The amount of stimulation required for ejaculation increased with age (often a benefit to men who experienced difficulties with premature ejaculation in their youth), and elevation of the testes before ejaculation decreased. Subjective intensity of the ejaculation was reduced, as was the volume of ejaculate. Aged men often experienced less physical imperative to ejaculate, and many men in their seventh and eighth decades found intercourse stimulating and satisfying without ejaculation at each coital opportunity. After ejaculation, the rapidity of detumescence increased and the period necessary to achieve another erection often extended to 24 hours or longer (*9*).

"It can be said with confidence that impotency is never a consequence of chronological age alone" (*10*). Loss of sexual functioning or interest among the aged is not attributable to an inevitable loss of physiological responsiveness. Rather, it is the result of other medical and social problems common to the elderly.

Risks from Age-Frequent Medical Illness

Relatively few of the illnesses that become increasingly common with advanced age present a direct threat to sexual functioning. The challenge to sexual adjustment is more indirect—through depression, self-fulfilling fears of lost performance or satisfaction, loss of general health, iatrogenic dyfunctions from medication, and decreased availability of an interested or interesting partner.

Diabetes mellitus is probably the preponderant age-frequent illness presenting a direct physiological challenge to sexual functioning. Current wisdom suggests that 50 per cent of diabetic men experience some impairment in erectile response. It is unclear whether this impairment results from peripheral neuropathy or vascular insufficiency associated with diabetes. Although the incidence of erectile dysfunction increases with age among diabetic men above 60, it is not certain whether age or duration of illness is the crucial variable (*11*). There is no physiological basis for impaired orgasmic capacity or libido in diabetic men, although retrograde ejaculation may be experienced by 1 or 2 per cent (*5*). The arousal potential, orgasmic capacity, and libidinal drive of diabetic women is also undisturbed by the disease (*5,12*). Psychological distress in respone to diabetes is usually present, and sexual counseling can often relieve anxiety and improve sexual functioning and satisfaction (*13*). It should never be assumed that the diagnosis of diabetes establishes a physiological basis for sexual dysfunction. Persons with diabetes are just as susceptible (if not more so) as nondiabetics to sexual problems of psychogenic etiology.

Similarly, the impact of *prostatectomy* involves a complex interaction of physiological and psychological factors. The transurethral prostatectomy offers the least risk to sexual functioning since nerve fibers that control erection and blood flow to the penis are not disrupted. Only 5 per cent of men undergoing the transurethral procedure later report erectile dysfunction. Suprapubic and retropubic surgical approaches to prostatectomy yield impaired erectile functioning in 10 to 20 per cent of such cases. Most post-operative cases of erectile dysfunction from these three methods are thought to be primarily psychogenic. Fear, ignorance, emotional reaction to ejaculatory changes, and avoidance of sexual performance demands are common psychological sources of dysfunction. Since retrograde ejaculation is experienced by 80 to 90 per cent of prostatectomy patients, psychological counseling around this change in functioning is likely to forestall untoward emotional response (*14*). The perineal procedure, more likely associated with radical surgical intervention for prostatic cancer, offers greater risk with 98 per cent of men reporting erectile difficulties (*5*). The greater incidence of dysfunction associated with this procedure is attributed to disruption of neurological functioning.

A comparative study of patients undergoing transurethral procedures highlighted the importance of psychological factors in later sexual functioning (*13*). Not one of the transurethral patients who received post-operative sexual counseling experienced erectile difficulties, whereas 62 per cent of similar patients who did not receive counseling experienced loss of erection and an additional 25 per cent experienced increased erectile difficulty. Although this complication rate is higher than usually reported for this procedure, this study illustrates that psychological causes must not be dismissed in situations that offer ready physiological explanations.

Similar patterns are evident among women undergoing *hysterectomy and oophorectomy*. Various studies report subsequent decreases in sexual activity of 10 to 40 per cent. Such decreases were highly correlated with the patient's negative expectations for post-operative adjustment. Reduction of endogenous estrogen from hysterectomy does not present a physiological challenge to sexual functioning, except indirectly through increased incidence of dyspareunia and infection secondary to vaginal atrophy. Although estrogen supplementation often ameliorates these complications, it does not directly increase sexual desire or enjoyment (*15*). Other studies indicate that some women report increased sexual activity and enjoyment after hysterectomy (*5*). Sexual counseling or therapy is often the approach of choice in cases of reduced sexual desire after surgical intervention. A study of women undergoing treatment for *gynecologic cancer* found that 84 per cent of patients who received two hours of sexual counseling returned to previous or higher levels of sexual functioning, compared with 43 per cent of uncounseled patients (*16*). The fact that 70 per cent of counseled patients returned to work in the following year, compared with only 36 per cent of uncounseled patients (although work was never discussed in the brief sex counseling sessions), presents a compelling cost-effective argument for inclusion of sexual counseling for optimal rehabilitation. It is necessary to obtain a thorough preoperative sexual history in order to assess the response to surgical procedures. Persons who previously were sexually active out of obligation rather than desire may seize upon the surgical intervention to avoid further sexual involvement.

Several other common illnesses and/or their treatment can indirectly disrupt sexual adjustment. In *breast cancer* and subsequent *mastectomy*, sexual complications stem from attendent depression and avoidance of sexual contact. Changes in body shape from surgical procedures, as well as hair loss from radiation and chemotherapy, may further decrease feelings of sexual desirability and desire. The impact of such procedures on the sexual adjustment of mastectomy patients and their partners is highly variable and more related to their expectations than to the severity of the illness. Husbands' negative reactions to their wives' mastectomies are strongly inversely correlated with the previous level of marital satisfaction (*17*).

The effects of *stroke* on sexual adjustment have not been well studied, and the little research to date has been conducted on patients under the age of 60. Existing data indicate that most stroke patients maintain an interest in sexual activity (*18*). However, reduced sexual contact due to their partner's concern about precipitating further neurological damage often occurs. Diminished libido is occasionally noted in dominant hemisphere impairment, and neurologically induced erectile, ejaculatory, or orgasmic difficulties are possible. However, these are relatively rare sequelae. Mechanical, emotional, and communication problems are the most common source of sexual difficulties (*5*). Concomitant drug treatment of hypertension or depression in stroke patients can impair sexual functioning or desire.

Similarly, the major sexual sequelae from *myocardial infarction,* decreased sexual desire and erectile dysfunction, stem from ignorance, anxiety, avoidance, depression, and poor self-esteem (*5*). Side effects of chemotherapy must be monitored as well. Studies of heart attack patients often indicate significant reductions in sexual behavior that are uncorrelated with age or severity of the attack. Many patients who have adequate work capacity or who otherwise resume normal activities fail to reinstitute sexual contact (*19,20*). In the absence of specific counseling, patients determine their sexual behavior in keeping with their limited knowledge, fears, and superstitions (*20*).

Arthritis may present mechanical barriers to sexual activity, and some related syndromes (e.g., Sjogren's syndrome) can create reduced mucosal secretions, oral or genital ulcers, aesthetic concerns, and body image conflicts. *Chronic pain syndrome* often intensifies at night, when partner availability is greatest, and remits during early morning, when partner availability is often problematic. Depression, irritability, and pain may distract and inhibit sensate focusing and consequently diminish sexual gratification.

Since psychological reaction and drug side effects account for most of the sexual response to the syndromes discussed thus far, the potential for amelioration of these risk factors to sexual adjustment is significant. The need for rapid intervention in the sexual component of the convalescent process is highlighted in the catch phrase "use it or lose it." *Disuse atrophy,* common to many body functions, is a particular problem for geriatric sexuality. It is vital that sexual sequelae of medical illness receive prompt attention and intervention. Common urinary infections, to which elderly females are particularly predisposed due to vaginal changes after menopause, can cause dyspareunia and lead to sexual withdrawal. Prolonged abstention from sexual intercourse imposes a greater threat to maintaining genital functioning at senescence than during youth. Men who abstain from intercourse often experience erectile difficulties when attempts at coitus are resumed. Women who abstain experience greater vaginal shrinkage than comparably aged women who remain coitally active. Masturbation appears to maintain vaginal lubricative response in women. However, it does not mitigate vaginal shrinkage or maintain a man's erectile response during coitus (*5*). Frequent vaginal containment of a phallus or reasonable substitute appears to preserve continued vaginal elasticity.

PSYCHOLOGICAL RISK FACTORS

As noted in the discussion of physiological risk factors, a person's psychological reaction to natural and pathological physiological changes profoundly affects his or her sexuality:

> Human behavior, be it sexual or otherwise, is influenced by interactions between physiological state, physical and social environment, an individual's personal learning history, the psychological meaning one attaches to one's experiences, and the immediate situation. Human *sexual* behavior, because of the powerful role it plays in the lives of most people, is particularly susceptible to the influence of these factors.(*8*)

Sexual Ignorance and Misinformation

Public school sex education did not become a local option in all 50 states until 1980. Many of today's senior citizens grew up in an era in which sex was not a topic for public (or private) discussion. Those who depend solely on personal experimentation and the popular media to learn about sexuality (as most of us do) are at a disadvantage when confronted with realistic situations of adult life.

Ignorance of normal changes in sexual response due to advancing age is widespread. Comfort (*10*) has pointed out that "men whose stereotype of virility depends upon hurried erection followed by hurried intercourse may interpret these changes as a loss of function, and the consequent anxiety may induce failure of erection." Retarded ejaculation, inhibited sexual desire, avoidance of intimacy, and depression are also possible difficulties that ignorance can yield if an older man expects to become erect as rapidly as he did at age 18 (assuming he experienced no sexual difficulty at that time). Men who considered themselves sexual athletes in their youth often compete with their own earlier prowess, to the detriment of their performance and satisfaction in later life. Women and men who are unaware of healthy, age-related changes in sexual response in both sexes place unrealistic performance pressure on themselves and their partners. Couples who have restricted female sexual participation to passive roles may have difficulty tolerating or providing the increased direct penile stimulation an aging man requires to establish or maintain an erection.

Widespread *ignorance of the sexual behavior and sexual interest of elderly people* is also potentially debilitating. In seven years' experience as a sex therapist, I have yet to have patients request help to make them sexually satisfied; they request help to make them "normal." Historically, men and women have always been willing to modify their sexual behavior and preferences to conform to the prevailing "normality" of the times. In the absence of knowledge about sexuality in advanced age, many persons today assume abstinence to be the norm. Although inaccurate, such expectations become self-fulfilling prophecies.

Society assumes that the elderly are not sexually active because they do not generally volunteer information to the contrary. In truth, research data collected over decades indicate that more than half of married couples over 60 remain coitally active (*6*). There is a general reduction in coital behavior as age increases, although the point at which this pattern begins is not clear. Some investigations suggest that coital frequency begins to decline in the early 20s, with relative frequency patterns established in early adulthood continuing in later years. Other studies support the finding that coital frequency declines considerably in the middle of the seventh decade (*8*).

Research suggests that, although sexual activity may decrease with advanced age, sexual interest does not (*21*). About 50 per cent of men in their 80s and 90s report continued sexual interest, although an increasing gap between frequency of interest and continued sexual behavior is noted after age 50. Masturbation is reported by about 25 per cent of men even into the 80s and 90s (*8*), and about 20 per cent of men in this group report continued coital activity (*22*). Generally fewer women report continued sexual interest than do men, with only about a third of women over age 60 reporting interest, compared with three quarters of men. Women show less gap between interest and behavior than do men. Women's interest level, albeit lower than that reported by men, tends to remain stable over time (*23*).

There are several explanations for gender differences in report of sexual interest. Men may give overly optimistic reports because of perceived social pressure to express continued interest. Societal gender roles that link masculinity wth unflagging sexual interest may well outweigh social pressure to deny sexual interest in old age. Analogous female gender role pressures may cause women to understate their sexual interest.

The reasons married couples cease coital activity may further clarify gender differences in sexual interest. The central importance of an interested and interesting partner to continued sexual activity has been stressed before (*5*). A study of 241 women and 261 men over age 45 revealed that women who were married but not coitally active attributed this pattern to their husband's decisions (*24*). Such decisions were attributed to the husband's lack of interest, erectile difficulties, or poor health. It is noteworthy that 71 per cent of the men who ceased coital activity attributed this pattern to their own decision, which was based on lack of interest, erectile difficulties, or poor health. Implicit in this pattern is the possibility that these women were more sexually interested than their male partners but their sexual behavior was determined by male preference.

Most investigations of sexual interest during later life have relied upon direct reports, as well as reports of sexual thoughts, dreams, and fantasies. However, these are all basically self-report data. Mager (*4*) suggested that attitudinal interest is more accurately assessed by the approach or avoidance of specific behavior than by self-report. Male sexual interest may actually be equivalent to, or perhaps below, that of females as age advances and male erectile performance declines. Men may tend to present themselves as more sexually interested than in fact they are and thus may report more sexual interest than do women when asked. Frustration in the bedroom and male bravado in the living room may actually contribute to reduced interest among women.

Marital status has minor impact on male sexual behavior and interest, but unmarried women report negligible frequency of sexual contact (*22*). Men may enjoy relatively stable availability of partners due to the male/female mortality differential and may secure willing partners outside marriage. Some men report increased sexual contact in their geriatric years. Whereas in some cases increased coital activity may reflect improved physical health in later life, it more commonly indicates the lessening of sexual inhibitions, reconciliation with life goals, economic success, and the increased availability of time, a partner, and a suitable social setting.

Increased geriatric male sexual activity may also reflect increased relative desirability among the remaining pool of available men. The reported decline in female sexual behavior and interest may indicate that unmarried women are unable to secure partners in the increased competition for men, are unable to do so within the context of a desired commitment to a relationship, or are unwilling to settle for less desirable partners than they were previously able to attract. In any of these possible situations, declining female sexual interest may reflect a self-protective disinvestment from an unsatisfying situation.

What can be done to maintain sexual interest and behavior among women? It has been suggested that the best way to maintain female sexual interest and behavior in senescence is to increase the life-span and sexual vigor of more men (*23*). Alternatively, since neither male longevity nor potency is likely to increase in the near future, efforts to reduce destructive social attitudes that encourage men to abandon sexual activity because of reduced erectile functioning may increase the number of interested and interesting sexual partners available to women.

Previous sexual experience is another important determinant of senescent sexual behavior. Sexual interest and behavior among elderly men correlate highly with levels of interest and behavior during earlier years. In contrast to sexual mythology, which suggests that sexual potency is finite and requires rationing to preserve functional abilities in later life, utilization tends to maintain later involvement. Among elderly women, sexual behavior and interest are highly related to previous enjoyment of sexual activity, but independent of earlier levels of such activity (*22*). Women who previously engaged in obligatory sexual behavior may seek refuge in societal prescriptions of diminished geriatric sexual activity, whereas women whose behavior was motivated out of desire may feel increasing freedom to express and explore their sexuality as older adults.

Physical and emotional health also affect sexual patterns in the elderly. The frequency of intercourse is correlated with physical health. However, sexual interest and enjoyment are more related to subjective assessment of health and feelings of well-being (*23*).

Social Attitudes and Stereotypes

In ways analogous to societal ignorance, social attitudes and stereotypes are a potential threat to satisfying adjustment in later life. Butler and Lewis (*14*) outline several common social attitudes that inhibit recognition of sexual potential in later life:

Old people have no sexual desires.
They couldn't make love even if they wanted to.
They are too fragile physically, and it might hurt them.
They are physically unattractive and therefore sexually undesirable.
The whole notion is shameful and decidedly perverse.

Implicit in these attitudes is a pervasive societal *preoccupation with sexual performance and body functioning.* As breasts and erections tend to be less statuesque, men and women withdraw from the sexual arena. Those who felt they were not among the top contenders in their youth often drop out early in the competition. Preoccupation with sexual performance is so pervasive that it is fairly common for persons to place performance ahead of sexual satisfaction. A number of geriatiric men who seek treatment for erectile difficulties actually have struggled for years with premature ejaculation. Common attempts to increase ejaculatory latency by reducing or abandoning foreplay and distracting themselves during coitus can culminate in erectile difficulty as a man's need for stimulation to achieve an erection increases in later life.

Views of the function of sexuality that focus on specific behavior rather than on the needs that motivate it further threaten healthy senescent sexuality. Many (if not most) adults equate sex with intercourse and use the two words interchangeably. Self-image of being "sexually active" is frequently totally dependent on sexual activity with a partner. People who engage in self-stimulation are usually described in negative terms, and such attitudes perpetuate reduced sexual satisfaction and the myth of sexless senescence.

As a society, we ignore the nongenital aims of sexuality and intimacy, which motivate behavior in young and old alike. These include

A sense of belonging and relatedness
Familiarity and recognition
Repetition, linking the past with hope for the future
Maintaining identity, permanence, and timelessness
Sharing emotion, including the capacity to give pleasure and worthiness to receive it
Exercise
Recreation and escape from boredom and loneliness (*17*)

These motives exist from womb to tomb and are undiminished by changes in marital, employment, or reproductive status.

Societal prohibitions are subtly but powerfully transmitted in sexual humor about the elderly, which predominantly focuses on diminished sexual performance or the inappropriateness of sexual prowess or interest.

Lack of Early Intervention

It is little wonder that the elderly develop self-rejecting attitudes that preclude sexual behavior or diminish sexual satisfaction. The *absence of lifelong sex education and sexual attitude clarification* facilitates the perpetuation of destructive sexual ignorance and debilitating stereotypes. Educating the elderly may help, but long-held attitudes toward geriatric sex are resistant to modification. Each generation eventually falls victim to the antigeriatric biases directed to the preceding generation. Knowledge of age-related changes in sexual response and behavior patterns is needed during young adulthood if it is to be appreciated and utilized in senescence. Sex education in the home and recognition of parents' and grandparents' sexual potential might be powerful role models for children. Recognition that sexual attitudes that were workable and appropriate for age 13 might not be so at age 30 would facilitate flexibility in expressing sexuality at age 80.

Inattention to early warning signs of sexual maladjustment, often mistakenly accepted as age-appropriate behavior, is another risk factor. These warning signs include extreme possessiveness, avoidance of opportunities for closeness and affection, social withdrawal, embarrassment and shame, anger at "sexy senior citizens," sexual acting out, and depression (*22*). The difficulty of resuming sexual functioning after prolonged abstinence necessitates timely intervention in the sexual concerns of the elderly.

Active Suppression and Benign Neglect of Senescent Needs

Many children do not believe that their parents are sexually active. When parents reach senescence, their children's denial resurfaces as a demand that parents conform to a nonsexual image. This expectation is particularly strong when a parent is not married or when the children have custodial responsibility for the parent. Perhaps it is ironic retribution for past parental attempts to inhibit adolescent sexuality when the circumstances were reversed.

Health care facilities and religious institutions often ignore or inhibit the sexual needs of the elderly. Physical structure, lack of privacy, scheduling of activities, and administrative procedures in nursing facilities can be unintentional or purposeful barriers to maintaining physical and emotional intimacy. Silence from religious representatives can be as powerful a prohibition of sexuality as silence from parents during childhood. Religious beliefs often become increasingly meaningful in the later years of life. Thus, the clergy have a unique opportunity to facilitate healthy sexual adjustment. Masturbatory prohibitions, originally aimed at facilitating reproduction and discouraging avoidance of the conjungal relationship, may not be appropriate for the elderly who lack partners or do not desire them.

CONCLUSION

Avoidance of sexual discussion by physicians and other health professionals is a significant risk to geriatric sexual adjustment. Patients with age-related diseases often receive no counseling for commonly observed sexual sequelae. Two thirds of a sample of men recuperating from myocardial infarcts reported receiving no sexual counseling, and the remaining third reported receiving vague and nonspecific advice. Two thirds of this sample had reduced coital activity to half their previous level, and such reductions were unrelated to physical ability (*25*). Another study of post-coronary males found 30 per cent to have erectile difficulty (*26*). Health care providers cannot rely on the guidelines of "when indicated" for raising the topic of sexuality because personal attitudes about who and what is sexual interfere with this judgment. Physicians are products of the current society and thus subject to prevalent biases about sexuality. Relying on patients to ask questions pertaining to sexuality is impractical, since most will not. Patients rely on physicians to indicate when questions on sexual concerns or interest are appropriate. Waiting for the patient to ask places the burden on the person with the lesser knowledge to ask the right question in the right way at the right time.

REFERENCES

1. S. E. Monroe and K.M.J. Menon, Changes in reproductive hormone secretion during the climacteric and postmenopausal periods, *Clin. Obstet. Gynec.* **20:**113 (1977).
2. G. Wagner and J. P. Semmens, Vaginal function (blood flow, fluid, pH, and electropotential) in postmenopausal women before and during estrogen substitution: A pilot study, *Excerpta Medica,* in press.
3. R. B. Weg, The physiology of sexuality in aging, in *Sexuality and Aging* (R. L. Solnick, ed.) University of Southern California Press, Los Angeles, 1978.

4. R. F. Mager, *Developing Attitudes Toward Learning.* Pitman, Belmont, Calif., 1972.
5. R. C. Kolodny, W. H. Masters, and V. E. Johnson, *Textbook of Sexual Medicine.* Little Brown, Boston, 1979.
6. W. H. Masters, and V. E. Johnson, *Human Sexual Response.* Little Brown, Boston, 1966.
7. D. G. Bartuska, Physiology of aging: Metabolic changes during the climacteric and menopausal periods, *Clin. Obstet. Gynec.* **20:**105 (1977).
8. J. Raboch, J. Mellam, and L. Starka, Plasma testosterone in male patients with sexual dysfunctions, *Arch. Sexual Behav.* **4:**541 (1971).
9. N. Corby and R. Solnick, Psychological and physiological influences on sexuality in the older adult, in *Handbook of Mental Health and Aging* (J. E. Burden and R. B. Sloane, eds.). Prentice-Hall, Englewood Cliffs, N.J., 1980.
10. A. Comfort, Sexuality in later life, in *Handbook of Mental Health and Aging* (J. E. Burden and R. B. Sloane, eds.). Prentice-Hall, Englewood Cliffs, N.J., 1980.
11. R. L. Braddom, J. B. Hollis, and D. O. Castell, Diabetic peripheral neuropathy: A correlation of nerve conduction studies and clinical findings, *Arch. Physical Med. Rehab.* **58:**308 (1977).
12. M. Ellenberg, Lack of effect of diabetes on sexual function of females, *Med. Aspects Human Sexuality* **15:**109 (1981).
13. J. Zohar, D. Meiraz, and N. Durst, Factors influencing sexual activity after prostatectomy: A prospective study, *J. Urol.* **116:**332 (1976).
14. R. I. Bulter, and M. I. Lewis, *Aging and Mental Health: Positive Psychological Approaches.* Mosby, St. Louis, 1973.
15. L. Dennerstein, C. Wood, and G. D. Burrows, Sexual response following hysterectomy and oophorectomy, *Obstet. Gynecol.* **13:**97 (1975).
16. M. A. Capone, R. S. Good, K. S. Westie, and A. F. Jackson, Psychosocial rehabilitation of geneological oncology patients, *Arch. Physical Med. Rehab.* **61:**128 (1980).
17. D. K. Wellisch, K. R. Jamison, and R. O. Pasnau, Psychosocial aspects of mastectomy: II. The man's perspective, *Am. J. Psychiatry* **135:**543 (1978).
18. A. B. Ford, and A. P. Orfifer, Sexual behavior and the chronically ill patient, *Med. Aspects Human Sexuality* **1:**51 (1967).
19. A. Bloch, J. Maeder, and J. Haissly, Sexual problems after myocardial infarction, *Am. Heart J.* **90:**536 (1975).
20. W. B. Tuttle, W. L. Cook, and F. Fitch, Sexual behavior in postmyocardial infarction patients, *Am. J. Cardiol.* **13:**140 (1964).
21. J. T. Freeman, Sexual capacities in the aging male, *Geriatrics* **16:**37 (1961).
22. A. Verwoerdt, *Clinical Geropsychiatry,* 2nd edn. William & Wilkins, Baltimore, 1981.
23. E. Pfeiffer, and G. C. Davie, Determinants of sexual behavior in middle and old age, *J. Am. Geriatrics Soc.* **20:**151 (1972).
24. E. Pfeiffer, A. Verwoerdt, and G. C. Davis, Sexual behavior in middle life, *Am. J. Psychiatry* **128:**1262 (1972).
25. W. B. Tuttle, W. L. Cook, and E. Fitch, Sexual behavior in postmyocardial infarction patients, *Am. J. Cardiol.* **13:**140 (1964).
26. E. Weiss, and O. S. English, *Psychosomatic Medicine,* 3rd edn. Saunders, Philadelphia, 1957, p. 216.

17 Risk Factors and Aging

Leonard Hayflick

The risk factors for senility, like those for other chronic pathologies of the elderly, result from the effects of time on cell function. Yet time alone does not produce functional decrements in cells. For example, we have arrested normal human cells at subzero temperatures for decades with no observable time-dependent effect on their functional ability (*1*). Yet, when these cells are reconstituted and permitted to function in vitro, they, like their unfrozen ancestors, incur over 100 biological decrements as they age. Many of these decrements are characteristic of aging human cells in vivo (*2*).

In order to consider the risk factors for any age-associated chronic disease, it is important to recognize the fact that aging, in its extreme manifestations, occurs only in the human species. On the evolutionary scale, it has been extended only recently to include the domestic and zoo animals that man has chosen to protect. Feral animals do not exhibit aging changes because, soon after sexual maturation, their normal age-associated physiological decrements quickly increase their vulnerability to predators and disease. When feral animals run less fast, leap less high, or see less well, they become easier prey for predators. When their immune system incurs decrements soon after sexual maturation, their vulnerability to disease and pathology increases. It is for these reasons that old animals rarely survive under natural conditions. In fact, aging even in humans is a relatively new phenomenon, at least in respect to the proportion of the total population that it affects.

In very recent evolutionary times, humans essentially have eliminated their animal predators. Within the past century, we have discovered how to eliminate virtually all causes of death attributable to diseases that occur in the early years. These deaths were caused substantially by accidents and infectious diseases. Figure 17-1 shows that the increase in life expectation at birth in the United States that has occurred in the last 80 years is

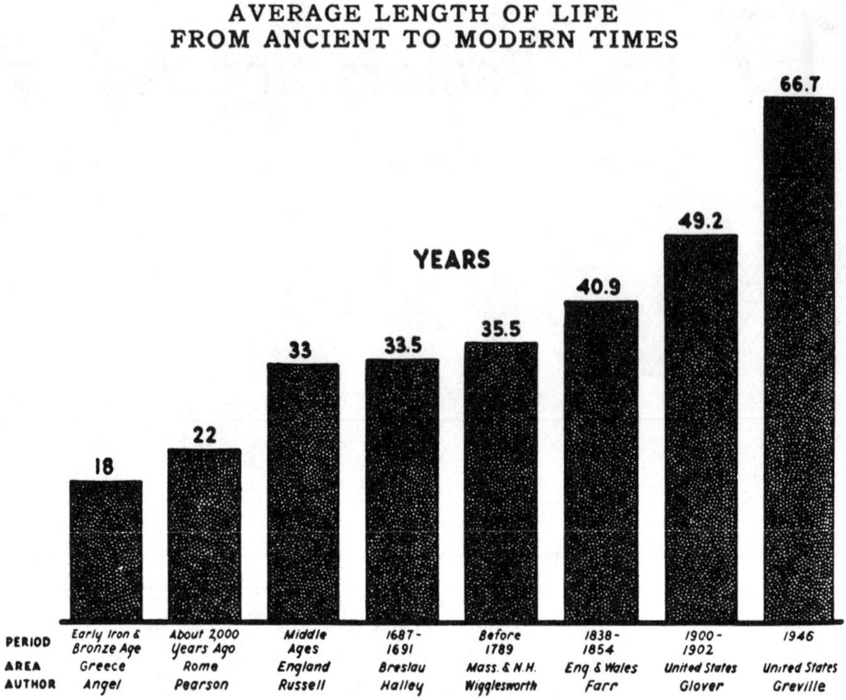

Figure 17-1. Average length of life from ancient to modern times. (From L.I. Dublin, A.J. Lotka, and M. Spiegelman, *Length of Life,* Ronald Press, New York, 1949.)

equivalent to the entire increase that has occurred from the early Iron and Bronze ages to 1900. In 1982 life expectation at birth in the United States was 70 for males and 77 for females (*3*). The 20-year increase in life expectation at birth that has occurred since 1900 in this country has benefited almost entirely those individuals in the younger groups. For example, if you were 65 or older in 1900, your life expectation then would not be much different from what it is today (Figure 17-2). Human aging is a relatively recent quantitative phenomenon. The age group over 75 in the United States, and in most other developed countries, is increasing faster than any other age group. The proportion of old people in the total population in developed countries is increasing rapidly and will continue to do so into the next century.

Teleologically, one might argue that our success in eliminating animal predators and infectious diseases has resulted in our ability to live so far beyond sexual maturation that a plethora of physiological decrements have been revealed that were never intended to be experienced. With respect to the survival of a species, there is no advantage in having its members living much beyond the age of reproductive ability and rearing of offspring. Evidence for this in humans is the fact that life-expectation

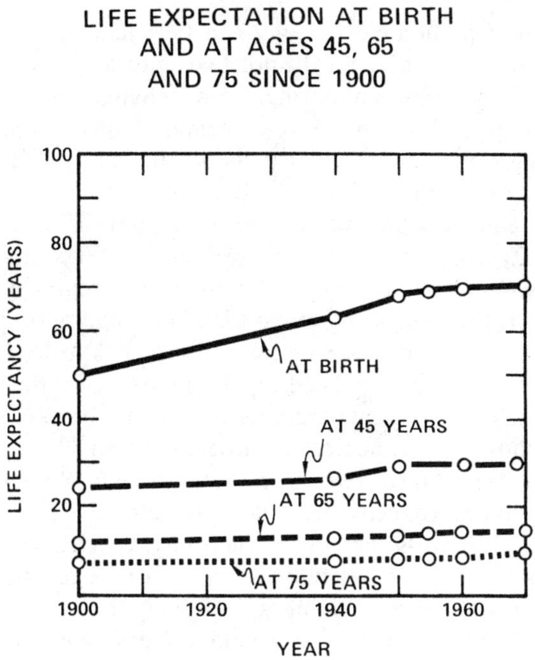

Figure 17-2. Life expectation at birth and at ages 45, 65, and 75 are depicted since 1900. The gain in life expectation of about 24 years since 1900 has occurred mostly in the younger age groups.

at birth was only 18 years in the early Iron and Bronze ages and 22 years during the early Roman Empire (Figure 17-1). That is not to say that some individuals at that time did not survive beyond those ages. Many did, but the survival of the human species did not and does not depend on any of its members living beyond, say, the age of 30.

Aging, therefore, might be regarded as an artifact of civilization. Its extreme biological manifestations, or increasing risk factors, were brought about by man himself. The expression of those risk factors on the scale currently being experienced is a new biological phenomenon. Never in the history of the human species has the proportion of old people to young people been as great as it is today. The risk factors for senility, like those for other age-associated pathologies, might be regarded as the price that we must pay for learning how to survive so long that we reveal biological changes that, perhaps teleologically, were never intended for us to experience.

DEATH DUE TO "NATURAL" CAUSES

Risk factors for any age-associated pathology are by their very definition rooted in the statistical analysis of a particular data base. The data base for age-associated pathologies usually can be challenged because of the strong probability that the data do not take into account the distinction that must be made between normal aging changes and the increased vulnerability to pathology that those normal changes produce. Normal biological changes that occur in virtually all the cells of an aging animal result in an increased vulnerability to those pathologies. For humans, the end result is death attributable to causes written on death certificates.

In 1825, the English actuary Gompertz discovered the important mathematical expression that governs the likelihood of death in humans. He found that, from the age of 30 onward, the probability of dying doubles every 7 years (*4*). Thus after sexual maturity the risk factors for dying are exponential with increasing age. Of equal importance is the finding that a variety of human physiological functions, although subject to some individual variation, show a slow, nearly linear decline from 30 years of age. The rate constants for this linear loss occur at about 0.8 to 0.9 per cent loss per year of the functional capacity present at 30 years (*5*).

It is important to stress that the normal physiological decrements that occur in virtually all organs as humans age must be regarded as normal events. Many of these normal changes, especially those known to occur in the immune system and in the neuroendocrine system, simply increase our vulnerability to disease and pathology. One might well argue that the leading causes of death written on death certificates—cardiovascular diseases, stroke, and cancer—are not the primary causes of death at all. The causes are the normal age-associated physiological decrements that increase vulnerability to those pathologies.

The importance of this concept is that increasing risk factors with advancing age to senility, or any age-associated pathology, is rooted not in the pathology itself but in normal age-associated decrements. These decrements may number in the tens of thousands. They are exemplified by such age-associated normal decrements as the graying of hair, loss of skin elasticity, loss of hearing and visual acuity, stature decrease, reaction-time changes, and hand grip strength decrease. They extend to normal losses in, for example, immune and neuroendocrine functions, undoubtedly triggered by events at the molecular level. None of these changes is considered to be a disease, yet the occurrence of many such changes results in increased risk or vulnerability to pathologies such as senility.

Fifty years ago many death certificates written for many old humans stated the reason for death as "natural causes." In more recent years this previously substantial "cause" of death has been virtually eliminated. This cause of death is the only one that has been resolved with no expenditure of funds or the dedicated efforts of skilled biomedical researchers. In fact, the discoverer of the cause—and presumably the cure—of this once popular cause of death continues to go unrecognized. This situation is unique in the annals of biomedical research, for the modesty of the discoverer remains unparalleled.

For the reasons just given, the three major causes of death that now appear on death certificates (cardiovascular diseases, stroke, and cancer) might well be replaced, more accurately, by "natural causes." Thus the risk factors for age-associated causes of death are factors intrinsic, perhaps, to all aging cells. Since the rates of change in physiological decrements vary from person to person, it is self-evident that the increased risk to such pathologies as senility will vary as well.

MEAN TIME TO FAILURE

A useful analogy can be made between aging biological systems and complex machines. Engineers use the term "mean time to failure" to express the increasing risk over time that a machine will ultimately fail. Without repairs, an automobile may have a mean time to failure of three years, a television set five years, and a refrigerator seven years. The risk factors involved may range from abuse and normal wear and tear to metal fatigue, effect of repeated temperature fluctuations on vulnerable parts, and oxidation or other chemical reactions.

For both animals and machines the risk factors may be environmental and/or intrinsic.

CELLULAR AGING

The notion that aging occurs in animals that reach a fixed size after maturity is beyond dispute, but is the inevitability of the risk factors for aging and death of individual cells composing that organism predetermined? A superficial consideration of this thought may provoke incredulity since it is intuitively obvious that a dead or age organism must consist of dead or aging cells. Nevertheless, whatever causes aging changes and death in the whole organism undoubtedly does not produce similar changes, and at the same rate, in each cell composing that organism. If the rates of aging vary among organs, tissues, and cells, then the root causes of aging may occur as a consequence of decrements in some few cell types where the rate is fastest and the effects greatest.

There are at least two ways in which this question has been put to the test. First, vertebrate cells have been grown and studied in cell culture, and, second, eukaryotic cells containing specific markers allowing them to be distinguished from host cells have been serially transplanted to isogenic laboratory animals. The goals of such studies have been directed toward answering the fundamental question, Can normal vertebrate cells, functioning and replicating under ideal conditions, escape the risk factors of aging and death that are universally characteristic of the whole animals from which they were derived?

Of central importance to this question is whether the cell populations studied in vitro are composed of normal or abnormal cells. Clearly the aging of animals occurs in normal cell populations. If we are to equate the behavior of normal cells in vivo to similar cells in vitro, then the latter must be shown to be normal as well. For this reason the "immortal" cell lines, of which HeLa, 3T3, BHK 21, and L cell populations are prototypes, must be excluded from consideration because they are composed of cells that are abnormal in one or more important properties. The widespread use of these cell lines throughout the world is subject to the criticism that they are not characteristic of any cell type found in human or animal tissue. Much experimental data generated from the use of such cell populations cannot be extrapolated to apply to cells that characterize the animal species from which the cells originally descended.

This fundamental flaw in interpreting normal cell behavior in vitro can in fact be circumvented. Cell populations entirely typical of normal cells found in vivo can be cultured and, with respect to gerontological inquiry, findings with these cells are profoundly different from the findings with abnormal cell lines.

Twenty-two years ago, Moorhead and I (*6*) found that cultured normal human embryonic fibroblasts underwent a finite number of serial subcultivations, or population doublings, and then died. We demonstrated that, when such cells are grown under the most favorable conditions, death is inevitable after about 50 population doublings (the Phase III Phenomenon). We also showed that the death of the normal cells is not due to some trivial explanation involving medium components or cultural conditions but that death of cultured normal cells is an inherent property of the cells themselves (*6,7*). That observation has now been confirmed in hundreds of laboratories in which variations in medium components and cultural conditions have been as numerous as the laboratories themselves.

Since normal diploid cell strains have a limited doubling potential in vitro, studies on any single strain would be severely curtailed were it not possible to preserve these cells at subzero temperatures for apparently indefinite periods of time. The reconstitution of frozen human fetal diploid cell strains has revealed that, regardless of the doubling level reached by the population at the time it is preserved, the total number of doublings that can be expected is about 50 when those made before and after preservation are combined (*6,7*).

As of this writing, we have reconstituted about 130 ampules of our human diploid cell strain WI-38, which was placed in liquid nitrogen storage 22 years ago. Since 1962 one ampule has been reconstituted approximately each month, and all have yielded cell populations that have undergone 50 ± 10 cumulative population doublings. This represents the longest period of time that viable normal human cells have been arrested at subzero temperatures (*1*).

Since normal human embryo fibroblasts can undergo only a fixed number of reproductive cycles in vitro, we postulated that this observation might be interpreted as representing aging at the cellular level. Although we and others were skeptical of this interpretation at first, subsequent experimental data have tended to support its validity.

Because cultured normal human cells derived from embryonic tissue have a finite proliferative capacity of about 50 population doublings and because this may represent cellular aging, it was important to determine the proliferative capacity of normal cells derived from human adults of various ages. Our first report of such studies did indeed show a diminished proliferative capacity for cultured normal human adult fibroblasts, in which 14 to 29 doublings occurred in cells derived from eight adult donors (*7*). The range of doublings found in cells cultured from 13 human embryos was 35 to 63.

Subsequently, reports from several other laboratories (*8–12*) not only confirmed the principle we observed but extended it significantly. Thus, it is now generally believed that there is an inverse relationship between the age of human donors and the in vitro proliferative capacity of several kinds of their cells.

IN VIVO STUDIES

If all animal cell types were continually renewed, without loss of function or capacity for self-renewal, the organs composed of such cells would function normally indefinitely and the organism would live forever. Renewal cell populations do not occur in most tissues; however, when they do, proliferation is often finite. The important question, then, is: Is it possible to circumvent experimentally the aging and death of normal animal cells that result from the aging and death of the host by transferring marked cells to younger animals seriatum? If such experiments could be conducted, then an in vivo counterpart of in vitro experiments would be available and we would predict that normal cells transplanted serially to proper inbred hosts would, like their in vitro counterparts, age and die. Such experiments would largely rule out those objections to in vitro findings that are based on the artificiality of cell replication in vitro. The question could be answered by serial orthotopic transplantation of normal somatic tissue to new, young, inbred hosts each time the recipient approaches old age. Under these conditions, do transplanted normal cells of age-chimeras proliferate indefinitely?

Data from seven different laboratories in which mammary tissues (*13–15*), skin (*16*), hematopoietic cells (*17–21*), and single antibody-forming cell clones (*22*) were used indicate that normal cells serially transplanted to isogenic hosts do not survive indefinitely. Furthermore, the trauma of transplantation does not appear to influence the results (*16*). Finally, in heterochronic transplants, survival time is related to the age of the grafted tissue (*16*). It is well known that, under similar conditions of tissue transplantation, cancer cell populations, like immortal cell lines, can be serially passed indefinitely.

The fact that normal transplanted cell populations may function beyond the normal life span of the host species is in keeping with speculation that the risk factors for aging are not necessarily timed at the same rate in all tissues. Furthermore, aging may be due not to the loss of cell division capacity but to other functional decrements known to occur prior to the loss of ability to replicate (*2, 23*).

FUNCTIONAL LOSSES

The possibility that animals age because one or more important cell populations lose their proliferative capacity is unlikely. It is more probable that, as we have shown, even though normal cells have a finite capacity for replication in vitro, this limit is rarely, if ever, reached in vivo. We suggest that functional losses that occur in cells prior to the cessation of division capacity produce physiological decrements in animals long before their normal cells reach maximum proliferative capacity. Indeed, we are now aware of more than 100 functional changes taking place in normal human cells grown in vitro and expressed well before the cells lose their capacity to replicate (*2*). It is more likely that these changes, which herald the approaching loss of division capacity, play the central role in the expression of aging and result in death long before cells fail to divide.

Cells incapable of division in mature animals (e.g., neurons, muscle cells) may play a greater role in the expression of age changes than cells in which division commonly occurs. It is important, therefore, to indicate that cessation of mitotic activity is only one of many functional decrements and that its genetic basis may be similar to that of functional decrements known to occur in nondividing cells. It is supposed that the same gene action that results in physiological decrements in aging nondividing cells also occurs in aged cells that can divide.

It is our contention, therefore, that age changes result not necessarily from losses in cell division capacity but simply from losses of function in any class of cells. That function could be measured as reduced division capacity or as any other of the myriad functional decrements characteristic of aging cells. The genetic changes leading to these decrements are postulated to be the common denominator, so that the cause of loss of dividing potential in vitro may have the same basis as the loss of other cell functions characteristic of nondividing cells. It follows therefore that an understanding of the mechanism by which cultured normal cells lose their capacity to replicate could provide insights into the causes of decrements in other functional properties, which are characteristic of nondividing cells and which may even more directly increase the risk factors that lead to biological aging.

Thus, the loss of cell function and cell death, which are intrinsic parts of development, may be intrinsic parts of aging. Developmental changes may simply continue on to become age changes with no clear delineation. The underlying genetic basis for developmental sequences could be the same mechanism that produces aging changes.

Acknowledgment

This work was supported in part by Grant AG 03478 from the First National Advisory Council on Aging, National Institutes of Health, Bethesda, Md.

REFERENCES

1. L. Hayflick, Survival of normal human cells for 21 years at subzero temperatures, in preparation.
2. L. Hayflick, Cell aging, in *Annual Review of Gerontology and Geriatrics* (C. Eisdorfer, ed.). vol. 1. Springer, New York, 1980.
3. Bureau of the Census, *Population Characteristics of the United States,* PC-80-S1-1. U.S. Department of Commerce, Washington, D.C., 1982.
4. B. Gompertz, On the nature of the function expressive of the law of human mortality and on a new mode of determining life contingencies, *Phil. Trans. Roy. Soc. London,* series A **115:**513 (1825).
5. B. L. Strehler and A. S. Mildvan, General theory of mortality and aging, *Science* **132:**14 (1960).
6. L. Hayflick, and P. S. Moorhead, The serial cultivation of human diploid cell strains, *Exp. Cell Res.* **25:**585 (1961).
7. L. Hayflick, The limited in vitro lifetime of human diploid cell strains, *Exp. Cell Res.* **37:**614 (1965).
8. G. M. Martin, C. A. Sprague, and C. J. Epstein, Replicative life-span of cultivated human cells: Effects of donor's age, tissue and genotype, *Lab. Invest.* **23:**86 (1970).
9. Y. LeGuilly, J. Simon, P. Lenoir, and M. Bourel, Long-term culture of human adult liver cells: Morphological changes related to in vitro senescence and effect of donor's age on growth potential, *Gerontologia* **19:**303 (1973).
10. E. L. Bierman, The effect of donor age on the in vitro life-span of cultured human arterial smooth-muscle cells, *In Vitro* **14:**951 (1977).
11. E. L. Schneider, and Y. Mitsui, The relationship between in vitro cellular aging and in vivo human age, *Proc. Natl. Acad. Sci. USA* **73:**3584 (1976).
12. R. L. Walford, S. Q. Jawaid, and F. Naeim, Evidence for in vitro senescence of T-lymphocytes cultured from normal human peripheral blood, *Age* **4:**67 (1981).
13. C. W. Daniel, Finite growth span of mouse mammary gland serially propagated in vivo, *Experientia* **29:**1422 (1973).
14. C. W. Daniel, K. B. deOme, J. T. Young, P. B. Blair, and L. J. Faulkin Jr., The in vivo life span of normal and preneoplastic mouse mammary glands: A serial transplantation study, *Proc. Natl. Acad. Sci. USA* **61:**53 (1968).
15. C. W. Daniel and L.J.T. Young, Influence of cell division on an aging process, *Exp. Cell Res.* **65:**27 (1971).
16. P. L. Krohn, Review lectures on senescence: II. Heterochronic transplantation in the study of aging, *Proc. Royal Soc. London,* series B **157:**128 (1962).
17. G. Cudkowicz, A. C. Upton, G. M. Shearer, and W. L. Hughes, Lymphocyte content and proliferative capacity of serially transplanted mouse bone marrow, *Nature* **201:**165 (1964).
18. C. E. Ford, H. S. Micklem, and S. M. Gray, Evidence of selective proliferation of reticular cell clones in heavily irradiated mice, *Br. J. Radiol.* **32:**280 (1959).
19. D. E. Harrison, Normal production of erythrocytes by mouse marrow continuous for 73 months, *Proc. Natl. Acad. Sci. USA* **70:**3184 (1973).
20. D. E. Harrison, Normal function of transplanted marrow cell lines from aged mice, *J. Gerontol.* **30:**279 (1975).
21. L. Siminovitch, J. E. Till, and E. A. McCulloch, Decline in colony-forming

ability of marrow cells subjected to serial transplantation into irradiated mice, *J. Cell. Comp. Physiol.* **64**:23 (1954).

22. A. R. Williamson, and B. A. Askonas, Senescence of an antibody-forming cell clone, *Nature* **238**:337 (1972).
23. L. Hayflick, The cellular basis for biological aging, in *Handbook of the Biology of Aging* (C. Finch and L. Hayflick, eds.). Van Nostrand Reinhold, New York, 1977.

Index